Calcium hydroxylapatite soft tissue fillers: expert treatment techniques

This comprehensive reference provides a focused yet in-depth overview of calcium hydroxylapatite (CaHA) use in aesthetic and regenerative medicine. It explores the evolution of Radiesse and other CaHA formulations, core rheological principles, and clinical protocols for both on- and off-label facial and body indications. With an emphasis on anatomy, injection techniques, and complication management, the book includes advanced applications ranging from ligament lifting to skin quality improvement protocols and rejuvenation techniques. This guide equips aesthetic physicians and dermatologists with the knowledge to deliver safe, effective, and versatile CaHA treatments.

Advanced injection techniques
Refined expert techniques to optimize facial and non-facial CaHA use
Updated complication protocols
Updated CaHA complication algorithms with expanded ultrasound-guided applications
Formulation-driven practice
Rheology-based protocols for improved tissue integration and sustained outcomes

UMA Academy is founded on a simple, strongly felt belief: that cosmetic medicine is a growing force for good. We exist to help other doctors in our unique field to develop the judgement and knowledge to transform lives, not just looks—so ever more people can look and live the way they want.

Our curriculum of book publications, webinars, discourses, and hands-on training is created by some of the people who developed The Netherlands' medical specialty of aesthetic medicine. Tailor-made for the digital age, our courses combine a solid theoretical background with clinical training and unprecedented access to the expertise of some of the industry's top practitioners.

knowledge is beautiful

UMA Academy Series in Aesthetic Medicine

Botulinum Toxin in Aesthetic Medicine
Jani van Loghem

Calcium Hydroxylapatite Soft Tissue Fillers: Expert Treatment Techniques, Second Edition
Jani van Loghem

Soft Tissue Filler Complications: Prevention and Management
Jani van Loghem and Philippe Snozzi

For more information on this series, please visit routledge.com/UMA-Academy-Series-in-Aesthetic-Medicine/book-series/UMA

Calcium hydroxylapatite soft tissue fillers: expert treatment techniques

second edition

Edited by
Jani van Loghem
UMA Institute
Amsterdam, The Netherlands

CRC Press
Taylor & Francis Group
Boca Raton London New York

CRC Press is an imprint of the
Taylor & Francis Group, an **informa** business

Second edition published 2026
by CRC Press
2385 NW Executive Center Drive, Suite 320, Boca Raton FL 33431

and by CRC Press
4 Park Square, Milton Park, Abingdon, Oxon, OX14 4RN

CRC Press is an imprint of Taylor & Francis Group, LLC

ISBN: 978-1-041-01961-9 (hbk)
ISBN: 978-1-041-15927-8 (pbk)
ISBN: 978-1-003-61712-9 (ebk)

DOI: 10.1201/9781003617129

Typeset in Minion
by Apex CoVantage, LLC

Access the Support Material: Visit routledge.com/s/VanLoghem/p/book/9781041019619

Contents

Preface

Calcium Hydroxylapatite Soft Tissue Fillers: Expert Treatment Techniques, Second Edition, is a hands-on reference book, created with the input of the world's leading experts on the use of calcium hydroxylapatite (CaHA). It can be used by doctors, nurses, and other professional injectors to study the relevant anatomy, aesthetic target sites, and injection techniques and to review the safest and most effective treatment protocols available for this versatile product. As a training aid, the book contains multiple photo sequences aided by filmed injection techniques as well as schematic diagrams to help clarify the proposed techniques. We have not only chosen to include the official on-label indications, but we also asked various internationally renowned experts to share their ways of adapting the standard protocols to new indications and sharing their innovations. As a disclaimer, therefore, many of the techniques discussed are off-label and should be used at the practitioner's own discretion.

Injection of soft tissue fillers is the second most frequently requested aesthetic medical procedure in the United States and The Netherlands. Only botulinum toxin is injected more than dermal fillers, partly because neuromodulators have a shorter longevity than fillers. As the relatively young medical field of aesthetic medicine is maturing, products and techniques are constantly changing to improve patient safety and satisfaction. While hyaluronic acid is the current gold standard and most frequently injected soft tissue filler, biostimulators have taken up a very prominent place in the arsenal of most aesthetic practitioners. There are a few commercially available biostimulatory products on the market such as CaHA, poly-L-lactic acid (PLLA), polycaprolactone (PCL), and more. In this book we focus on the use of CaHA, currently the most used biostimulatory product—acting both as a scaffold and releasing pro-regenerative cues—and injected for many facial and body indications. While the product is relatively safe, there are complications and risks involved, widely discussed in the current text.

To achieve beautiful results, practitioners must combine an aesthetic eye with a deep understanding of anatomy and injection depths. Around the globe, international experts also share their insights at congresses or seminars on newly developed techniques and emerging indications. These contributions continuously enrich our collective knowledge and shape clinical practice. The demand for high-quality aesthetic training is immense, with hundreds of congresses, workshops, and masterclasses taking place each week. However, some of the general protocols shared by pharmaceutical companies may be more influenced by marketing priorities than by revolutionizing indications. In this book, we aim to provide unbiased, non-commercial guidance grounded in expert consensus and real-world experience. This is a multispecialty collaboration, designed to benefit aesthetic physicians, surgeons, and nurses across a range of disciplines and subspecialties.

Jani van Loghem

Contributors

EDITOR

JANI VAN LOGHEM, MD PHD
Aesthetic physician KNMG at UMA Clinic;
Medical director at UMA Clinic;
Founder of UMA Clinic and UMA Academy (The Netherlands)

CONTRIBUTORS

NABILA AZIB, MD
Plastic Surgeon at Dr. Nabila Azib Plastic Surgery;
Head of the Aesthetic Medicine Department at ECAMS (Ireland)

SHINO BAY AGUILERA, DO
Cosmetic Dermatologist at Shino Bay Cosmetic Dermatology & Laser Institute;
Volunteer Professor at NOVA Southeastern University, Broward General and Larkin Hospital (U.S.A.)

AINA CERVERA-BAREA, DVM, MSC
Head of Research Department at UMA Academy (The Netherlands)

YATES YEN-YU CHAO, MD
Cosmetic Dermatologist;
Founder of Chao Institute of Aesthetic Medicine (Taiwan)

NIAMH CORDUFF, MBBS, FRACS
Specialist Plastic Surgeon at RiverEnd Aesthetics (Australia)

SEBASTIAN COTOFANA, MD, PHD, PHD
Associate Professor of Anatomy and Surgery at Albany Medical College (U.S.A.)

ANNA DANIILOVNA LOKASTOVA, MD
Cosmetic Dermatologist at Professor Yutskovskaya's Clinic (Russia)

STEVEN DAYAN, MD
Facial Plastic Surgeon;
Clinical Assistant Professor at University of Illinois (U.S.A.)

TOM DECATES, MD PHD
Assistant Professor at Department of Dermatology in Erasmus MC Rotterdam (The Netherlands)

NABIL FAKIH-GOMEZ, MD, MSC
Cranio-Maxillo-Facial Surgery Specialist at FACEXPERT Clinic & Academy;
Vice-President of the Spanish Society of Facial Plastic Surgery (Spain)

ALESSANDRO GENNAI, MD
Reconstructive and Aesthetic Plastic Surgeon at Studio Gennai (Italy)

KATE GOLDIE, MD
Medical Director at Henley Clinic (U.K.)

FADI HAMADANI, MD, MSC, BMEDSCI, HON. FACCSM (SURG/MED)
Senior Plastic Surgeon at H Clinic Hospital;
Founder and Medical Director at FTH Plastic and Aesthetic Clinic (Palestine)

THUY-VAN TINA HO, MD
Double Board-Certified Facial Plastic and Reconstructive Surgeon at Tina Ho MD Facial Plastic Surgery (U.S.A.)

POLINA HOLOVINA, MD
Aesthetic Physician at UMA Clinic (The Netherlands)

JONATHAN KADOUCH, MD, PHD
Cosmetic Dermatologist at ReSculpt Clinic (The Netherlands)

JOHN LEONARDO, MD
President of Leonardo Medicine Professional Corporation (Canada)

ALEC D. MCCARTHY, PHD
Director of Regenerative Aesthetics at Merz Aesthetics (U.S.A.)

FABRIZIO MELFA, MD
Founder and Scientific Director at Mediaging Group and Mediaging Clinic Center (Italy)

TATJANA PAVICIC, MD PHD
Board-Certified Dermatologist at Tatjana Pavicic Private Practice (Germany)

WOUTER J. PEETERS, MD
Plastic, Reconstructive, and Aesthetic Surgeon at Vriesdonk Clinic (Belgium)

VIVIANA PERICO, MD
Aesthetic Physician;
Author of the Bionutriblend technique;
Founder of Dra. Viviana Perico Medicina Estética Especializada Clinic (Colombia)

PEEROOZ SAEED, MD, PHD
Orbital and Oculoplastics Surgeon;
Professor of Orbital Surgery at University of Amsterdam (The Netherlands);
Head of Orbital Center Amsterdam, Department of Ophthalmology at Amsterdam University Medical Center (The Netherlands)

LEONIE W. SCHELKE, MD, PHD
Associate Professor at Department of Dermatology in Erasmus MC Rotterdam (The Netherlands)

PIETER SIEBENGA, MD, PHD
Aesthetic Physician KNMG;
Founder of ROCA Clinics Amsterdam (The Netherlands)

PHILIPPE SNOZZI, MD
Medical Director at Smoothline Clinics (Switzerland);
PhD candidate at Department of Ophthalmology in Amsterdam University Medical Center (The Netherlands)

LUIS SORO, DO, FAAD
Board-Certified Dermatologist at Shino Bay Cosmetic Dermatology & Laser Institute (U.S.A.)

JOB THUIS, MD
Aesthetic Physician KNMG at UMA Clinic (The Netherlands)

PETER VELTHUIS, MD, PHD
Co-Founder of CutaneoUS (The Netherlands);
Cosmetic Dermatologist Trainer at CutaneoUS (The Netherlands)

YANA A. YUTSKOVSKAYA, MD, PHD
Cosmetic Dermatologist;
Founder of Professor Yutskovskaya's Clinic Network (Russia)

Abbreviations

CaHA calcium hydroxylapatite
CMC carboxymethylcellulose
ECM extracellular matrix
HA hyaluronic acid
NCTF New Cellular Treatment Factor
SMAS superficial musculoaponeurotic system

Calcium Hydroxylapatite

1

Radiesse and Other CaHA Products: The Story of Calcium Hydroxylapatite

KATE GOLDIE, NIAMH CORDUFF, ALEC D. McCARTHY, JANI VAN LOGHEM, WOUTER J. PEETERS, AND PHILIPPE SNOZZI

1.1 THE HISTORY OF CAHA

Calcium hydroxyapatite (CaHA) is a naturally occurring mineral found in stone as well as in the bones and teeth of animals, including humans. Primarily composed of calcium and phosphate, CaHA represents the active component of Radiesse, a soft-tissue filler that will be thoroughly discussed in this book. Initially, CaHA had several other regenerative therapeutic indications, including dental, orthopedic, ear, nose, and throat procedures. It successfully underwent rigorous safety and efficacy evaluations by the European Medicines Agency (EMA) and the US Food & Drug Administration (FDA) before being approved for aesthetic applications [1]. This new use of CaHA in regenerative aesthetics—a distinct branch of regenerative medicine—aims to restore tissue architecture through biomechanical and biostimulatory effects, rejuvenating the aesthetic appearance of tissues primarily affected by aging processes.

In the early 1990s, a CaHA product marketed as Coaptite (developed by Bristol-Myers Squibb) was used to treat urinary incontinence. In 1999, the technology was acquired by U.S.-based BioForm Medical, which expanded its application to facial treatments. By 2001, the first patients received this improvised treatment. Subsequently, in 2003, FDA granted clearance for a product marketed as Radiance that was later rebranded as Radiesse. In 2004, Radiesse received initial approval by the EMA as a medical device for aesthetic purposes. In 2006, it received a CE mark for plastic and reconstructive surgery, to be used for deep dermal and subdermal soft-tissue augmentation of the facial area. In the same year, the FDA approved Radiesse for treating moderate-to-severe rhytids and folds, such as the nasolabial fold. Additionally, it was authorized for the restoration and/or correction of lipoatrophy in patients with human immunodeficiency virus (HIV) [2]. In 2009, BioForm Medical was acquired by German pharmaceutical company Merz Pharma, which relaunched Radiesse in various global markets, leading to a significant surge in sales. In 2015, the FDA expanded the approval of Radiesse for use in non-facial indications, such as hand augmentation. The patented formulation of Radiesse resulted in a ten-year monopoly. Since its initial introduction in 2003, no changes were made to the Radiesse formulation until 2016, when a lidocainized version, Radiesse+, was released into the U.S. market and further rolled out globally. In 2018, at least two other manufacturers began producing CaHA products according to the specifications of Radiesse. In 2021, Radiesse(+) was launched as the only injectable specifically designed for improving moderate to severe jawline contour deficiencies. Furthermore, in 2024, Merz Aesthetics secured EU approval to use hyperdiluted Radiesse for treating moderate to severe wrinkles on the décolleté.

Since most of the research and experience conducted so far has focused on Radiesse, the techniques and research discussed in this book pertain to the use of that specific product. However, it is important to note that other CaHA products with similar properties can also be utilized when employing the various techniques described in this book.

1.2 BACKGROUND

Radiesse is a CaHA-based filling product used for volumizing indications and administered through subdermal, subcutaneous or supraperiosteal injections, with the additional benefit of skin quality enhancement via [2]. Calcium is a mineral component found in nails, teeth, and bones (averaging about 1 kg in a medium-sized adult) as well as in the skin and soft tissues (about 10 g). Moreover, calcium plays an essential role in many metabolic and physiologic processes such as cell differentiation, regulation of gene transcription, muscle contraction, and cell adhesion. Especially, CaHA–CMC is biocompatible due to the similarity with the endogenous hydroxyapatite in human tissues (CaHA chemical formula $Ca_{10}(PO_4)_6(OH)_2$); hence it does not need allergy testing prior to injection [3].

Radiesse is made up of two main components: CaHA microspheres and a gel carrier in the volumetric proportion of 30% and 70%, respectively. CaHA microspheres are predominantly hydrophilic, aiding in moisture retention. The CMC gel carrier is composed of saline, glycerin, and sodium carboxymethylcellulose

DOI: 10.1201/9781003617129-1

(CMC). CMC is a water-soluble anionic cellulose derivative, with shear-thinning properties allowing for application through small-diameter needles and cannulas, preserving the shape of the microspheres and self-assembling after removal of shear stress via non-covalent crosslinking [4]. Lack of chemical crosslinking in CMC disperses easily when mixed or diluted, reducing the risk of clumping and subsequent swelling post-injection, making Radiesse an ideal candidate for hyperdiluting [5]. The high viscosity combined with the pseudoplastic nature of CMC ensures a smooth application and uniform dispersion of the microspheres within the carrier, making the CaHA–CMC gel a reliable, effective, and well-tolerated option in aesthetic treatments. Recognized by the FDA as safe, CMC is preferred in pharmaceutical applications for its drug-binding capabilities, pH sensitivity, and ability to efficiently deliver active ingredients. Therefore, CMC not only increases the shelf life but also acts as a humectant, explaining the frequent post-injection edema observed with CaHA [6].

CMC, together with other cellulosic materials, is also known for being nontoxic, nonallergic, biocompatible, and biodegradable [7,8]. Other interesting properties from antibacterial polymers is their capacity to mimic the amphiphilic host defense peptides by creating electrostatic interactions that disrupt the bacterial membrane [9,10]. This property has also been researched in CMC, with the conclusion that this biopolymer has a low biofilm-forming ability [4,8,11], most likely reducing filler-derived infections.

1.3 THE SCIENCE BEHIND CAHA BIOSTIMULATION AND TISSUE REGENERATION

Upon thorough mixing and injection, Radiesse combines the CMC gel and CaHA spheres, resulting in an immediate 1:1 correction. The CMC gel tends to dissociate easily, avoiding clogging and thus reducing post-injection swelling [12]. In approximately three months' time, the CMC gel will be resorbed, while at the same time, the CaHA particles will attract and stimulate fibroblasts to produce collagen fibers. The CMC gel will provide an immediate effect, while the CaHA microspheres act as a scaffold and induce collagenesis, thereby offering a long-term effect (Figures 1.1–1.2). The CaHA microspheres are manufactured in the size range of 25–45 μm, with micropores of 2–5 μm in diameter, and are designed to be spherical and smooth in order to minimize skin trauma during injection and reduce the occurrence of serious side effects, such as the formation of granulomas [13,14]. Further, the larger size of the microsphere prevents macrophage phagocytosis, as macrophages are unable to phagocytose particles larger than 10 μm [15]. Various studies investigated the degradation of CaHA particles, with differing observations. The dissolution of these microspheres may occur through various mechanisms. Upon completion of the degradation and resorption process, the released calcium and phosphate ions, which are identical to those naturally occurring in the body, are processed through metabolic pathways and naturally eliminated [16]. Therefore, CaHA is a nonpermanent filler that is fully resorbable.

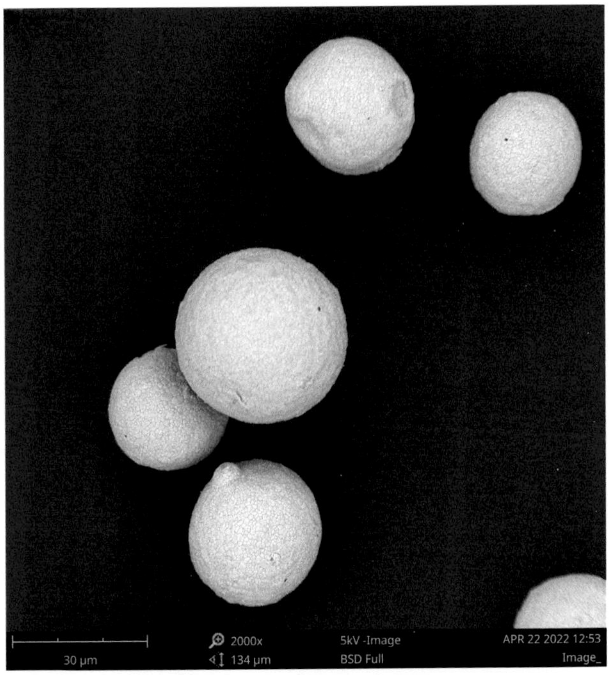

Figure 1.1 Scanning electron microscopic image of CaHA–CMC microspheres. (Image courtesy of Dr. Kleiton Cunzler.)

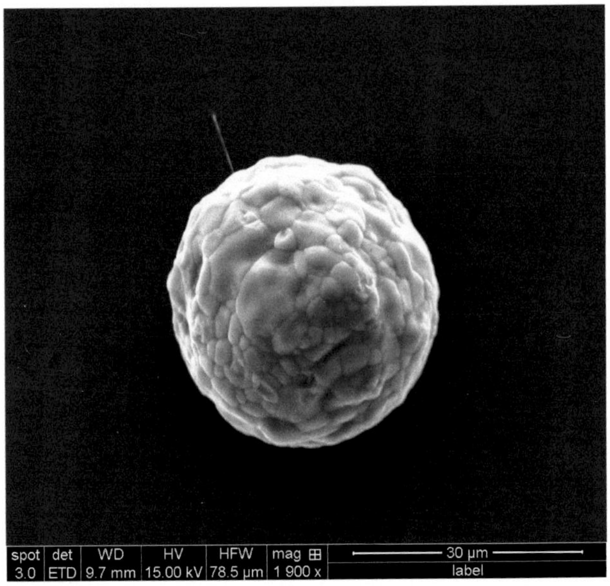

Figure 1.2 Scanning electron microscopic image of sputter-coated CaHA–CMC microspheres. (Image courtesy of Dr. Alec D. McCarthy.)

1.3.1 Biodegradation of CaHA–CMC

The interactions between the Radiesse biomaterial and its interface with the immune system are complex and not yet fully elucidated. Since CaHA–CMC microspheres are larger than 10 μm, individual macrophages are unable to engulf these particles, resulting in their degradation through the fusion of macrophages into multinucleated giant cells (MNGCs). The biomaterial interaction results in different types of MNGCs, some of which lead to foreign body response and fibrosis and others to more regenerative responses, driven by multiple factors which are outside the scope of the chapter [17]. Studies demonstrated that CaHA microspheres undergo degradation [18–23] with or without the involvement of MNGCs, including foreign body giant cells (FBGCs) [14,16]. For instance, histological analysis observed a pronounced foreign body reaction involving giant cells enveloping the CaHA particles in tissue samples from patients at various post-injection intervals. Additionally, analysis from 25 patients revealed consistent occurrences of mauve-to-gray or beige spheres within giant cells. These spheres were also surrounded by lymphocytes following treatments with CaHA filler [19–22]. Comparative research with injectable silk particles also noted similar immune responses in rodent models [24]. Kim demonstrated that macrophages initially do not engulf CaHA particles. However, over time, these microspheres are gradually degraded and absorbed by MNGCs. This absorption process typically spans approximately nine months and does not lead to the formation of granulomas or chronic inflammation (Figure 1.3) [20]. MNGCs contain many acidic vacuoles in their cytosol, which use vacuolar-type H^+-ATPase (V-ATPase) proton pumps to acidify these areas, thus dissolving hydroxyapatite coatings [25]. Therefore, a similar process might be involved in breaking down soft tissue fillers like CaHA microspheres, although direct evidence is still missing.

Interestingly, other electron microscopic studies observed no FBGCs or phagocytosis following injections of CaHA filler. Instead, they have demonstrated big, flattened cells abutting the microspheres. These are proposed to be fused cells derived from monocytes that release vesicles containing hydrolytic enzymes into the cytoplasm, where they degrade microspheres into microgranules and eventually into calcium and phosphate ions [14,26]. The resulting soluble Ca^{2+} ions then diffuse or are actively transported out of the cells into the surrounding medium. The local increase in Ca^{2+} concentration directly influences fibroblasts via specific calcium channels, such as transient receptor potential (TRP) channels (Figure 1.4).

1.3.2 Mechanism of Tissue Regeneration

Regenerative aesthetics aims to renew both the structure and function of aging tissues through regeneration of many of the elements that make up the ecosystem of the extracellular matrix (ECM). This is quite different to fibrotic replacement of volume loss. Radiesse is a three-dimensional matrix designed to replicate the biophysical signals and mechanical cues found in the ECM [27,28]. It offers both physical and biochemical cues that encourage the flourishing and proliferation of fibroblasts. Histological studies have demonstrated the ability of Radiesse to induce production of type I and type III collagen [29], organized perivascular elastin,

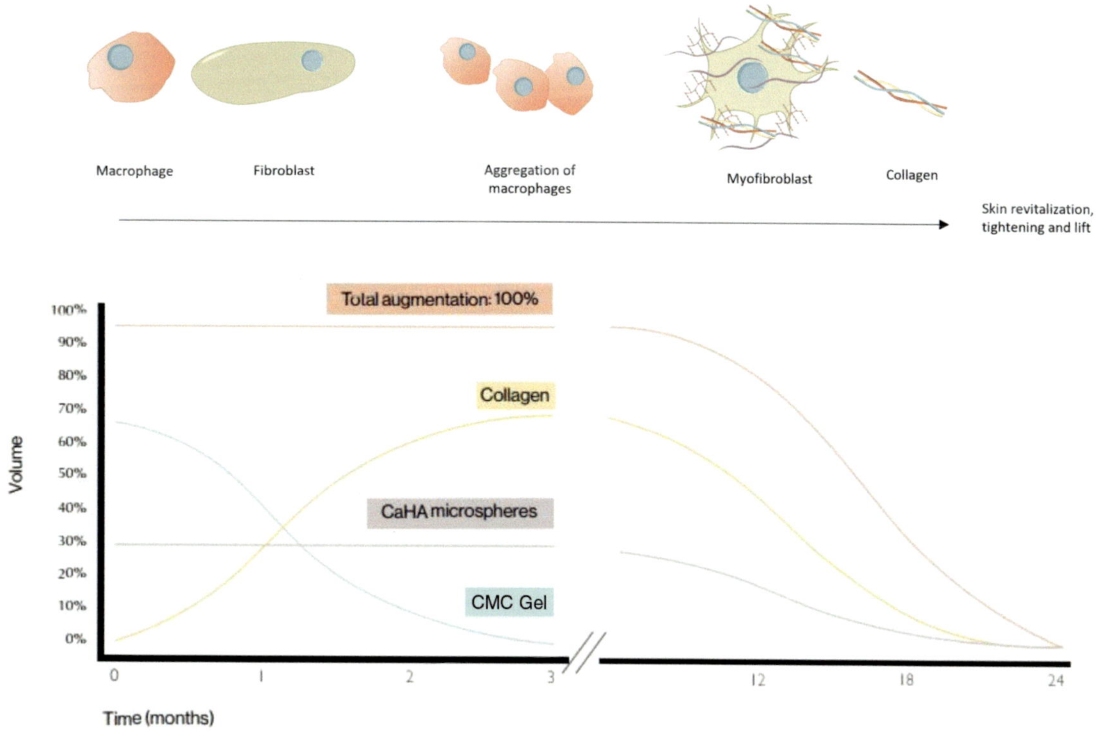

Figure 1.3 **Proposed timeline of CaHA–CMC degradation:** Graphic representation of the proposed gel and collagen behaviors in time. Note: This is the authors' interpretation.

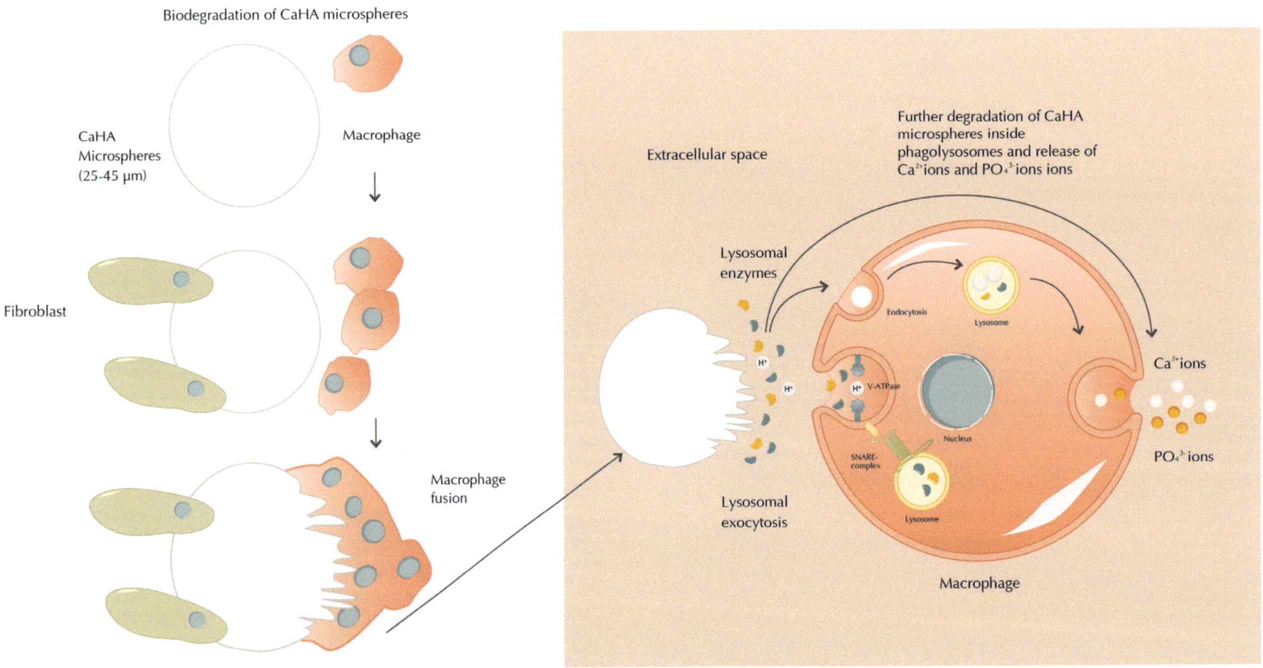

Figure 1.4 Proposed mechanism of CaHA–CMC degradation: Over time, CaHA–CMC microspheres are surrounded by multinucleated giant cells formed by the fusion of macrophages. The magnified view of CaHA biodegradation shows that multinucleated cells facilitate extracellular degradation by releasing hydrolytic lysosomal enzymes, such as acid phosphatases. This process is aided by the V-ATPase in the plasma membrane, which creates an acidic environment in the extracellular hydrolytic compartment, known as the lysosomal synapse. As the microspheres become small enough, they are endocytosed by macrophages and further degraded intracellularly through phagocytosis into Ca^{2+} and PO_4^{3-} ions.

proteoglycans [30], and glycosaminoglycans [31,32], all components of the ECM, as well as functional improvement in dermal thickness and skin pliability. Along with the functional stimulation of the fibroblast to synthesize new collagen and elastin, CaHA also acts on the structural aspect of the fibroblast. Human wrinkle fibroblasts have different functional behavior compared with normal fibroblasts, with significantly lower contractile forces. When in direct contact with fibroblasts, CaHA increases the contractility of a senescent wrinkle fibroblast to a level almost equivalent to normal skin fibroblasts (Figure 1.5) [33].

Fibroblasts in adult tissues are usually quiescent but turn into active myofibroblasts upon stimuli and secrete ECM proteins to help in tissue remodeling. Upregulation of fibroblasts is initially conducted through mechanotransduction pathways, both indirect via stretching up of the lax ECM fibers and direct by spreading and attachment of the fibroblasts by integrins to the microspheres [34,35]. The optimal spacing of CaHA microspheres is crucial for activating fibroblasts and initiating collagen production [5]. Biochemical stimulation also plays a key role in fibroblast activity, involving changes in intracellular calcium levels. Calcium enters cells through TRP channels, especially the transient receptor potential vanilloid 4 (TRPV4) channels, increasing intracellular calcium and activating pathways essential for ECM synthesis (Figure 1.5) [36]. These cytokines promote fibroblast migration to areas with higher calcium concentrations, leading to their transformation into myofibroblasts. These myofibroblasts actively participate in ECM remodeling and cell contraction, driven by synchronized calcium oscillations [37–39].

Calcium also has an indirect action on collagen production, involving an enzymatic action that slows its degradation [40]. Collagen, a vital element of youthful skin, is degraded by the enzyme collagenase I by lysing collagen fibers. It is synthesized by basal keratinocytes in the deepest layer of the epidermis. During the skin aging process, the proliferation of keratinocytes and their renewal slow down, resulting in a thinning of the epidermis. The physiological calcium gradient regulates the renewal and differentiation of keratinocytes [38,39]. Once differentiated, the keratinocytes move from the basal layer to upper layers of the skin, where the calcium environment is more concentrated. This process of differentiation and migration decreases the synthesis and secretion of collagenase 1 (Figure 1.5) [41]. Following injection of CaHA, the increase in calcium concentration in the epidermis stimulates keratinocyte differentiation [39], and in the presence of calcium, the cycle of keratinocyte transformation is accelerated, resulting in a faster renewal of the stratum corneum, thus explaining the improved radiance and skin tone that is observed clinically after CaHA injection.

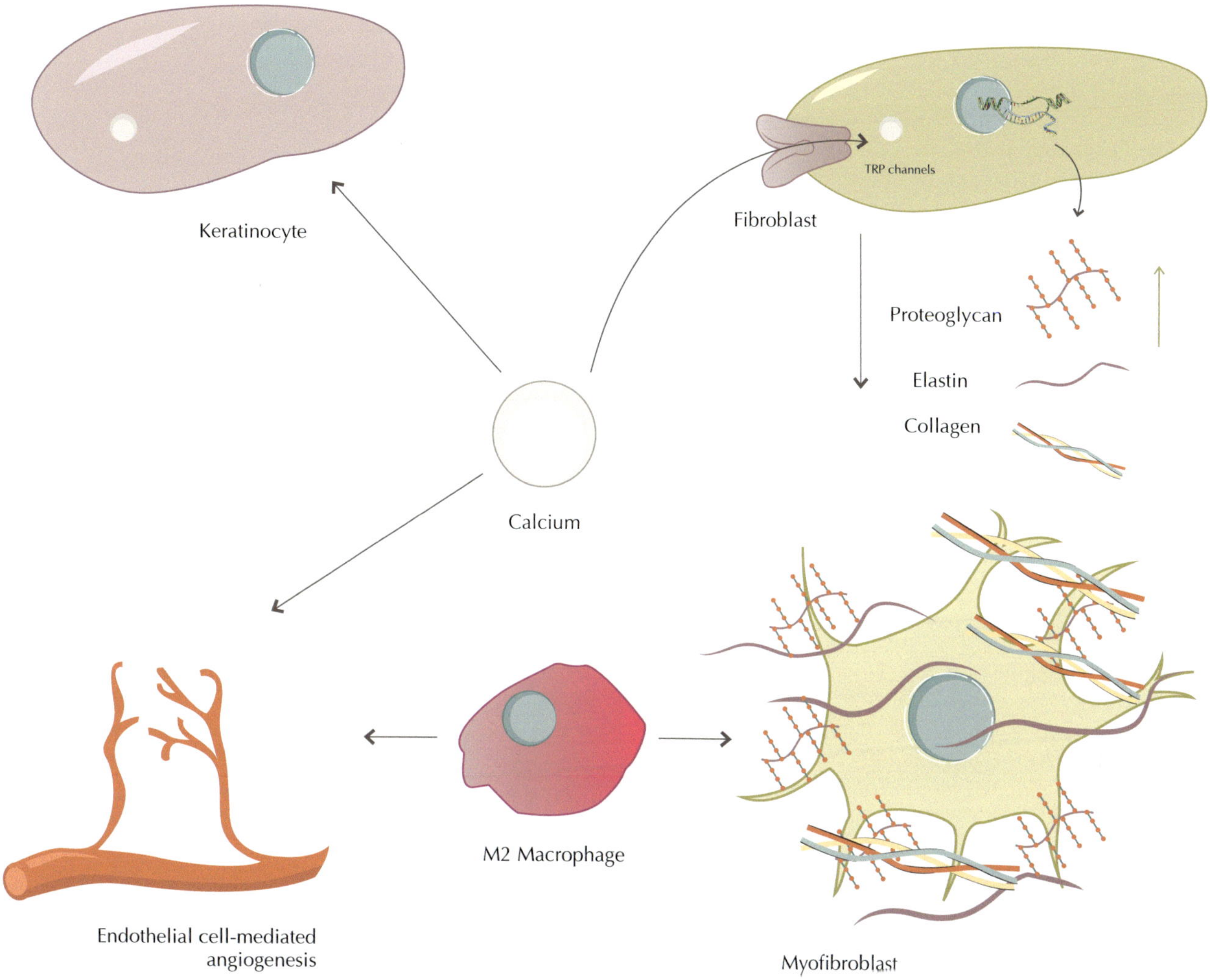

Figure 1.5 Role of calcium in driving tissue regeneration: Ca^{2+} ions are important secondary messengers in activating fibroblasts and initiating the transcription of genes for extracellular matrix (ECM) components like collagen, elastin, and proteoglycans. The movement of fibroblasts toward higher calcium gradients influences cellular signaling and the dynamics of the actin cytoskeleton, promoting essential processes such as actin polymerization and stress fiber formation, necessary for fibroblast differentiation into myofibroblasts. Furthermore, interactions with M2 macrophages, which stimulate fibroblast migration and VEGF release, highlight the cooperative aspects of these processes in facilitating angiogenesis. Calcium's role in maintaining skin hydration and integrity through the regulation of lipid and ceramide production in keratinocytes further illustrates its significant, yet not solitary, impact on tissue regeneration.

In summary, initial adsorption of plasma proteins and the formation of a clot leads to signaling molecules that attract macrophages to the area. The biomaterial properties of CaHA (shape, surface topography, wettability, chemistry, electric charge, plasticity) and subsequent signaling molecules determine the polarization of macrophages toward an M2 phenotype (pro-repair) as opposed to an M1 phenotype which predetermines an inflammatory pathway. By leaning toward M2 polarization, and in concert with signaling from other resident tissue cell populations—such as stem cells—a pro-regenerative tissue pathway is initiated. These processes are aided by the calcium-rich environment that occurs as the microspheres degrade, reaching a Ca^{2+} threshold that serves as a biological cue that induces fibroblast activity, including M2 polarization and subsequent tissue regeneration (Figure 1.5). Therefore, we postulate that the regeneration process is initiated by the mechanical stimulation of fibroblasts and sustained through a regenerative immunological pathway supported by biochemical signaling via calcium release.

1.3.3 Angiogenesis and Neovascularization

In the context of skin rejuvenation, angiogenesis plays a pivotal role. Research has shown that both the angiogenic capacity and the vascular density in skin tissues diminish as part of the aging process [20]. Calcium plays a vital role as a signaling molecule in pathways that regulate angiogenesis, particularly through the activity of M2 macrophages, which utilize VEGF signaling [41–44]. Although the precise mechanisms remain partly undefined, evidence suggests that CaHA can stimulate angiogenesis via increased VEGF production in macrophages, which then activates endothelial cells. Supporting this, Oh *et al.* found that endothelial cells exhibit increased migration, proliferation, and vessel formation when exposed to macrophage-treated media containing CaHA [45]. Other studies documented increased vessel density and diameter, capillary numbers, and positive CD34 staining after CaHA–CMC injections [46]. These findings are reinforced by a randomized study showing significantly greater angiogenesis at four and nine months post-injection with CaHA–CMC compared to hyaluronic acid fillers [31]. These results indicate that CaHA treatments enhance angiogenesis through calcium modulation and macrophage-mediated VEGF pathways (Figure 1.5). Calcium, therefore, plays a major role in facilitating the long-term skin quality improvements observed after injection of Radiesse (Figure 1.5).

1.3.4 Resorption of the CMC Gel and CaHA Microspheres

Demonstrable duration of augmentation is believed to be usually in the range of 10–12 months [14,47], while other physicians have photographic evidence of persistent correction up to 24 months [48] and even 2.5 years examined with magnetic resonance imaging [49].

1.3.5 Rheology

As there are different CaHA products on the market, no single statement can be made about the general rheologic properties of CaHA-containing injectables. The main rheological characteristics of Radiesse CaHA are high elasticity (*G*′) and viscosity (η^*), which confer on it immediate filling effects at the site of injection. Radiesse has one of the highest viscosities when compared with other dermal fillers, which means it remains at the site of injection and does not spread into the surrounding tissue (Figure 1.6). It also has high elasticity—the ability of a gel to return to its initial shape after being subjected to pressure—providing it with greater lifting capacity than many other dermal

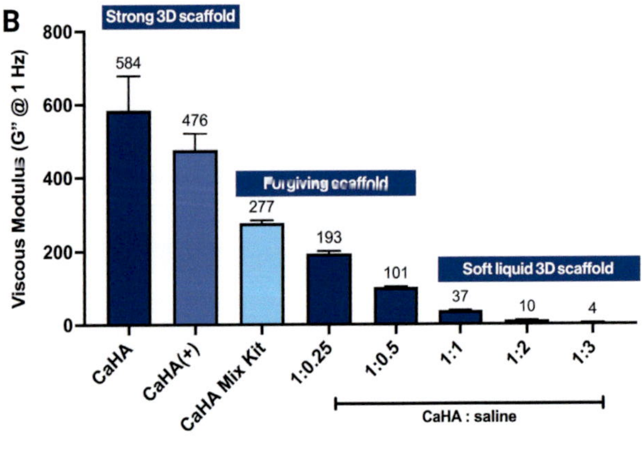

Figure 1.6 Comparison of viscous modulus (*G*") values for multiple CaHA filler formulations and in combination with gradual saline dilutions.

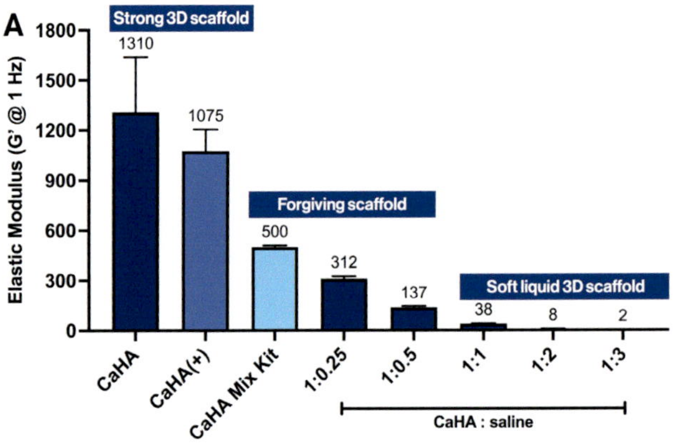

Figure 1.7 Comparison of elastic modulus (*G*′) values for multiple CaHA filler formulations and in combination with gradual saline dilutions.

fillers (Figure 1.7), making CaHA a very versatile product in the armamentarium of the aesthetic physician [12,50]. These physical properties make the product an economical one without dilution, as less material is needed to provide the same aesthetic result as competitive HA products on the market that have a lower viscosity and elasticity. Using dilution with lidocaine and/or saline, the CaHA viscoelasticity can be reduced (Figure 1.8).

1.4 SAFETY PROFILE OF CAHA

Based on the results of a published review of the literature, CaHA appears to have an overall good safety profile. However, skin discoloration, edema, infection, nodule formation, and vascular compromise are the most common adverse events [51]. Several treatment approaches exist for managing CaHA complications, which will be further discussed in Chapter 42.

1.4.1 Granuloma Formation

Extensive research has been conducted on the safety and tolerability of CaHA. Very few granulomas have been recorded in patients treated exclusively with CaHA products. In contrast, cross-linked hyaluronic acid (HA) products have a higher prevalence of granuloma formation. Sanchez and others showed that fragmented HA fibers from filler can signal tissue damage to the immune system. In other words, when HA filler fibers (low molecular weight) are free, the body sees them as broken-down tissue [52]. The surface of the CaHA spheres is smooth, and therefore the chance of granuloma formation is smaller than if their surface were irregular or spiky. There are some reports of granuloma formation after CaHA injection, but, as Lemperle *et al.* observed, Radiesse appears to cause the lowest rate of granuloma formation among all filler substances [14].

1.4.2 Bone Formation

Nonporous, ceramic CaHA, and macroporous CaHA (which has a highly organized pore structure ranging from 10–500 μm) permit osseointegration.

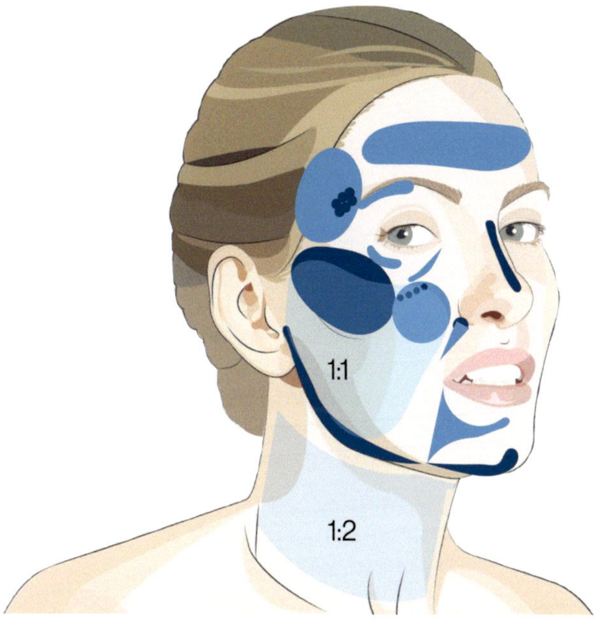

Figure 1.8 Injection schematics of CaHA for rheomodulation purposes in face and neck. The different shades of blue indicate the elastic properties achieved with different formulations. Yale blue (darkest) areas are preferred for creating strong 3D scaffold effects, with CaHA+ conferring ligament lifting, volumizing, and contouring properties; undiluted CaHA is preferred in these areas. Azure blue represents areas accepting of mildly diluted CaHA formulations, enabling forgiving scaffolds for skin fold filling, volumizing, and improving skin regeneration. Uranian blue (lightest) areas tolerate CaHA hyperdilutions that create soft liquid scaffolds, in turn mediating skin regeneration.

The large pores of macroporous CaHA readily permit fibrovascular ingrowth, whereas nonceramic CaHA cement is used widely in reconstructive surgery to repair bony defects, with gradual replacement by new bone growth [29,53]. In Radiesse, CaHA microspheres are microporous, with particles featuring pores of only 2–5 µm, which are too small to promote fibrovascular ingrowth and bone formation. Importantly, there are no documented cases to date of subdermally injected Radiesse causing bone formation in the subcutaneous tissues. The possibility of stimulating longer augmentation and bone formation when injecting it along the periosteum remains speculative, as no articles definitively demonstrate this potential. In fact, researchers have shown that CaHA must be placed subperiosteal to induce bone formation, although periosteal placement will not generate bone [54,55].

Normally, osteoblasts are necessary to produce bone matrix, and therefore injection of CaHA products in soft tissue will not result in bone formation. Additionally, a study shows that mesenchymal stem cells can be stimulated by biphasic CaHA products (BCPs), depending on their physical features and chemical composition [56]. The products modulate stem cell behavior, and stem cells from different origins are inherently distinct in their gene expression profile and can be triggered toward osteochondrogenic fate by BCPs [56]. This study used specific CaHA products that were designed for osteogenesis and had the specific surface features and necessary pores to produce bone matrix. Soft tissue filler products have smooth particles and do not have pores and have not been associated in any study with the formation of bone matrix.

Bone cannot be formed, as CaHA is not bone; it is a mineral component found in bones and teeth. No osteoprogenitor cells or bone morphogenic proteins are present in the dermis or subcutaneous tissue. Moreover, micromotion present in the soft tissue prevents osteogenesis. Extensive literature describing the use of CaHA in a variety of soft tissue applications describes no osteogenesis [14].

1.4.3 Radiologic Visibility

Carruthers *et al.* looked at plain X-ray films and computed tomography (CT) scans immediately after injection. They found a light hazy appearance on plain X-ray films among 13% to 56% of cases. On CT scans, however, a more definitive white haziness was clearly seen in 96.7% to 100% of the cases [57] Tzikas showed CT scan persistence of the product seven months after injection of the lips [47], whereas Pavicic and others showed complete biodegradability of CaHA after 2.5 years in an MRI study [49].

1.5 DILUTION AND INJECTION TECHNIQUE

1.5.1 Introduction

Soft tissue fillers have been used for decades to correct wrinkles and folds and soft-tissue volume loss. Used as a volumetric filler, CaHA can be injected in different tissue layers: supraperiosteal, subdermal, and deep dermal. In a more diluted version, it may also be injected more superficially for dermal rejuvenation. CaHA is a well-known soft tissue filler product. After injection in the subcutis, CaHA induces a histiocytic and fibroblastic response, acting as a scaffold for new tissue formation and stimulating collagen and elastin formation around the filler for sustained aesthetic improvements [16,29,31,58].

Amselem, Cogorno-Wasylkowski, and colleagues published the first reports about skin improvement after injection of diluted CaHA in the superficial dermis of arms, abdomen, and thighs [59,60]. Increased interest in the collagen-stimulating capacity of CaHA led to the development of subdermal injection techniques to stimulate dermal regeneration without a direct volumizing effect [32,61–63]. Therefore, current evidence suggests that titrated aqueous dilutions of CaHA can be tailored to achieve customized rheological properties that move along a resiliency–regeneration continuum, with immediate volumization at one end and biostimulation at the other [34,35] (Figure 1.8).

A global panel of expert aesthetic physicians reviewed available evidence for the safe and effective use of diluted and hyperdiluted CaHA in the face and body and compared personal experience (Table 1.1) [64].

1.5.2 Dilution or Hyperdilution Rationale

The concept of dilutional rheomodulation is widely used in dermal fillers applied in the clinical arena and proven to be effective and safe for regenerative strategies [35]. As shown in Figures 1.6–1.7, CaHA can be injected in different dilutions. Undiluted, the filler is highly viscoelastic and ideally suited for periosteal implantation and volume augmentation [64–66]. CaHA is regularly used as Radiesse and Radiesse+ (CaHA with lidocaine) formulations. As for Radiesse, it is most often diluted at a 1:1 or 1:2 ratio. The dilution makes the product more manageable for more superficial injection without altering its efficacy [67]. While low dilution ratios create a volumizing and contouring effect, dilution ratios at 1:1 or greater present a direct filling effect (*G′*) that is diminished, and thus, the aesthetic correction observed is the direct results of biostimulation and remodeling features alone. In the consensus paper published in 2018, an overview is given on different areas in the body along with the preferred dilution in terms of safety and efficacy (Figure 1.8) [65]. The authors suggest delivering approximately 1.5 mL of CaHA/100 cm^2. In normal skin, a 1:1 to 1:2 dilution is advised. In fragile, thin skin, it is safer to use a 1:2 or an even higher dilution (Table1 1.2).

1.5.3 Product Mixing

Sterility or "clean mixing" is essential in the dilution process. Other than in the "classic" 5:1 mixture ratio (1.5 mL CaHA mixed with 0.3 mL lidocaine/saline),

Table 1.1 Best Practices for Using CaHA in Aesthetic Procedures.

Indication	Average Volume of Undiluted CaHA	Dilution Ratio	Injection Plane/ Technique	Proposed Needle/ Cannula
Correcting bone resorption, lifting ligaments, contouring, and projecting	1.5 mL	1:0	Periosteal boluses or retrograde linear threads. Subcutaneous retrograde linear threads	At injector's discretion
Folds, areas with thin tissue envelope (like temples, forehead)	1.5 mL	1:0.17	Subcutaneous, interfascial, or periosteal retrograde linear threads	At injector's discretion
Pan-facial skin quality improvement	1.5 mL/side	Most commonly 1:1 to 1:2	Subdermal. Retrograde linear threads	25G, 50 mm
Scars	1.5 mL per session	1:1	Subcision followed by subcutaneous retrograde linear threads	23–27G sharp needle
Neck	1.5 mL/side	1:2 to 1:3	Immediate subdermal. Retrograde linear threads	22G, 50 mm
Décolletage	1.5–3 mL	1:1 to 1:2	Immediate subdermal. Retrograde linear threads	22G, 70 mm
Breasts	3–4.5 mL/side	1:1 to 1:2	Subdermal vectoring	25G, 50 mm, or sharp needle 27G, 40 mm
Mild laxity of the upper arm	3 mL/arm	1:2	Immediate subdermal. Retrograde linear fanning	22G, 70 mm
Abdomen	1.5 mL/100 cm2	1:1 to 1:2	Subdermal. Crosshatching or fanning	Sharp needle 27G, 40 mm; cannula 22G, 70 mm
Buttocks: gluteal sagging and mild dermal irregularities	1.5 mL/100 cm2	1:1 to 1:2	Subdermal crosshatching	22G, 70 mm
Mild laxity of the legs	1.5 mL/100 cm2	1:1 to 1:2	Immediate subdermal	22G, 70 mm
Cellulite dimples	1.5 mL per 100 cm^2		Subdermal crosshatching	27G, 18mm sharp needle. Subcision of dimples with 18G needle
Striae distensae	1.5–3 mL per session		Subcutaneous retrograde linear threads	27G sharp needle

Note: Initially, a 1:1 dilution is advised for optimal regenerative outcomes. However, for areas with thinner skin, a greater dilution is recommended to prevent unevenness and visible deposits. It is suggested to limit the retrograde injection volume to no more than 0.1 mL.

Table 1.2 Total Volume after Dilution

Undiluted CaHA	Lidocaine	Saline	Dilution Ratio	Total Volume/100 cm² Injected
1.5 mL	-	0 mL	1:0	1.5 mL
	-	0.375 mL	1:0.25	1.875 mL
	0.5 mL	0.25 mL	1:0.5	2.25 mL
1.5 mL	0.5 mL	1 mL	1:1	3 mL
	0.5 mL	2.5 mL	1:2	4.5 mL
3.0 mL	0.5 mL	2.5 mL	1:1	6 mL
	0.5 mL	5.5 mL	1:2	9 mL

Formulation: 1.5–3.0 mL/100 cm² (area of 10 × 10 cm)
Note: The counter syringe for a 1.5 mL of CaHA should be at least 5 mL, and for a 3 mL of CaHA, a counter-syringe of 10 mL is needed for appropriate mixing (see Figure 1.5).

make sure the counter syringe is large enough to contain the combined filler and diluent. To avoid prolonged numbness in the treated area and lipotoxic effects due to lidocaine, limit the amount of lidocaine to a maximum of 1 mL, and add saline to the desired amount of diluent (Table 1.2).

Several gentle passes between both syringes (at least 10 times each way) are needed to ensure product homogeneity. In dilutions greater than 1:1, the mixture tends to separate quickly after mixing. Remixing immediately before injection is advised. See further Video 1.1.

Video 1.1 How Radiesse is mixed.

Recently, innovations with the use of Radiesse have resulted in various blends of CaHA with HA gels. Where earlier reports describe improved patient satisfaction after the combination of Radiesse CaHA and Restylane (NASHA HA) in the same facial areas [68,69], actual mixing (blending) of Radiesse and hyaluronic acid gels in one syringe was published as from 2019 [70–72] and is now seeing a fast increase in global usage. In Chapter 3, different blends created upon mixing with Radiesse are discussed, further indicating fluidification changes (Figure 3.4) acquired after diluting the CaHA product.

1.5.4 Sharp Needle versus Blunt Cannula

As in other indications for dermal fillers, the choice of sharp needle or blunt cannula depends on the area to be injected and personal comfort or preference. The authors strongly advise the use of blunt cannulas to minimize bruising and to avoid product visibility. When CaHA is injected to improve skin quality, mostly large areas are treated. Blunt cannulas are associated with less postinjection pain and bruising compared to needles [73–75], an important consideration when injecting extensive areas of the body, for example, extremities.

In contrast to the use of CaHA in volume augmentation, where deep dermal and periosteal placement is advised, the hyperdiluted version is injected in the superficial dermal layers. In very thin skin, sharp needles can cause a too superficial placement of the product, which leads to product visibility and small nodules that lasts for months. When cannulas are used, the product will end automatically in the right layer of the skin, even when this skin is ultrathin, like in the upper arm or the neck area.

The goal of dermal injection of CaHA is to deliver a thin, uniform coating to the entire surface of the area of concern. With the (hyper)diluted product, skin irregularities, lines, or wrinkles are not targeted. When the product is placed in the superficial dermal plane, the process of neocollagenesis, neovascularization, and neoelastogenesis will start. This is a slow process that will take at least three months to show results which are clinically significant [76].

1.5.5 Treatment Intervals

CaHA stimulates dermal remodeling due to neocollagenesis, whereby collagen type I gradually replaces collagen type III [76]. Histological examination suggests a cycle in which the highest deposition of new collagen and elastin occurs around four months after injection, with stability achieved by nine months.

In patients under 40 years, the neocollagenesis and neoelastogenesis is so strong that one single treatment results in a significant clinical improvement within four months. In those cases, reinjecting can be proposed after 18 to 24 months (Table 1.3).

In patients older than 40 years, where neocollagenesis is a slower process, retreatment is proposed after

Table 1.3 Treatment Intervals for CaHA Reapplications

Level of Response	Steps
Good	Re-apply after 12–18 months
Moderate	Re-apply after 4–6 months; then re-apply after 12–18 months

three to four months to enhance dermal remodeling. Sometimes a third treatment session is needed to achieve optimal aesthetic effect, with maintenance injections every 12 to 18 months hereafter (Table 1.3).

1.6 RADIESSE INJECTABLE IMPLANT: INSTRUCTIONS FOR USE

1.6.1 Description

Radiesse injectable implant is a steam-sterilized, latex-free, nonpyrogenic, semisolid, cohesive, and completely biodegradable deep subdermal implant. The principal component is synthetic calcium hydroxylapatite, a biomaterial with over 20 years of use in orthopedics, neurosurgery, dentistry, otolaryngology, and ophthalmology. Calcium hydroxylapatite is the primary mineral constituent of bone and teeth. The semisolid nature of the implant is created by suspending calcium hydroxylapatite in a gel carrier that consists primarily of water (sterile water for injection USP) and glycerin (USP). The gel structure is formed by the addition of a small amount of sodium carboxymethylcellulose (USP). The gel is dissipated in vivo and replaced with soft tissue growth, while the calcium hydroxylapatite remains at the site of injection. The result is long-term yet non-permanent restoration and augmentation. Radiesse injectable implant is classified as a Class III Medical Device according to Annex IX of the Medical Device Directive. Radiesse injectable implants at 3.0 mL, 1.5 mL, 0.8 mL, and 0.3 mL have a particle size range of 25–45 μm and can be injected with a 25G outer diameter (O.D.) to 27G inner diameter (I.D.) or larger needle with a standard Luer fitting. Use of needles smaller than 27G I.D. may increase the incidence of needle occlusion.

1.6.2 Intended Use/Indication

Radiesse injectable implant is indicated for plastic and reconstructive surgery, including deep dermal and subdermal soft tissue augmentation of the facial area, and is also intended for restoration and/or correction of the signs of facial fat loss (lipoatrophy) in people with human immunodeficiency virus.

1.6.3 Contraindications

- Radiesse injectable implant is contraindicated in the presence of acute and/or chronic inflammation or infection when these involve the area to be treated.
- Radiesse injectable implant is contraindicated in patients with known hypersensitivity to any of the components.
- Radiesse injectable implant is contraindicated in patients prone to developing inflammatory skin conditions or those patients with a tendency to develop hypertrophic scars. Do not implant in the epidermis or use as a skin replacement. Implantation into the epidermis or superficial dermis could lead to complications such as fistula formation, infections, extrusions, nodule formation, and induration.
- Radiesse injectable implant is not intended to be used for the correction of glabellar folds. A higher incidence of localized necrosis has been associated with glabellar injection. Complications associated with other injectables indicate that forceful injection into superficial dermal vessels of the glabellar area could cause retrograde movement into the retinal arteries resulting in vascular occlusion.
- Radiesse injectable implant is contraindicated in the presence of foreign bodies such as liquid silicone or other particulate materials.
- Radiesse injectable implant should not be used in areas where there is inadequate coverage of healthy, well-vascularized tissue.
- Radiesse injectable implant should not be used in patients with systemic disorders which cause poor wound healing or will lead to tissue deterioration over the implant.
- Radiesse injectable implant is contraindicated for patients with bleeding disorders.

1.6.4 Warnings

- Implant should not be injected into blood vessels. Injection into blood vessels may cause platelet aggregation, vascular occlusion, infarction, embolic phenomena, or hemolysis, leading to ischemia, necrosis, or scarring. This has been reported to occur in the lips, nose, and glabellar or ocular area.
- Implant should not be injected into organs or other structures that could be damaged by a space-occupying implant.
- Implant should not be implanted in patients while the patient is on an aspirin regimen or while taking other medications that could inhibit the healing process.
- Implant should not be implanted in infected or potentially infected tissue or in open cavities because infection or extrusion may occur. A significant infection may result in damage or loss to the skin overlying the implant. Hematomas or seromas may require surgical drainage. In the event of hypersensitivity or allergic reaction, a significant inflammation or infection may occur, requiring the removal of the implant.
- Some injectable implants have been associated with hardening of the tissues at an injection site, migration of particles from an injection site to other parts of the body, and/or allergic or autoimmune reactions. Based on clinical usage, animal studies, and supporting literature, this has not been observed nor is it expected with Radiesse injectable implant.
- As with any implant material, possible adverse reactions that may occur include, but are not limited to, the following: inflammation, infection, fistula formation, extrusion, hematoma, seroma, induration formation, inadequate healing, skin discoloration, and inadequate or excessive augmentation.

- Safety and effectiveness during pregnancy or in lactating females has not been established.
- The safety and efficacy of Radiesse injectable implant for use in the lip mucosa has not been established.

1.6.5 Precautions

- Radiesse injectable implant requires soft tissue for easy percutaneous injection. Scar tissue and significantly compromised tissue may not accept the implant appropriately.
- Infection requiring treatment may occur at the injection site. If such infection cannot be corrected, it may become necessary to remove the implant.
- Injection-related reactions, including bruising, erythema, swelling, pain, itching, discoloration, or tenderness, may occur at the site of the injection. These usually resolve spontaneously within one to two days after the injection. Nodule(s) may form requiring treatment or removal.
- Irregularity of the implant may occur which may require a surgical procedure to correct.
- Do not overinject the area to be treated. In extreme cases, site rupture could occur. Radiesse injectable implant can be easily added in subsequent injections but cannot be easily removed.
- The Radiesse injectable implant injection procedure, like similar injection procedures, has small but inherent risks of infection and/or bleeding. The patient may experience slight discomfort during and following the procedure. Therefore, anesthetic techniques common with this treatment should be considered. The usual precautions associated with percutaneous injection procedures should be followed to prevent infection.
- Do not re-sterilize. Radiesse injectable implant is supplied sterile and nonpyrogenic in a sealed foil pouch and is intended for single-patient, single-treatment use only.
- The foil pouch should be carefully examined to verify that neither the pouch nor the syringe has been damaged during shipment. Do not use if the foil pouch is compromised or the syringe has been damaged. Do not use if the syringe end cap or syringe plunger is not in place. There is a small amount of moisture normally present inside the foil pouch for sterilization purposes; this is not an indication of a defective product. To help avoid needle breakage, do not attempt to straighten a bent needle. Discard it and complete the procedure with a replacement needle.
- Do not reshield used needles. Recapping by hand is a hazardous practice and should be avoided.
- The safety of Radiesse injectable implant with concomitant dermal therapies such as epilation; UV irradiation; or laser, mechanical, or chemical peeling procedures has not been evaluated in controlled clinical trials.
- If laser treatment, chemical peeling, or any other procedure based on active dermal response is considered after treatment with Radiesse injectable implant, there is a possible risk of eliciting an inflammatory reaction at the implant site. This also applies if Radiesse injectable implant is administered before the skin has healed completely after such a procedure.
- Injection of Radiesse into patients with a history of previous herpetic eruption may be associated with reactivation of the herpes.
- Safety of Radiesse injectable implant beyond three years has not been investigated in clinical trials.

1.6.6 Adverse Events

The following adverse events were reported during clinical trials performed with Radiesse injectable implant: ecchymosis, edema, erythema, nodule, pain, pruritus, soreness, tenderness, numbness, contour irregularity, lumps, irritation, rash, needle jamming, discoloration, hardness, headache, scab, tightness, bloodshot eyes, black eye, abrasions, spots, nerve sensitivity, dry burning sensation, warmth, felt stretched skin, pimples, flushing, fever, ear running, backed-up salivary glands, firmness, hearing loss, and puffiness.

1.6.7 Post-Market Surveillance

The following adverse events were received from post-marketing surveillance for Radiesse injectable implant inside and outside the United States and were not observed in the clinical trials with Radiesse injectable implant: infection, overinjection, underinjection, loss of effect, product displacement, allergic reaction, necrosis, granuloma, exposed material, hair loss, tingling, ptosis, abscess, paralysis, superficial injection, herpetic infection, hematoma, blanching, blistering, bluish color, dark circles, undesirable results, dizziness, double vision, festoons, flu-like symptoms, grey discoloration, Guillain–Barre syndrome, hyper-ventilating, inflammation, ischemic reaction, lymphoid hyperplasia, nausea, pallor to skin, prior medical condition worsened, pericarditis, possible blood clot, scarring, sensitivity to cold, skin texture changed, tissue mass developed, vascular compromise, and ocular ischemia. The most commonly reported serious adverse events (with a frequency greater than five reported events) were necrosis, allergic reaction, edema, and infection. The following describes these serious adverse events:

- Necrosis was generally preceded by pain and blanching of the skin at the time of injection accompanied by stinging or tingling and bruising, redness, and swelling.

- Onset of necrosis ranged from immediately at time of injection to 12 days after injection. Treatment for necrosis generally consisted of a combination of nitroglycerin ointment/vasodilatation, ibuprofen, acetaminophen or aspirin, antibiotics, steroids, nonsteroidal wound treatment ointment, and warm compresses. For cases where information was available, patients had recovered or were recovering with minimal to no scarring at last contact. Few cases required consultation with a plastic surgeon for possible excision and revision surgery to correct the defect resulting from the necrosis.
- Allergic reaction was identified by itchiness and severe swelling, including swelling of the face and tongue. Onset ranged from immediately after injection to two days after injection. Allergic reaction was generally treated with antihistamines and steroids. Some cases required hospitalization. All patients recovered from the allergic reaction with no permanent adverse outcome.
- Serious edema has been reported with an onset ranging from one day to three weeks (inflammation related to nodule formation). Treatment generally consisted of administration of antibiotics, antihistamines, and steroids. In some cases, patients sought treatment in an emergency room or were hospitalized. Generally, events resolved within one to two days, but a few patients have been reported as having intermittent or persistent edema related to a reoccurring infection. For cases where information was available, most patients have recovered or are recovering.
- Infection, often identified as cellulitis, was accompanied by swelling, hardened areas, redness, pustules, and pain. The onset of infection ranged from one day to two months and generally lasted two days but in one case persisted for six months. Infections were generally treated with antibiotics. For cases where information was available, patients had recovered or were recovering. Few patients experienced scarring that may require corrective surgery or discoloration at the site of the infection.

1.6.8 Individualization of Treatment

Before treatment, the patient's suitability for the treatment and need for pain relief should be assessed. The outcome of treatment will vary between patients. In some instances, additional treatments may be necessary depending on the size of the defect and the needs of the patient. Additional injections may be performed but only after sufficient time has passed to evaluate the patient. The patient should not be reinjected sooner than seven days after the previous treatment.

1.6.9 Directions for Use

1.6.9.1 General

The following are required for the percutaneous injection procedure:

- Radiesse injectable implant syringe(s) (provided separately)
- Appropriate size needle(s) with Luer lock fittings. The preferred size is a 25G O.D. to 27G I.D., or larger needle with a standard Luer fitting. Use of needles smaller in diameter than 27G I.D. may increase the incidence of needle occlusion.

1. Prepare patient for percutaneous injection using standard methods. The treatment injection site should be marked by a surgical marker and prepared with a suitable antiseptic. Local or topical anesthesia at the injection site or sedation should be used at the discretion of the physician. After anesthetizing the site, apply ice to the area to decrease local swelling/distention.
2. Prepare the syringes and injection needle(s) before the percutaneous injection. A new injection needle may be used for each syringe, or the same injection needle may be connected to each new syringe for same-patient treatment.
3. Remove foil pouch from the carton. The pouch can be opened and the syringe dropped onto the sterile field when required. There is a small amount of moisture normally present inside the foil pouch for sterilization purposes; this is not an indication of a defective product.
4. Peel or twist apart the needle packaging to expose the hub. For use of needles other than the needle(s) provided with this package, follow the directions provided with the needle(s).
5. Remove the Luer syringe cap from the distal end of the syringe prior to attaching the needle. The syringe can then be twisted onto the Luer lock fitting of the needle. The needle must be tightened securely to the syringe and primed with Radiesse injectable implant. If excess implant is on the surface of the Luer lock fittings, it will need to be wiped clean with sterile gauze. Slowly push the syringe plunger until the implant material extrudes from the end of the needle. If leakage is noted at the Luer fitting, it may be necessary to remove the needle and clean the surfaces of the Luer fitting or, in extreme cases, replace both the syringe and the needle.
6. Locate the initial site for the implant. Scar tissue and cartilage may be difficult or impossible to inject. Avoid, if at all possible, passing through these tissue types when advancing the injection needle. NOTE: Do not inject into a blood vessel.
7. The depth of the injection and the amount injected will vary depending on the site and extent of the restoration or augmentation. Radiesse injectable implant should be injected sufficiently deeply to prevent nodular formation at the surface of the skin or ischemia of the overlying tissue.
8. DO NOT OVERCORRECT THE INJECTION SITE. Use a 1:1 correction factor. Mold or massage the injected implant periodically during

the injection process to maintain a smooth contour of the implant.

9. If significant resistance is encountered when pushing the plunger, the injection needle may be moved slightly to allow easier placement of the material. If significant resistance is still encountered, it may be necessary to pull the needle entirely out of the injection site and try again in a new position. If significant resistance continues to persist, it may be necessary to try a different injection needle. If this is not successful, replace the syringe and injection needle.
10. Advance the needle into the deep dermis to the starting location. (Refer to additional instructions subsequently for augmentation of specific facial areas.) Carefully push the plunger of the syringe to start the injection and slowly inject the implant material while withdrawing the needle, placing a line of material in the desired location. Continue placing additional lines of material until the desired level of augmentation is achieved.

1.6.10 Augmentation of Cheeks, Chins, Face, or Corner of the Mouth

1. Insert needle with bevel down at approximately a 30° angle to the skin. The needle should slide into the deep dermis to the point you wish to begin the injection. This should be easily palpable with the nondominant hand.
2. Apply slow continuous even pressure to the syringe plunger to inject the implant as you withdraw the needle, leaving behind a single thin thread or strand of implant material. The thread of implant material should be completely surrounded by soft tissue without leaving globular deposits.
3. Individual threads of implant material should be placed parallel and adjacent to each other and layered when deeper folds are corrected. As an option, the threads can be cross-layered in a deeper plane for structural support.
4. After injection, use the index finger and thumb to smooth the areas and better distribute the implant in case of any slight nodular deposition of material.
5. Injection can be made in the subcutaneous tissue or muscle but not adjacent to bone or in the epidermis.

See further Video 1.2.

1.6.11 Patient Counseling Information

The patient should be instructed about appropriate postprocedural care, which may include the following, to promote normal healing and avoid complications.

- Apply ice or cool compresses to areas of injection for approximately 24 hours.
- Avoid the sun, tanning (ultraviolet) lights, sauna, and intense facial treatments postoperatively.
- Massage area if palpable nodules become present.
- Promote facial rest for one week by encouraging patients to limit talking, smiling, and laughing.

Inform the patient that postoperative swelling and numbness are common. Swelling will usually resolve within 7–10 days but may persist for several weeks. Numbness should resolve within 4–6 weeks.

1.6.12 How Implant Is Supplied

Radiesse injectable implant is provided sterile and nonpyrogenic in a syringe packaged in a foil pouch and boxed for convenient storage. Each unit consists of one prefilled syringe containing either 3.0 mL, 1.5 mL, 0.8 mL, or 0.3 mL of Radiesse injectable implant and one or two 25G–27G needle(s). The degree of accuracy of syringe graduations is ±0.025 mL for 1.5 mL, 0.8 mL, and 0.3 mL volumes. The degree of accuracy of syringe gradations is ±0.5 mL for the 3.0 mL volume. Do not use if packaging and/or syringe are damaged or if the syringe end cap or syringe plunger is not intact.

The contents of the syringe are intended for single-patient, single-treatment use only and cannot be resterilized. Reuse may compromise the functional properties of the device and/or lead to device failure. Reuse may also create a risk of contamination of the device and/or cause patient infection or cross-infection including but not limited to transmission of infectious disease(s) and blood transfer between patients, all of which, in turn, may lead to patient injury, illness, or death.

1.6.13 Storage

Packaged Radiesse injectable implant should be stored at a controlled room temperature between 15 and 32°C (59 to 90°F). Do not use if the expiration date has been exceeded. The expiration date is printed on the product labels.

1.6.14 Disposal

Used and partially used syringes and injection needles could be biohazardous and should be handled and disposed of in accordance with facility medical practices and local, state, or federal regulations.

1.6.15 Consultation: Expectations

Before the onset of the treatment, you should always ensure that a patient has realistic expectations in regard to the result of the treatment. It is essential that a patient know what is and is not possible. A thorough understanding of the patient's preferences and desires allows the treating physician to manage the expectations of the patient.

1.7 OTHER BRANDS

1.7.1 Crystalys

Crystalys is CaHA-based dermal filler that is designed to restore facial volume and natural contours by promoting endogenous collagen. Crystalys offers immediate and long-lasting effects, with clinical results visible for up to two years. The product is composed of 55.7% CaHA, glycerin, sodium carboxymethylcellulose, and phosphate buffer and is available with or without 0.3% lidocaine. Crystalys has been marketed in Israel from September 2011 for facial soft tissue augmentation.

Crystalys stands out due to its round, smooth, non-porous CaHA microspheres, sized 25–45μm in diameter, which ensure easy extrusion and minimize the risk of particle migration and phagocytosis, leading to a smoother appearance. The microspheres form a scaffold that supports fibroblast ingrowth, which in turn produces new collagen, ensuring a lasting, natural, and youthful look. This mechanism of action provides an immediate filling and lifting effect, with long-term results that develop in harmony with the material's degradation. Clinical data shows high patient satisfaction, with 93% of patients recommending the treatment, 92% satisfied with the treatment, 90% experiencing superior post-treatment results, and 90% likely to return for future treatments. Adverse events were low in frequency, with no serious adverse events observed; all side effects were mild, temporary, and correctable, typically related to the injection site rather than the filler itself. Crystalys is provided in a box containing 2 × 1.25–mL syringes, and its benefits include minimal discomfort during treatment due to lidocaine, biocompatibility, and biodegradability, along with a volumizing, lifting effect backed by extensive clinical experience and a sound safety profile.

1.7.2 Novuma

Novuma is also a CaHA-based dermal filler, originally developed by Burgeon Biotechnology, which strategically partnered with Laboratoires Vivacy (France) to deploy across Europe [77]. Its concentration of CaHA particles is in the same range as Crystalys, with 55–60% (w/w) CaHA microspheres by weight in the CMC gel. Novuma is currently indicated for facial volumizing procedures and skin quality improvement, while additional indications such as neck, décolletage, extremities, abdomen, or hips are under evaluation. It is marketed for its immediate filler effect, combined with long-term skin rejuvenation, lifting, and contouring effects through fibroblast-mediated collagen and elastin stimulation [78].

1.7.3 HArmonyCa

HArmonyCa is a soft tissue filler developed by Panaxia, an Israel-based company. Its formulation is derived from the CE marked devices, Crystalys lidocaine and Hydrayalix deep lidocaine. In terms of composition, HArmonyCa is a hybrid filler consisting of 70% hyaluronic acid (HA) gel (20 mg/mL) and 30% CaHA microspheres (55.7%, 25–45 μm in diameter) [79]. The Israeli Ministry of Health granted marketing approval for HArmonyCa lidocaine in September 2016. This was followed by approval in Brazil in April 2020. In October 2020, Allergan aesthetics, a subsidiary of AbbVie Company, acquired HArmonyCa. Subsequently, the product received its CE mark in November 2020, and the HArmonyCa lidocaine variant achieved the same in May 2021.

The rationale behind the development of HArmonyCa was to combine the attributes of HA and CaHA in a single pre-filled syringe. HA is intended to provide immediate volume upon injection, while CaHA is to serve as a biostimulant, promoting the production of endogenous collagen for a sustained effect over time. Previous studies have evaluated the safety and efficacy of combining HA and CaHA filler products for aesthetic treatments in various facial areas [70,72]. However, these studies focused on blended products where HA and CaHA were mixed on-site and lacked standardized methodology. In contrast, HArmonyCa is a ready-to-use hybrid product. The manufacturer claims that there are some benefits using a hybrid product over a blended product because blending can potentially alter the original properties of the fillers, affecting cohesivity and rheology; on-site blending requires the use of multiple syringes, leading to concerns about sterility and contamination, and increases the risk of medical liability in the event of procedural errors. A recent single-center, prospective, quasi-experimental study involving 15 participants aged between 32 and 63 years aimed to assess the efficacy of HArmonyCa and reported significant patient satisfaction and an increase in dermal thickness at 90 and 120 days post-treatment [80]. These findings add weight to the manufacturer's claims that HArmonyCa offers a dual mode of action for facial soft-tissue augmentation. However, it remains unclear whether hybrid products offer an advantage over blended products, and further research is needed to provide additional data.

REFERENCES

[1] C. A. Garrido, T. C. F. V. S. Sampaio, "Use of bioceramics in filling bone defects," *Revista Brasileira de Ortopedia (English Edition)*, vol. 45, no. 4, pp. 433–438, 2010.

[2] "Radiesse injectable implant—instructions for use," *Radiesse* [online]: https://radiesse.com/app/uploads/2024/04/instructions-for-use-radiesse-wrinkles.pdf (accessed Nov. 2024).

[3] R. W. Evans et al., "Cultured human monocytes and fibroblasts solubilize calcium phosphate crystals," *Calcif Tissue Int*, vol. 36, no. 6, pp. 645–650, 1984.

[4] Y. Zhu et al., "A shear-thinning electrostatic hydrogel with antibacterial activity by nanoengineering of polyelectrolytes," *Biomater Sci*, vol. 8, no. 5, pp. 1394–1404, 2020.

[5] S. B. Aguilera et al., "The role of calcium hydroxylapatite (Radiesse) as a regenerative aesthetic treatment: A narrative review," *Aesthet Surg J*, vol. 43, no. 10, pp. 1063–1090, 2023.

[6] D. M. Varma et al., "Injectable carboxymethylcellulose hydrogels for soft tissue filler applications," *Acta Biomater*, vol. 10, no. 12, pp. 4996–5004, 2014.

[7] F. Salah et al., "Development, characterization, and biological assessment of biocompatible cellulosic wound dressing grafted Aloe vera bioactive polysaccharide," *Cellulose*, vol. 26, no. 8, pp. 4957–4970, 2019.
[8] H. Mohammadi et al., "Optimization of antimicrobial nanocomposite films based on carboxymethyl cellulose incorporating chitosan nanofibers and Guggul gum polysaccharide," *Scientific Rep*, vol. 14, no. 1, pp. 1–17, 2024.
[9] C. Zhang et al., "Poly(hexamethylene guanidine)-based hydrogels with long lasting antimicrobial activity and low toxicity," *J Polym Sci A Polym Chem*, vol. 55, no. 12, pp. 2027–2035, 2017.
[10] E. Olewnik-Kruszkowska et al., "Antibacterial films based on PVA and PVA–chitosan modified with poly(hexamethylene guanidine)," *Polymers*, vol. 11, no. 12, p. 2093, 2019.
[11] N. Jannatyha et al., "Comparing mechanical, barrier and antimicrobial properties of nanocellulose/CMC and nanochitosan/CMC composite films," *Int J Biol Macromol*, vol. 164, pp. 2323–2328, 2020.
[12] H. Sundaram et al., "Comparison of the rheological properties of viscosity and elasticity in two categories of soft tissue fillers: Calcium hydroxylapatite and hyaluronic acid," *Dermatol Surg*, vol. 36, no. Suppl 3, pp. 1859–1865, 2010.
[13] J. M. Lee, Y. J. Kim, "Foreign body granulomas after the use of dermal fillers: Pathophysiology, clinical appearance, histologic features, and treatment," *Arch Plast Surg*, vol. 42, no. 2, p. 232, 2015.
[14] G. Lemperle et al., "Human histology and persistence of various injectable filler substances for soft tissue augmentation," *Aesthetic Plast Surg*, vol. 27, no. 5, pp. 354–366, 2003.
[15] J. Van Loghem, "Calcium hydroxylapatite in regenerative aesthetics: Mechanistic insights and mode of action," *Aesthet Surg J*, vol. 45, no. 4, pp. 393–403, 2025.
[16] E. S. Marmur et al., "Clinical, histologic and electron microscopic findings after injection of a calcium hydroxylapatite filler," *J Cosmet Laser Ther*, vol. 6, no. 4, pp. 223–226, 2004.
[17] R. J. Miron et al., "Giant cells around bone biomaterials: Osteoclasts or multi-nucleated giant cells?," *Acta Biomater*, vol. 46, pp. 15–28, 2016.
[18] T. Daley et al., "Oral lesions associated with injected hydroxyapatite cosmetic filler," *Oral Surg Oral Med Oral Pathol Oral Radiol*, vol. 114, no. 1, pp. 107–111, 2012.
[19] A. M. Holzapfel et al., "Soft-tissue augmentation with calcium hydroxylapatite: Histological analysis," *Arch Facial Plast Surg*, vol. 10, no. 5, pp. 335–338, 2008.
[20] J. Kim, "Multilayered injection of calcium hydroxylapatite filler on ischial soft tissue to rejuvenate the previous phase of chronic sitting pressure sore," *Clin Cosmet Investig Dermatol*, vol. 12, pp. 771–784, 2019.
[21] P. R. Shumaker et al., "Calcium hydroxylapatite tissue filler discovered 6 years after implantation into the nasolabial fold: Case report and review," *Dermatol Surg*, vol. 35, no. Suppl 1, pp. 375–379, 2009.
[22] S. Shahrabi-Farahani et al., "Granulomatous foreign body reaction to dermal cosmetic fillers with intraoral migration," *Oral Surg Oral Med Oral Pathol Oral Radiol*, vol. 117, no. 1, pp. 105–110, 2014.
[23] I. Moulonguet et al., "Foreign body reaction to Radiesse: 2 cases," *Am J Dermatopathol*, vol. 35, no. 3, 2013.
[24] J. E. Brown et al., "Injectable silk protein microparticle-based fillers: A novel material for potential use in glottic insufficiency," *J Voice*, vol. 33, no. 5, pp. 773–780, 2019.
[25] B. Ten Harkel et al., "The foreign body giant cell cannot resorb bone, but dissolves hydroxyapatite like osteoclasts," *PLoS One*, vol. 10, no. 10, p. e0139564, 2015.
[26] N. Zerbinati et al., "Microscopic and ultrastructural evidences in human skin following calcium hydroxylapatite filler treatment," *Arch Dermatol Res*, vol. 309, no. 5, pp. 389–396, 2017.
[27] K. Goldie, "The evolving field of regenerative aesthetics," *J Cosmet Dermatol*, vol. 22, no. S1, pp. 1–7, 2023.
[28] N. Corduff, "Introducing aesthetic regenerative scaffolds: An immunological perspective," *J Cosmet Dermatol*, vol. 22, no. S1, pp. 8–14, 2023.
[29] A. L. Berlin et al., "Calcium hydroxylapatite filler for facial rejuvenation: A histologic and immunohistochemical analysis," *Dermatol Surg*, vol. 34, no. Suppl 1, pp. S64–S67, 2008.
[30] N. González, D. J. Goldberg, "Evaluating the effects of injected calcium hydroxylapatite on changes in human skin elastin and proteoglycan formation," *Dermatol Surg*, vol. 45, no. 4, pp. 547–551, 2019.
[31] Y. Yutskovskaya et al., "A randomized, split-face, histomorphologic study comparing a volumetric calcium hydroxylapatite and a hyaluronic acid-based dermal filler," *J Drugs Dermatol*, vol. 13, no. 9, pp. 1047–1052, 2014.
[32] Y. A. Yutskovskaya, E. A. Kogan, "Improved neocollagenesis and skin mechanical properties after injection of diluted calcium hydroxylapatite in the neck and décolletage: A pilot study," *J Drugs Dermatol*, vol. 16, no. 1, pp. 68–74, 2017.
[33] C. Courderot-Masuyer et al., "Evaluation of lifting and antiwrinkle effects of calcium hydroxylapatite filler: In vitro quantification

of contractile forces of human wrinkle and normal aged fibroblasts treated with calcium hydroxylapatite," *J Cosmet Dermatol*, vol. 15, no. 3, pp. 260–268, 2016.
[34] B. Nowag et al., "Calcium hydroxylapatite microspheres activate fibroblasts through direct contact to stimulate neocollagenesis," *J Cosmet Dermatol*, vol. 22, no. 2, pp. 426–432, 2023.
[35] A. D. McCarthy et al., "Comparative rheology of hyaluronic acid fillers, poly-L-lactic acid, and varying dilutions of calcium hydroxylapatite," *Plast Reconstr Surg Glob Open*, vol. 12, no. 8, p. e6068, 2024.
[36] D. Jiang et al., "The multifaceted functions of TRPV4 and calcium oscillations in tissue repair," *Int J Mol Sci*, vol. 25, no. 2, 2024.
[37] G. J. Fisher et al., "Looking older: Fibroblast collapse and therapeutic implications," *Arch Dermatol*, vol. 144, no. 5, pp. 666–672, 2008.
[38] L. Follonier Castella et al., "Regulation of myofibroblast activities: Calcium pulls some strings behind the scene," *Exp Cell Res*, vol. 316, no. 15, pp. 2390–2401, 2010.
[39] A. B. G. Lansdown, "Calcium: A potential central regulator in wound healing in the skin," *Wound Repair Regen*, vol. 10, no. 5, pp. 271–285, 2002.
[40] X. Pang et al., "Unraveling the role of calcium ions in the mechanical properties of individual collagen fibrils," *Scientific Rep*, vol. 7, no. 1, pp. 1–8, 2017.
[41] F. Moccia et al., "Endothelial Ca2+ signaling, angiogenesis and vasculogenesis: Just what it takes to make a blood vessel," *Int J Mol Sci*, vol. 20, no. 16, p. 3962, 2019.
[42] T. Subramaniam et al., "The role of calcium in wound healing," *Int J Mol Sci*, vol. 22, no. 12, p. 6486, 2021.
[43] N. Jetten et al., "Anti-inflammatory M2, but not pro-inflammatory M1 macrophages promote angiogenesis in vivo," *Angiogenesis*, vol. 17, no. 1, pp. 109–118, 2014.
[44] E. Zajac et al., "Angiogenic capacity of M1- and M2-polarized macrophages is determined by the levels of TIMP-1 complexed with their secreted proMMP-9," *Blood*, vol. 122, no. 25, p. 4054, 2013.
[45] S. Oh et al., "Poly-D, L-lactic acid stimulates angiogenesis and collagen synthesis in aged animal skin," *Int J Mol Sci*, vol. 24, no. 9, p. 7986, 2023.
[46] P. P. Rovatti et al., "Hyperdiluted calcium hydroxylapatite 1: 2 for mid and lower facial skin rejuvenation: Efficacy and safety," *Dermatol Surg*, vol. 46, no. 12, pp. E112–E117, 2020.
[47] T. L. Tzikas, "Evaluation of the radiance FN soft tissue filler for facial soft tissue augmentation," *Arch Facial Plast Surg*, vol. 6, no. 4, pp. 234–239, 2004.
[48] S. L. Silvers et al., "Prospective, open-label, 18-month trial of calcium hydroxylapatite (Radiesse) for facial soft-tissue augmentation in patients with human immunodeficiency virus-associated lipoatrophy: One-year durability," *Plast Reconstr Surg*, vol. 118, no. Suppl 3, 2006.
[49] T. Pavicic, "Complete biodegradable nature of calcium hydroxylapatite after injection for malar enhancement: An MRI study," *Clin Cosmet Investig Dermatol*, vol. 8, pp. 19–25, 2015.
[50] M. Meland et al., "Rheological properties of calcium hydroxylapatite with integral lidocaine," *J Drugs Dermatol*, vol. 15, no. 9, pp. 1107–1110, 2016.
[51] J. A. Kadouch, "Calcium hydroxylapatite: A review on safety and complications," *J Cosmet Dermatol*, vol. 16, no. 2, pp. 152–161, 2017.
[52] B. Sanchez et al., "Skin cell and tissue responses to cross-linked hyaluronic acid in low-grade inflammatory conditions," *Int J Inflam*, vol. 2023, no. 1, p. 3001080, 2023.
[53] P. D. Costantino et al., "Synthetic biomaterials in facial plastic and reconstructive surgery," *Facial Plast Surg*, vol. 9, no. 1, pp. 1–15, 1993.
[54] W. J. Parkes et al., "A preliminary report of percutaneous craniofacial osteoplasty in a rat calvarium," *Laryngoscope*, vol. 124, no. 7, pp. 1550–1553, 2014.
[55] A. Kaneko et al., "Hydroxyapatite nanoparticles as injectable bone substitute naterial in a vertical bone augmentation model," *In Vivo (Brooklyn)*, vol. 34, no. 3, pp. 1053–1061, 2020.
[56] S. E. Lobo et al., "Response of stem cells from different origins to biphasic calcium phosphate bioceramics," *Cell Tissue Res*, vol. 361, no. 2, pp. 477–495, 2015.
[57] A. Carruthers et al., "Radiographic and computed tomographic studies of calcium hydroxylapatite for treatment of HIV-associated facial lipoatrophy and correction of nasolabial folds," *Dermatol Surg*, vol. 34, no. Suppl 1, 2008.
[58] T. L. Tzikas, "A 52-month summary of results using calcium hydroxylapatite for facial soft tissue augmentation," *Dermatol Surg*, vol. 34, no. Suppl 1, 2008.
[59] M. Amselem, "Radiesse(®): A novel rejuvenation treatment for the upper arms," *Clin Cosmet Investig Dermatol*, vol. 9, pp. 9–14, 2015.
[60] V. C. Wasylkowski, "Body vectoring technique with Radiesse(®) for tightening of the abdomen, thighs, and brachial zone," *Clin Cosmet Investig Dermatol*, vol. 8, pp. 267–273, 2015.
[61] G. Casabona, P. Marchese, "Calcium hydroxylapatite combined with microneedling and ascorbic acid is effective for treating stretch marks," *Plast Reconstr Surg Glob Open*, vol. 5, no. 9, 2017.
[62] G. Casabona, G. Pereira, "Microfocused ultrasound with visualization and calcium hydroxylapatite for improving skin laxity and

cellulite appearance," *Plast Reconstr Surg Glob Open*, vol. 5, no. 7, 2017.

[63] N. G. Lapatina, T. Pavlenko, "Diluted calcium hydroxylapatite for skin tightening of the upper arms and abdomen," *J Drugs Dermatol*, vol. 16, no. 9, pp. 900–906, 2017.

[64] K. Goldie et al., "Global consensus guidelines for the injection of diluted and hyperdiluted calcium hydroxylapatite for skin tightening," *Dermatol Surg*, vol. 44, no. Suppl 1, pp. S32–S41, 2018.

[65] J. Van Loghem et al., "Calcium hydroxylapatite: Over a decade of clinical experience," *J Clin Aesthet Dermatol*, vol. 8, no. 1, pp. 38–49, 2015.

[66] A. Botsali et al., "The comparative dermal stimulation potential of constant-volume and constant-amount diluted calcium hydroxylapatite injections versus the concentrated form," *Dermatol Surg*, vol. 49, no. 9, pp. 871–876, 2023.

[67] M. Busso, R. Voigts, "An investigation of changes in physical properties of injectable calcium hydroxylapatite in a carrier gel when mixed with lidocaine and with lidocaine/epinephrine," *Dermatol Surg*, vol. 34, no. Suppl 1, 2008.

[68] M. S. Godin et al., "Use of Radiesse in combination with restylane for facial augmentation," *Arch Facial Plast Surg*, vol. 8, no. 2, pp. 92–97, 2006.

[69] T. Pavicic et al., "A novel, multistep, combination facial rejuvenation procedure for treatment of the whole face with incobotulinumtoxinA, and two dermal fillers-calcium hydroxylapatite and a monophasic, polydensified hyaluronic acid filler," *J Drugs Dermatol*, vol. 12, no. 9, pp. 978–984, 2013.

[70] J. W. Chang et al., "Facial rejuvenation using a mixture of calcium hydroxylapatite filler and hyaluronic acid filler," *J Craniofac Surg*, vol. 31, no. 1, pp. e18–e21, 2020.

[71] A. Moradi et al., "Nonsurgical chin and jawline augmentation using calcium hydroxylapatite and hyaluronic acid fillers," *Facial Plast Surg*, vol. 35, no. 2, pp. 140–148, 2019.

[72] N. Fakih-Gomez, J. Kadouch, "Combining calcium hydroxylapatite and hyaluronic acid fillers for aesthetic indications: Efficacy of an innovative hybrid filler," *Aesthetic Plast Surg*, vol. 46, no. 1, pp. 373–381, 2022.

[73] K. R. Beer, "Safety and effectiveness of injection of calcium hydroxylapatite via blunt cannula compared to injection by needle for correction of nasolabial folds," *J Cosmet Dermatol*, vol. 13, no. 4, pp. 288–296, 2014.

[74] J. Fulton et al., "Filler injections with the blunt-tip microcannula," *J Drugs Dermatol*, vol. 11, no. 9, pp. 1098–1103, 2012.

[75] D. Hexsel et al., "Double-blind, randomized, controlled clinical trial to compare safety and efficacy of a metallic cannula with that of a standard needle for soft tissue augmentation of the nasolabial folds," *Dermatol Surg*, vol. 38, no. 2, pp. 207–214, 2012.

[76] M. Amiri et al., "Skin regeneration-related mechanisms of calcium hydroxylapatite (CaHA): A systematic review," *Front Med (Lausanne)*, vol. 10, p. 1195934, 2023.

[77] Vivacy, Burgeon X Vivacy Sign Strategic Alliance [online] 2025: https://vivacy.com/en/hyaluronic-acid-injections-latest-research/burgeon-vivacy-partnership-skin-regeneration.

[78] Burgeon, Novuma CaHA Dermal Filler – Burgeon [online] 2025: https://burgeon.me/novuma-en/.

[79] Allergan, "HArmonyCATM lidocaine—injectable facial implant," [online], 2022: https://media.allergan.com/actavis/actavis/media/allergan-pdf-documents/HArmonyCa%E2%84%A2_with_lidocaine_IFU_GR.pdf.

[80] B. S. F. Bravo et al., "Dermal thickness increase and aesthetic improvement with hybrid product combining hyaluronic acid and calcium hydroxyapatite: A clinical and sonographic analysis," *Plast Reconstr Surg Glob Open*, vol. 11, no. 6, p. e5055, 2023.

Calcium Hydroxylapatite

2

Innovative Blends of CaHA

ALEC D. McCARTHY, VIVIANA PERICO, SHINO BAY AGUILERA, ALESSANDRO GENNAI, FABRIZIO MELFA, JONATHAN KADOUCH, NABIL FAKIH-GOMEZ, AND JANI VAN LOGHEM

2.1 BACKGROUND

In aesthetic medicine, the innovative blend of CaHA with other advanced methods marks a specialized and contemporary strategy for addressing facial aging. Because of their ability to simultaneously address various aspects of aging, these integrated treatments yield more comprehensive and enhanced results. Nonetheless, the effective and safe execution of these blended therapies necessitates in-depth knowledge of their individual and collective effects, highlighting the importance of expertise in this domain. In this chapter, we explore three innovative blended approaches utilizing CaHA, along with their respective treatment protocols.

2.2 CAHA: NCTF

The integration of CaHA with new cellular treatment factor (NCTF), a concoction of hyaluronic acid, vitamins, and other micronutrients, capitalizes on the micronutrient benefits of NCTF. Since micronutrient deficiencies in patients can affect treatment outcomes, supplementing amino acids and co-enzymes to CaHA, known for its regenerative properties, establishes a nutritional base for effective protein synthesis. The blended approach has been shown to significantly improve skin laxity, wrinkle severity, luminosity, and hyperpigmentation in all patients after a single session [1].

2.2.1 Step-by-Step Technique

1. Take equal volumes (1.5 mL) of Radiesse(+) and NCTF 135HA to achieve a 1:1 dilution in the facial region.

   For applications in the neck and décolletage areas, it is recommended to use a hyperdiluted mixture of 1:4 to avoid any risk of nodule formation.
2. Transfer each component into separate 5 mL syringes.
3. Connect the syringes via a female-to-female sterile adaptor. Ensure the adaptor is secure to prevent any leakage or contamination.
4. Pass the suspension back and forth between the syringes at least 20 times to ensure thorough mixing and homogenization of the two components.
5. Combine 2.5% lidocaine with 2.5% prilocaine to form a numbing cream and apply a thin, uniform layer of the cream to the mid and lower facial areas 30 minutes prior to the treatment.
6. Select a blunt-tip cannula 25G, 50 mm for the procedure.
7. Employ a three-point entry approach for the injection sites:
   i. The first insertion point is to be located 1 cm anterior to the zygomatic ligament.
   ii. Place the second insertion point 1.5–2 cm from the oral commissure.
   iii. Locate the third insertion point 1.0–1.5 cm anterior to the gonial angle.
8. Infiltrate 1% lidocaine with adrenaline solution (1:200000) at these points.
9. Administer the blended mixture using a retrograde fanning technique, moving from medial to lateral and placing 0.1 mL product in each retrograde passage.

See Video 2.1 to visualize the mixing technique of Radiesse and NCTF 135 HA.

Video 2.1 Mixing technique for Radiesse and NCTF 135 HA.

2.3 CAHA: GUIDED SEFFI

The guided superficial enhanced fluid fat injection (SEFFI) technique is an innovative advancement in aesthetic medicine, focusing on the rejuvenation of aging skin by utilizing the regenerative properties of autologous fat tissue. This minimally invasive method allows for the safe, effective, and standardized collection of superficial adipose tissue (SAT), which is particularly rich in mesenchymal and vascular stem cells, making it accessible even to practitioners without advanced surgical skills. The approach of integrating emulsified tissue prepared via the guided SEFFI technique with CaHA filler effectively addresses facial volume loss. This method not only achieves natural reharmonization but also ensures longer-lasting results [2,3].

2.3.1 Step-by-Step Technique

1. Administer local anesthesia using the microperforated cannula with 0.8 mm side port holes

DOI: 10.1201/9781003617129-2

mounted inside the unique patented guide (provided with the SEFFILLER kit) and wait for 10 minutes.
2. Gently aspirate adipose tissue from the abdomen or the trochanteric region using a back-and-forth fan movement using the microperforated cannula with 0.8 mm side port holes mounted inside the unique patented guide (provided with the SEFFILLER kit) (Figure 2.1).
3. Monitor the procedure and stop once 5 mL of superficial adipose tissue (SAT) has been collected (Figure 2.2).
4. Medicate the area using an adhesive wound strip and mildly compress with kinetic tape.

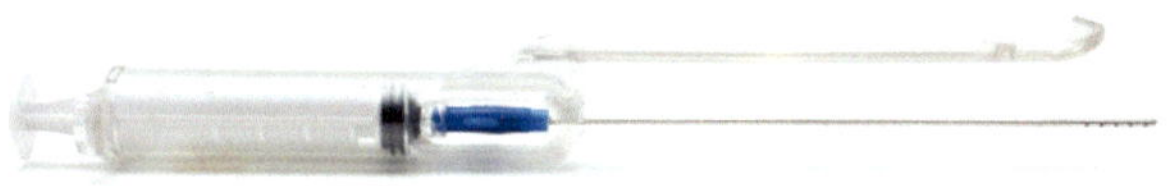

Figure 2.1 Guide with syringe and cannula.

5. Transfer the harvested adipose tissue into the reservoir syringes (blue plunger).
6. Fill the reservoir syringes with saline solution and allow them to stand vertically for five minutes, letting the contents separate via gravity into three layers: oil, tissue, and washing liquid in the bottom of the reservoir syringe (Figure 2.3).
7. Gently discard the washing liquid.
8. The microfragmented adipose tissue is ready for injection.
9. Prepare the CaHA dilution:
   i. Dilution (1:1)
      a. Connect the CaHA filler syringe to a 3 mL syringe using the Luer-lock transfer.
      b. Transfer the filler to the 3 mL syringe.
      c. Connect this syringe to another 3 mL syringe preloaded with 1.5 mL of sterile saline solution.

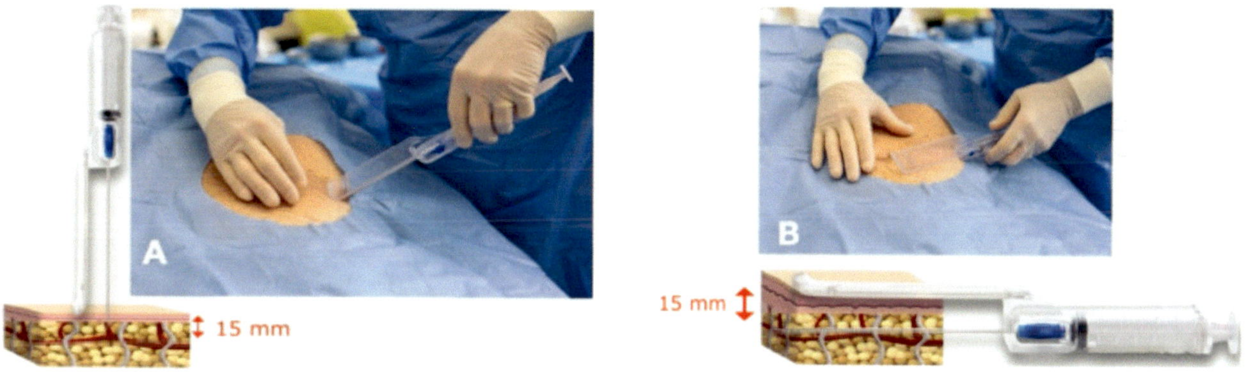

Figure 2.2 The guide ensures that the cannula does not go beyond 15 mm beneath the skin surface, targeting the collection of superficial adipose tissue (SAT) at the adequate depth. (A) The cannula's tip is designed to reach precisely 15 mm deep. The guide's blade prevents the cannula from going any deeper. (B) The guide's blade contacts the skin, enabling the cannula to harvest the SAT exactly at a 15 mm depth.

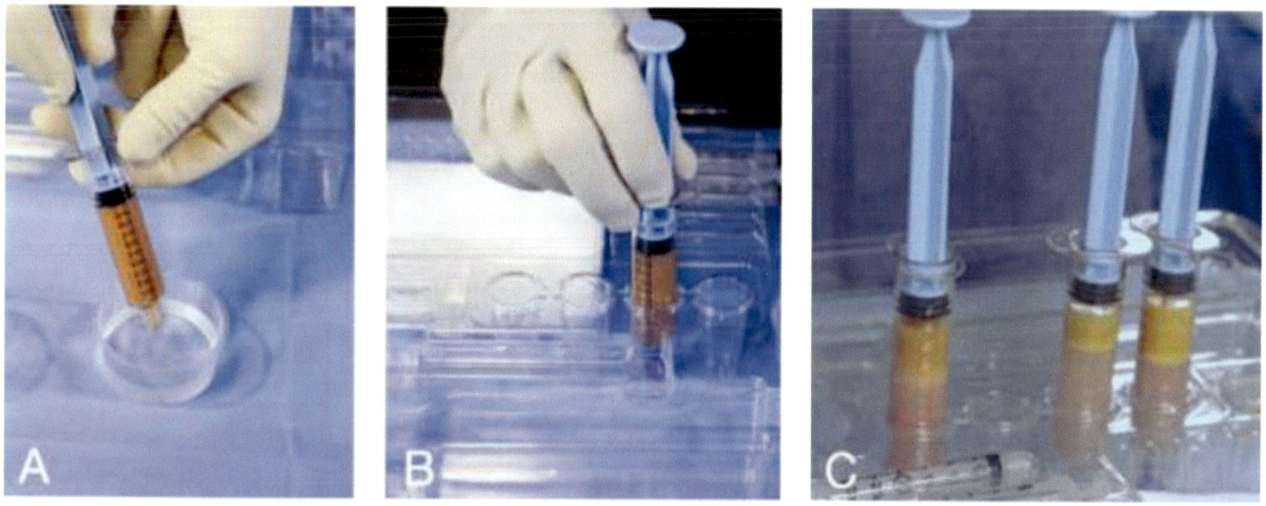

Figure 2.3 (A) Reservoir syringe filled with saline solution and capped. (B) Reservoir syringe positioned vertically in a holder for decanting. (C) Following a five-minute decanting, the tissue separates from the washing liquid, which is then set to be discarded.

d. Perform several transfers between the two syringes to achieve homogenous dilution.

ii. Hyperdilution (1:2, if required)

a. Transfer the CaHA filler to a 5 mL syringe.

b. Connect this syringe to another 5 mL syringe preloaded with 3 mL of sterile saline solution.

c. Perform multiple transfers between the two syringes to achieve a consistent hyperdilution.

10. If needed, perform minimal manipulation of the microfragmented adipose tissue by transferring the tissue between syringes (emulsification) to achieve the desired fluidity, especially for delicate facial regions (refer to fluidity chart in Figure 2.4).
11. Evaluate the patient in a standing position.
12. Use a marker to outline the facial areas designated for treatment.
13. Position the patient in a supine position.
14. Administer a small amount of local anesthesia at the entry points for the cannula.
15. Inject the prepared CaHA filler subcutaneously using a cannula and a linear retrograde fanning technique: 1:1 dilution for areas with thicker skin or 1:2 hyperdilution for thinner skin areas.
16. Gently massage the injected areas immediately after the procedure.
17. Next, using a cannula (20–21G), inject the processed adipose tissue sequentially. The injections should be made into the superficial subcutaneous layer, utilizing a linear retrograde fanning technique.
18. In the facial region with thicker skin, it is recommended to emulsify using three passes, achieving cluster dimension of approximately 600 μm. For thinner facial skin, a recommendation of six passes with cluster dimension of 500 μm is advised.
19. Gently massage the treated area.

See Figures 2.5–2.6 to visualize the before and after results with the SEFFI-CaHA technique.

2.4 CAHA: CPM–HA

The innovative combination of CaHA with cohesive polydensified matrix–hyaluronic acid (CPM–HA) represents another novel approach in facial rejuvenation. While HA is the gold standard for volumization, due to its strategic deposition, CaHA is primarily effective through neocollagenesis. Moreover, the blending of CaHA and HA can be accomplished via two distinct methods: layering the products in the same treatment area or injecting a premixed combination of the two. Layering involves the sequential application of each product, maintaining their distinct rheological properties, while the premixing approach blends the two fillers prior to injection, potentially altering their combined rheological characteristics. Premixing HA with CaHA not only introduces neocollagenesis properties to the HA filler but also leverages the high viscosity of HA to enhance CaHA's volumization effects, all while preserving tissue softness. Furthermore, premixing addresses the issue of early volume loss in CaHA treatments, as HA compensates for the rapid absorption of CaHA's gel carrier. Ultimately, premixing of CaHA and CPM–HA leads to longer-lasting effects and enhanced tissue lifting [4,5].

2.4.1 Step-by-Step Technique

1. Mix the contents of a CaHA syringe and a CPM–HA desired syringe range (CPM–HA R, CPM–HA B, CPM–HA I, CPM–HA V) using a Luer-lock connector, following the standardized protocols of hybrid filler application [6].
2. Transfer the contents into an empty mixing syringe.
3. For:
   i. Facial treatment, add 0.3–0.5 mL of 2% lidocaine for every 1.5 mL of CaHA.
   ii. Hand treatment, add 1.5 mL of 2% lidocaine for every 1.5 mL of CaHA.
   iii. Neck treatment, add 1.5 mL of saline.

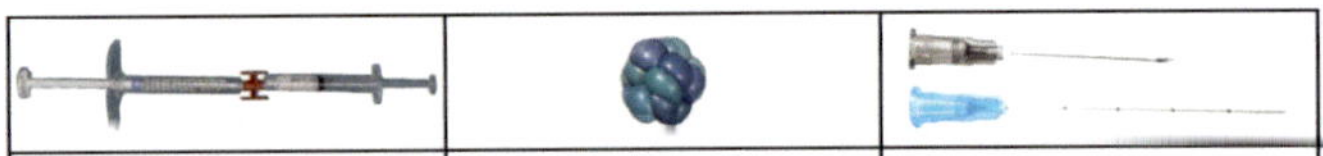

Number of passages	Clusters dimensions	Caliber of the cannula or needle
0	800 μm	18G (ID 0.83 mm)
2-3	600 μm	20G (ID 0.60 mm)
5-6	500 μm	21G (ID 0.51 mm)
10-11	400 μm	22G (ID 0.41 mm)
20-30	200 μm	27G (ID 0.21 mm)

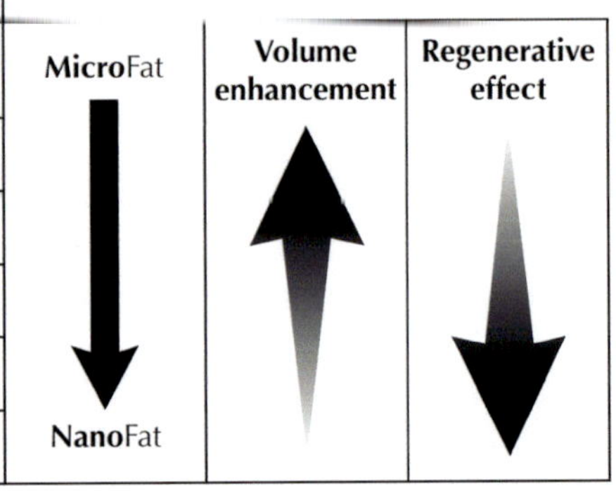

ID, internal diameter.

Figure 2.4 (A) Number of tissue passages between syringes via the transfer mechanism devoid of any filter. (B) Mean cluster dimensions following the transfers. (C) Typical dimensions of the cannula or needle employed to inject the tissue.

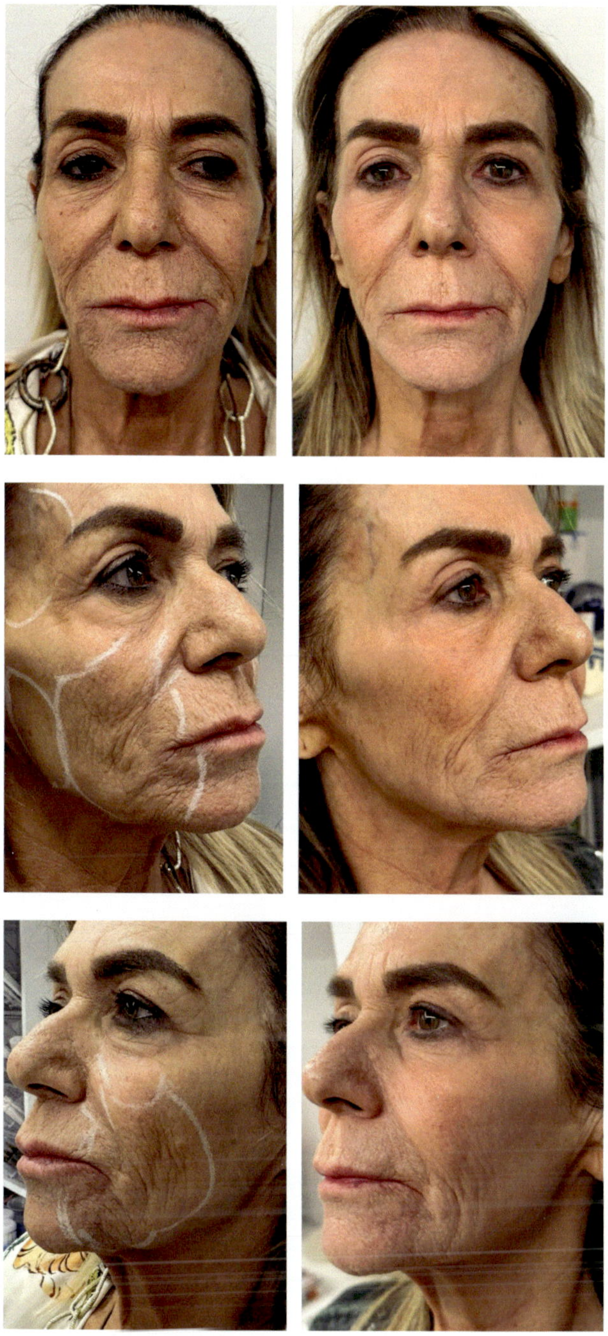

Figure 2.5 Before (left) and five months (right) post-treatment with SEFFI-CaHA.

4. Connect another empty mixing syringe to the filled syringe. Transfer the gels back and forth between the two syringes at least 20 times to ensure homogenization of the products.
5. The ratio of CaHA to HA depends on the treatment indication and severity. Face ratios can vary depending on the level of tissue laxity that needs to be addressed (CaHA:CPM–HA)
   i. Evident laxity, slight volume correction: 1:1 to 1:3
   ii. Mild laxity, mild volume correction: 1:4 to 2:4
   iii. Slight laxity, severe volume correction: 2:6 to 3:8

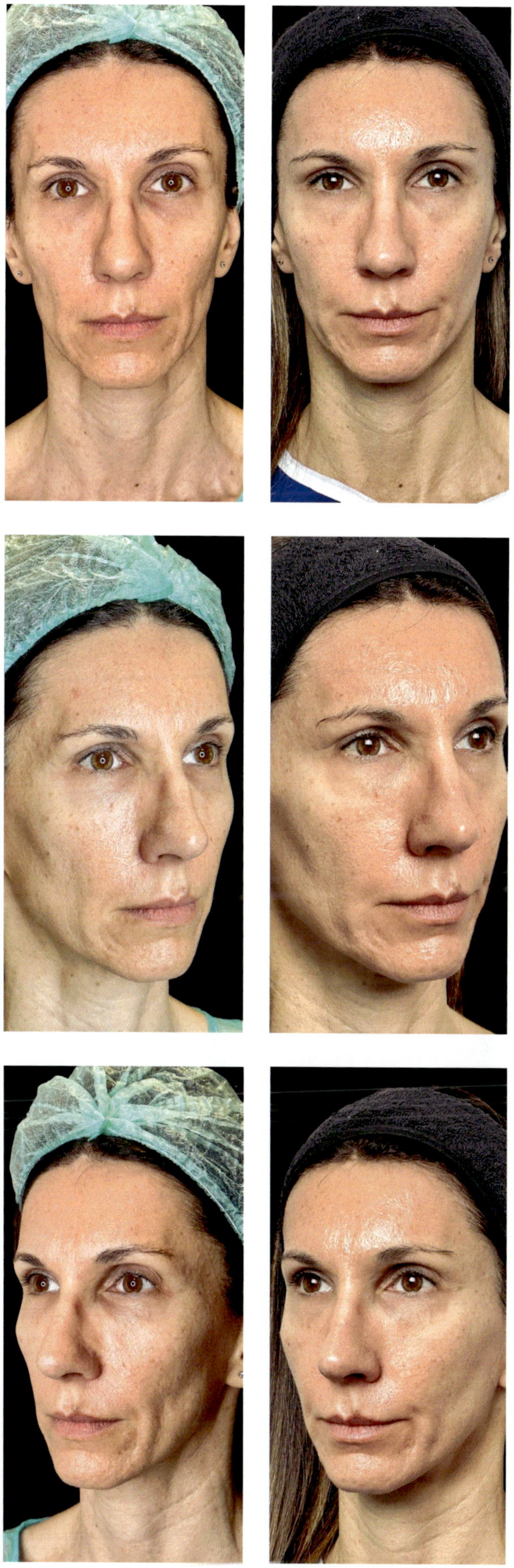

Figure 2.6 Before (left) and after (right) treatment with SEFFI-CaHA.

The ratios are based on the number of syringes, not volume.
6. Perform only subcutaneous injections (Mendelson's layer 2).
7. Use a fanning technique with a 22–25G, 50 mm cannula; inject 0.1–0.2 mL per trace.
8. Focus on the midface and lower face for injection.

See Video 2.2 to visualize the mixing technique of CaHA and CPM–HA.

Video 2.2 Mixing technique for CaHA and CPM–HA.

REFERENCES

[1] E. Theodorakopoulou et al., "Optimizing skin regenerative response to calcium hydroxylapatite microspheres via poly-micronutrient priming," *J Drugs Dermatol*, vol. 22, no. 9, pp. 925–934, 2023.
[2] A. Gennai et al., "Guided Superficial Enhanced Fluid Fat Injection (SEFFI) procedures for facial rejuvenation: An Italian multicenter retrospective case report," *Clin Pract*, vol. 13, no. 4, p. 924, 2023.
[3] F. Melfa et al., "Guided SEFFI and CaHA: A retrospective observational study of an innovative protocol for regenerative aesthetics," *J Clin Med*, vol. 13, no. 15, p. 4381, 2024.
[4] N. Fakih-Gomez, J. Kadouch, "Combining calcium hydroxylapatite and hyaluronic acid fillers for aesthetic indications: Efficacy of an innovative hybrid filler," *Aesthetic Plast Surg*, vol. 46, no. 1, p. 373, 2021.
[5] J. Kadouch, N. Fakih-Gomez, "A hybrid filler: Combining calcium hydroxylapatite and hyaluronic acid fillers for aesthetic indications," *Am J Cosm Surg*, vol. 39, no. 3, pp. 182–189, 2021.
[6] N. Fakih-Gomez et al., "Standarized protocols for hybrid filler application in aesthetic medicine," *Am J Cosm Surg*, 2024, vol. 0, no. 0. http://doi.org/10.1177/07488068241227278

Block Anesthesia of the Whole Face

3

JOHN LEONARDO AND JANI VAN LOGHEM

3.1 BACKGROUND

Local anesthesia is a medical technique that numbs a targeted area of the body, enabling surgical or diagnostic interventions without causing pain. The history of local anesthesia began with the use of cocaine as the first local anesthetic. In 1884, Carl Koller demonstrated its use in eye surgery [1]. The early 20th century witnessed the development of safer alternatives to cocaine such as procaine (Novocaine). In 1943, Nils Löfgren synthesized lidocaine, which showed a faster onset and longer duration of action than procaine. Today, lidocaine remains one of the most commonly used local anesthetics. Later, other agents like bupivacaine and ropivacaine were introduced. In the late 19th and early 20th centuries, techniques for regional nerve blocks, where local anesthetics were injected near major nerve trunks or plexuses to anesthetize targeted areas, were developed [2].

Local anesthetics can be categorized into two groups based on their chemical structures: esters and amides. Esters encompass drugs like procaine, chloroprocaine, tetracaine, cocaine, and benzocaine. They are hydrolyzed by the enzyme pseudocholinesterase. The amide group consists of substances like lidocaine, prilocaine, bupivacaine, and ropivacaine which are metabolized primarily in the liver.

Local anesthetics come in diverse forms, each tailored for specific applications. Creams and gels, which are non-invasive topical formulations, provide surface numbing, making them ideal for minor cosmetic treatments. Sprays, with their quick application, are beneficial for numbing superficial areas like the throat or oral mucosa during medical procedures. Patches, infused with local anesthetics, are adhesive and offer extended pain relief, making them suitable for managing chronic conditions or post-surgical pain. For deeper and more precise numbing, injectable anesthetics are introduced directly into tissues or near nerves, serving an essential role in surgeries, diagnostic procedures, and chronic pain management. The choice of anesthetic form is based on the nature of the procedure, the required depth of numbness, and individual patient considerations.

3.2 MECHANISM OF ACTION

Local anesthetics function by interrupting nerve signal transmission. Neurons communicate through changes in electric charges across their cell membranes, facilitated by the movement of sodium (Na^+) ions. These ions move through sodium channels which are either in resting, activated, or inactivated states. When a neuron is stimulated, these channels open, allowing Na^+ ions to rush into the cell, leading to depolarization and signal transmission. Local anesthetics exert their numbing effect by targeting and blocking these sodium channels, particularly in activated or inactivated states. This blockade prevents the neuron from depolarizing, pausing signal propagation, and resulting in temporary loss of sensation in the affected area.

3.3 ADMINISTRATION

Local anesthesia can be administered topically or via injectables based on the need and purpose. In aesthetic medicine, topical anesthetics are frequently used to numb the skin and reduce discomfort during various minimally invasive procedures. Lidocaine-containing products are the most commonly used topical anesthetics, as they are known to provide a numbing effect with minimal side effects.

Accurate dosing and precise administration of local anesthetics are important and must be performed by a certified practitioner. For safe application, dosage is often calculated based on the patient's weight.

- For injectable lidocaine without adrenaline, the maximum dose is 4 mg/kg of body weight.
- For a 70-kg patient, this equals 280 mg and can be prepared with 28 mL of 1% lidocaine (because 1% means 10 mg/mL) or 14 mL of 2% lidocaine (because 2% means 20 mg/mL).
- For injectable lidocaine combined with adrenaline, the maximum dose is 7 mg/kg of body weight.
- For a 70-kg patient, this equals 490 mg and can be prepared with 49 mL of 1% lidocaine + adrenaline or 24.5 mL of 2% lidocaine + adrenaline.
- For tumescent anesthesia, e.g. used in liposuction procedures, diluted lidocaine in saline, combined with sodium bicarbonate and adrenaline, the maximum dose is 55 mg/kg of body weight. For a 70-kg patient, this equals 3850 mg of total lidocaine.

Practitioners should also pay attention to the concentration and volume implications of local anesthetics. Injections with a higher concentration but lower volume require high accuracy to avoid a failed block. However, the injection site's anatomy remains undistorted. Conversely, a lower concentration with a higher volume allows broader diffusion and thereby

DOI: 10.1201/9781003617129-3

improves chances of successful application, albeit with the possibly of altering the anatomy at the injection site.

3.4 ADDITIVES TO LOCAL ANESTHETICS

Major drawbacks of local anesthetics include their short duration of action and dose-dependent side effects. Therefore, adjuvants or additives are often used in conjunction with local anesthetics to prolong their action and to limit the cumulative dose requirement (Figure 3.1). Such additives include:

- *Adrenaline:* When used as an additive, adrenaline can prolong the numbing effect of local anesthetic by vasoconstriction. It also minimizes the drug's absorption into the wider circulatory system, thereby decreasing potential systemic side effects. In solutions, the concentration of adrenaline varies, with 1:200000 containing 5 µg/mL and 1:100000 having 2.5 µg/mL. More dilute solutions of adrenaline are recommended for use in hypertensive patients. It's crucial to note that while adrenaline can enhance many anesthetics, it doesn't prolong the action of Ropivacaine.
- *Sodium bicarbonate:* When added to local anesthetics, it increases the pH, leading to an elevated unionized state of the anesthetic. This unionized form of the local anesthetic can more easily penetrate nerve membranes. The result is a faster onset and a reduction in the pain associated with the injection itself. Typically, a ratio of 1 mL of 8.4% sodium bicarbonate is added per 10 mL of local anesthetic, like lidocaine. However, it's important to note that sodium bicarbonate should not be mixed with bupivacaine, as it can lead to precipitation [3]. It is recommended to add sodium bicarbonate immediately prior to injection. The local anesthetic may denature if left unused for a prolonged period, rendering it ineffective.

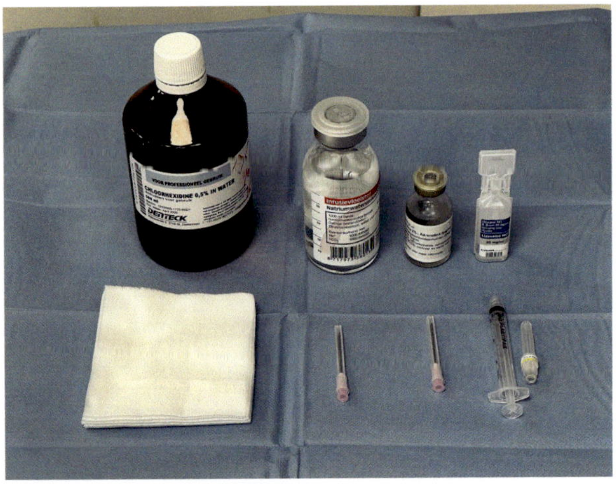

Figure 3.1 Materials used for administering local anesthesia.

3.5 TYPES OF NERVE BLOCKS

Nerve blocks involve placing the local anesthetic around specific nerve or nerve groups for pain management. In the context of aesthetic applications, these blocks are predominantly employed in the face and neck regions [4].

3.5.1 Trigeminal (Nerve V) Branch Block

The trigeminal nerve is the fifth cranial nerve and has three major branches: the ophthalmic (V1), maxillary (V2), and mandibular (V3) (Figure 3.2). Blocking any of these branches can be used for pain management, diagnostics, or surgical procedures.

3.5.2 Upper, Middle, and Lower Facial Blocks

Facial nerve blocks target the facial nerve branches, providing sensation and motor function to various face parts. The main branches include the zygomaticotemporal, supratrochlear, supraorbital, infraorbital, buccal, mandibular, and cervical branches (Figure 3.3). Some of these nerves can be found aligning vertically to the medial limbus line (Figure 3.4).

3.5.3 Neck Region

Nerve blocks of the posterior neck region typically target structures of the posterior mandible and anterior neck. The superficial cervical plexus innervates the skin of the anterolateral neck through the anterior primary

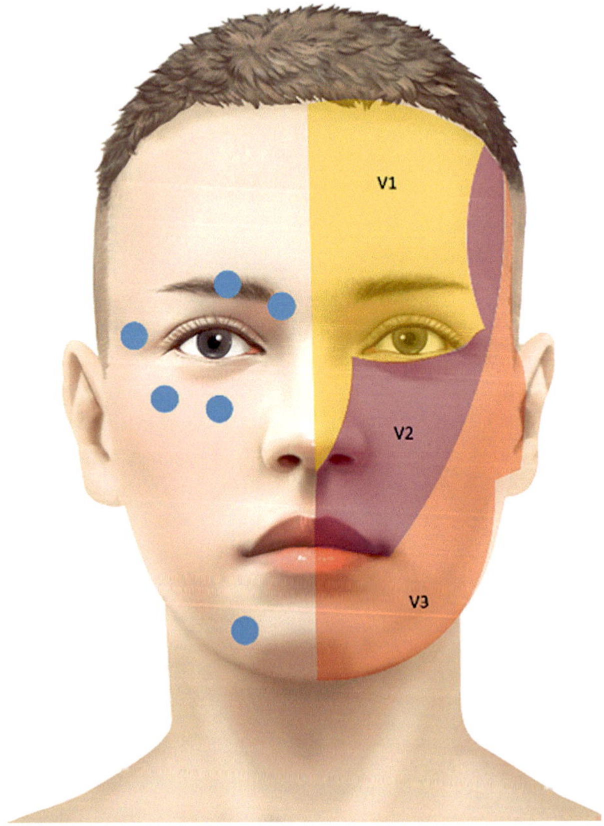

Figure 3.2 Overview of the regions that innervate the trigeminal nerve branches: the ophthalmic (V1), maxillary (V2), and mandibular (V3).

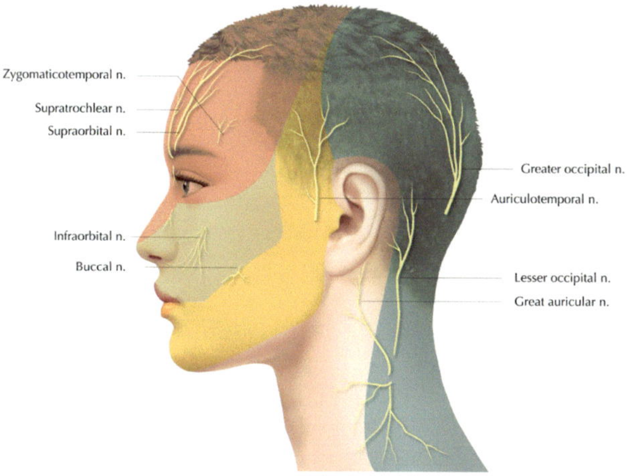

Figure 3.3 Innervation of the face, the neck, and the scalp.

rami of C2 through C4 [5]. These nerves converge at the midpoint of the sternocleidomastoid muscle at its posterior margin to provide sensory innervation to the skin of the lower mandible, neck, and supraclavicular fossa [6].

In this chapter, we explain in depth the step-by-step procedure for each nerve block along with the illustrations and videos. See Video 3.1 to visualize the nerve landmarks of the periorbital region.

Video 3.1 Nerve block landmarks.

3.5.3.1 Supratrochlear Nerve Block

- Disinfect.
- Determine injection location at the corrugator crease and the lower border of the head of the brow.
- Advance the needle softly to the periosteum.

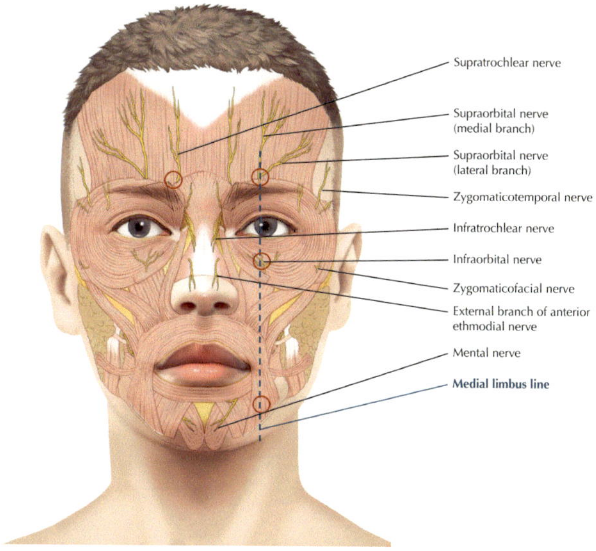

Figure 3.4 Vertical alignment of facial nerves to the medial limbus, contrary to traditional mid-pupillary descriptions.

- Aspirate and inject 0.2–0.5 mL.
- Consider injecting multiple smaller boluses.

See Figure 3.5 and Video 3.2 on how to perform a supratrochlear nerve block, Figure 3.6 to visualize the innervation area of the supratrochlear nerve, and Video 3.4 to observe the supratrochlear nerve block from a lateral view.

Video 3.2 Supratrochlear nerve block.

Video 3.3 Supraorbital nerve block.

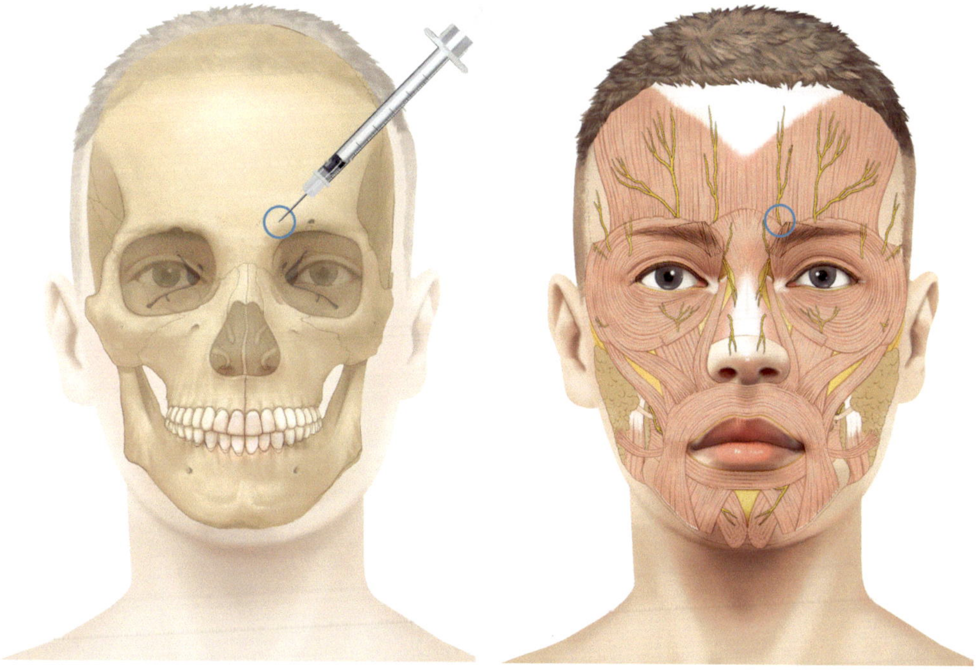

Figure 3.5 Supratrochlear nerve block.

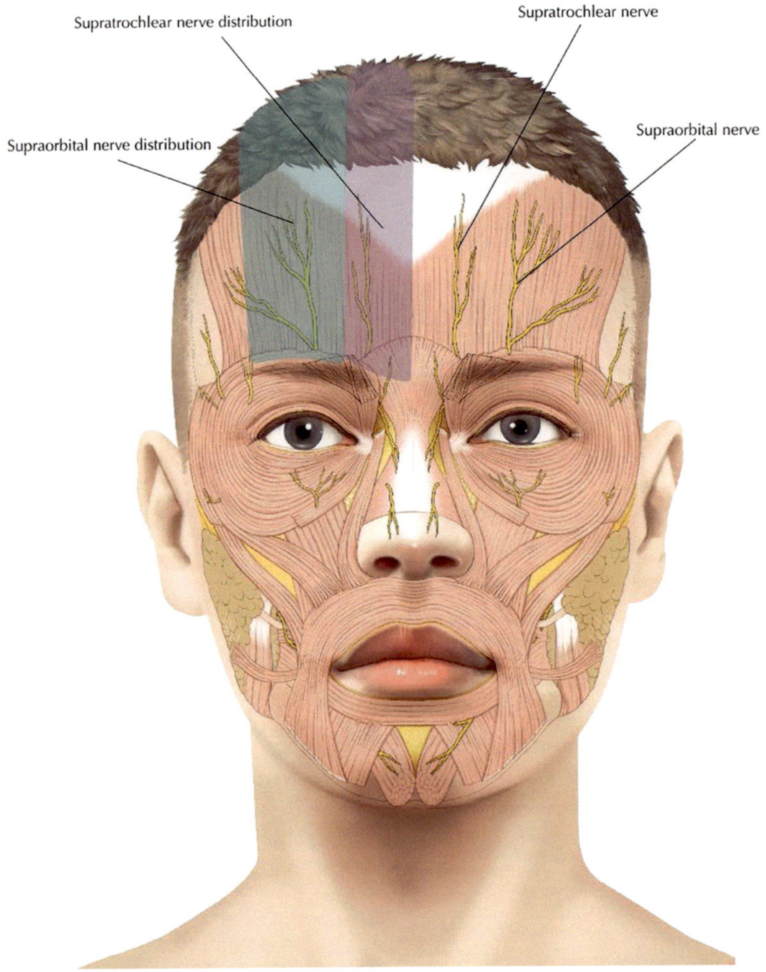

Figure 3.6 Innervation of the forehead by the supraorbital and supratrochlear nerves.

Video 3.4 Supratrochlear and supraorbital nerve block.

3.5.3.2 Supraorbital Nerve Block

- Disinfect.
- Determine injection location by palpating at the depression in the supraorbital rim.
- Advance from 45° latero-superior.
- Soft touch to the periosteum.
- Aspirate and inject 0.2–0.5 mL.
- Consider injecting multiple smaller boluses.

See Figure 3.7 and Video 3.3 on how to perform a supraorbital nerve block, Figure 3.6 to visualize the innervation area of the supraorbital nerve, and Video 3.4 to observe the supraorbital nerve block from a lateral view.

3.5.3.3 Zygomaticotemporal Nerve Block

- Disinfect.
- Determine the injection location by palpating the lateral orbital rim.
- Advance the needle at 45° from dorsally under the lateral orbital rim.
- Soft touch to the periosteum.
- Aspirate and inject 0.5–1 mL.
- Consider injecting multiple smaller boluses.

See Figure 3.8 and Video 3.5 on how to perform a zygomaticotemporal nerve block.

Video 3.5 Zygomaticotemporal nerve block.

3.5.3.4 Zygomaticofacial Nerve Block

- Disinfect.
- Palpate lateral orbital rim, about 5 mm inferior to the infraorbital rim.
- Soft touch with needle to the periosteum.
- Aspirate and inject 0.2–0.5 mL.
- Consider injecting multiple smaller boluses.

See Figure 3.9 and Video 3.6 on how to perform a zygomaticofacial nerve block.

Video 3.6 Zygomaticofacial nerve block.

3.5.3.5 Infraorbital Nerve Block

- Disinfect.
- Palpate with the fifth finger a depression 2–3 mm medial to mid-pupillary line and about 9 mm inferior to the infraorbital rim.
- Soft touch with the needle to the periosteum.

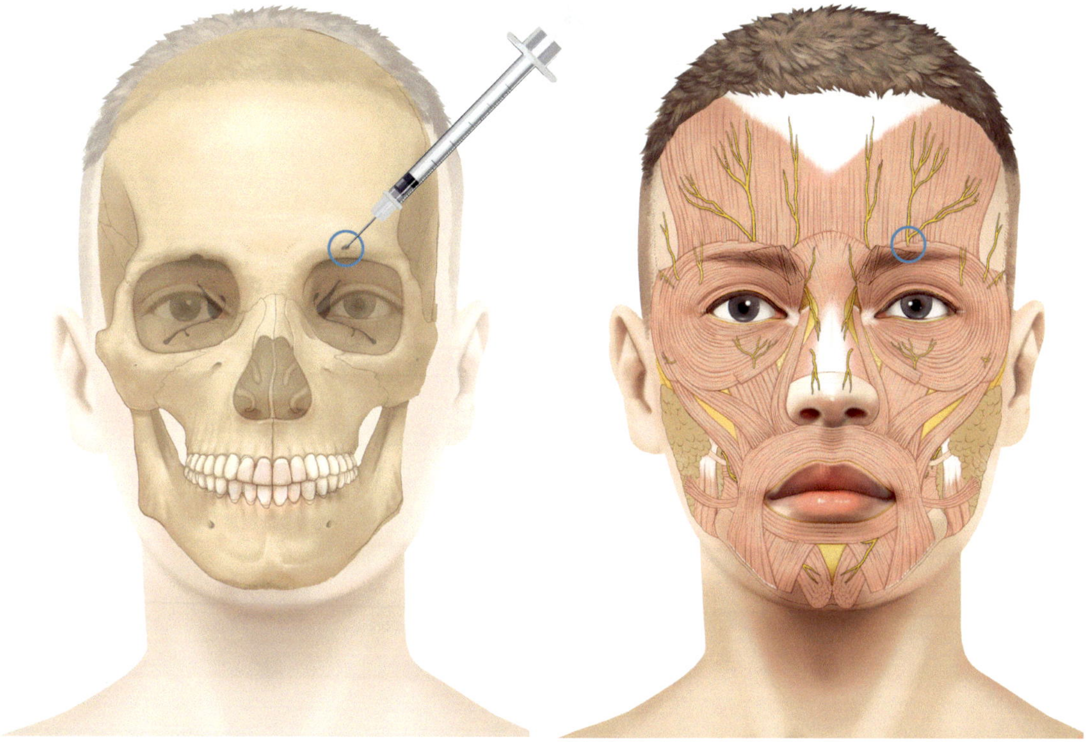

Figure 3.7 Supraorbital nerve block.

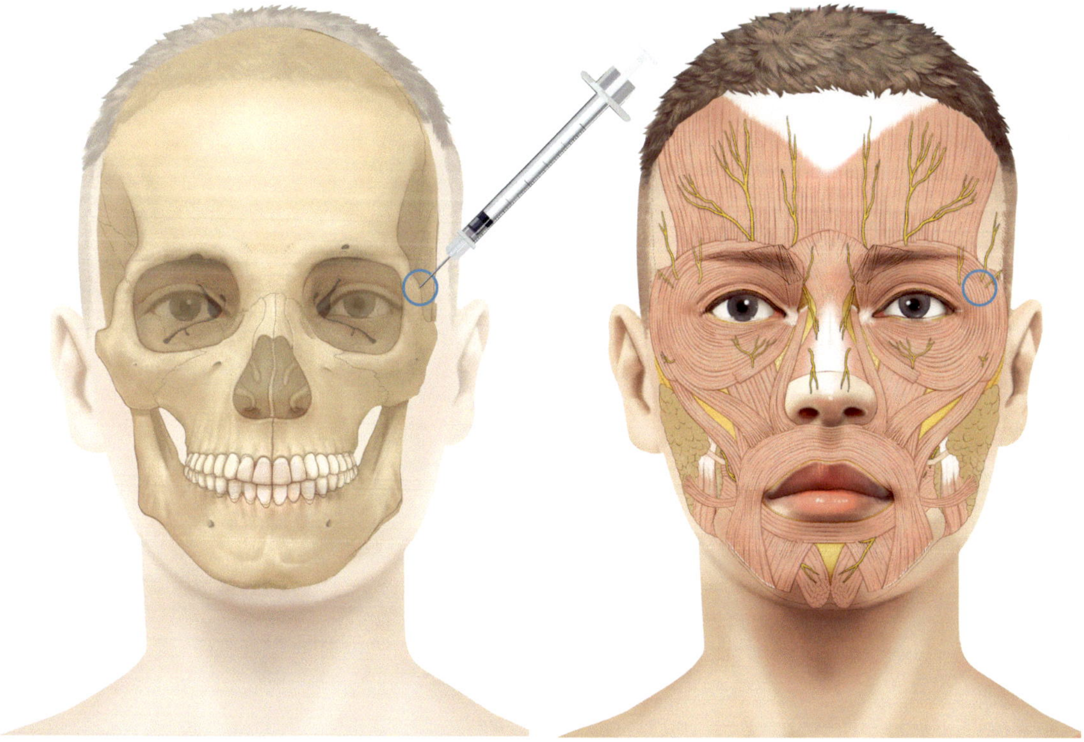

Figure 3.8 Zygomaticotemporal nerve block.

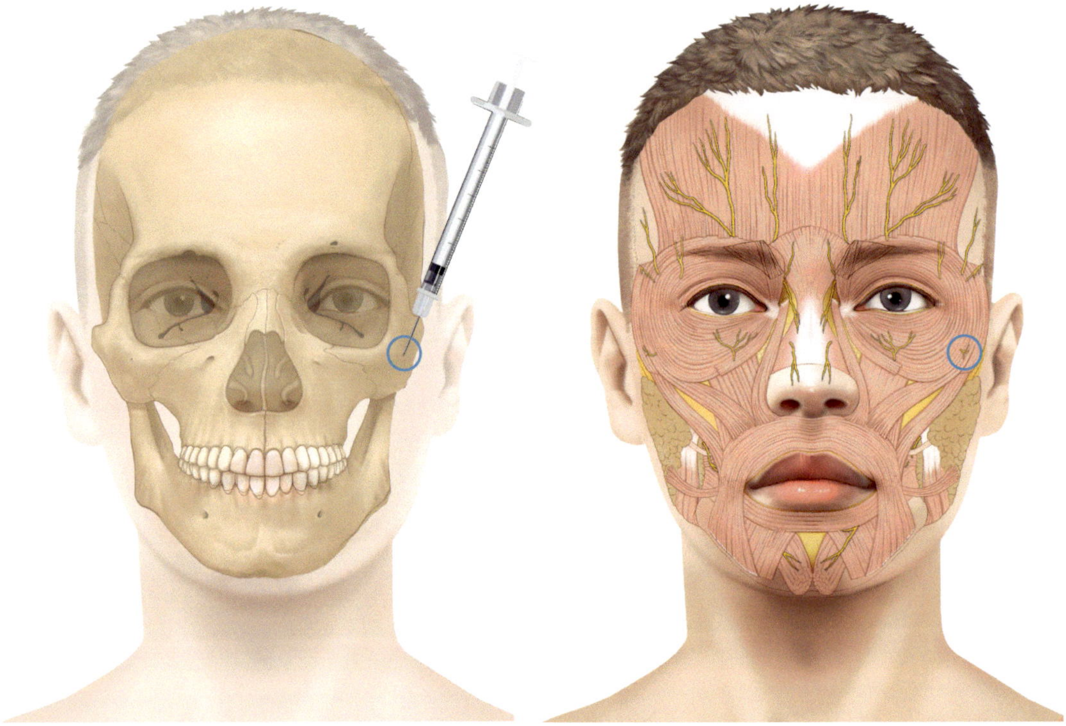

Figure 3.9 Zygomaticofacial nerve block.

- Aspirate and inject 0.2–0.5 mL.
- Consider injecting multiple smaller boluses.

See Figures 3.10–3.12 to visualize proximal, distal, and intraoral blocks of the infraorbital nerve and Video 3.7 on how to perform an infraorbital nerve block proximally.

Note: Block the philtrum just beneath the nose, at the columella, to anesthetize the medial upper lip.

This block targets terminal branches of the infraorbital nerve that may be missed in a more proximal infraorbital block (Figure 3.11).

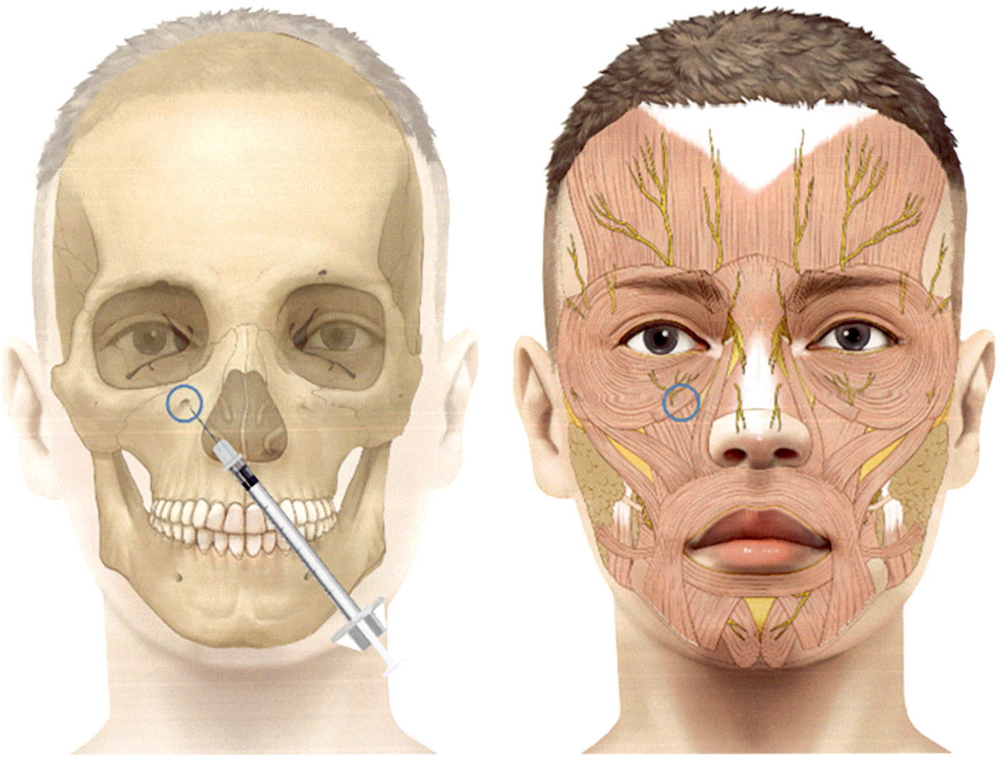

Figure 3.10 Infraorbital nerve block.

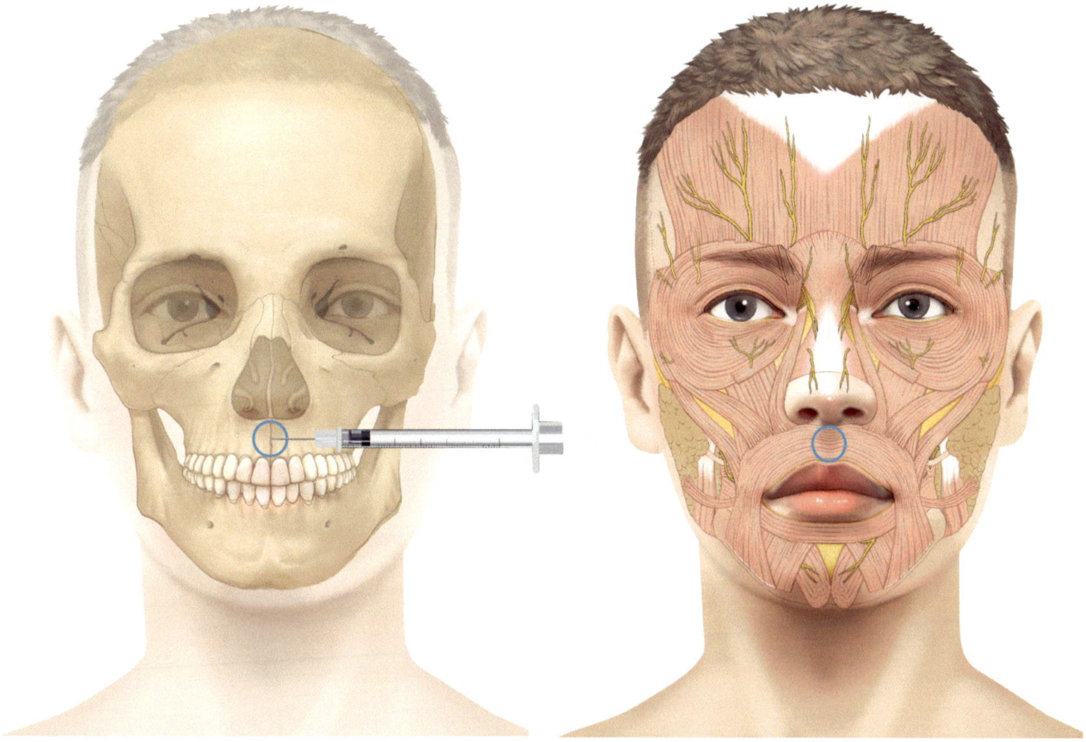

Figure 3.11 Philtrum nerve block.

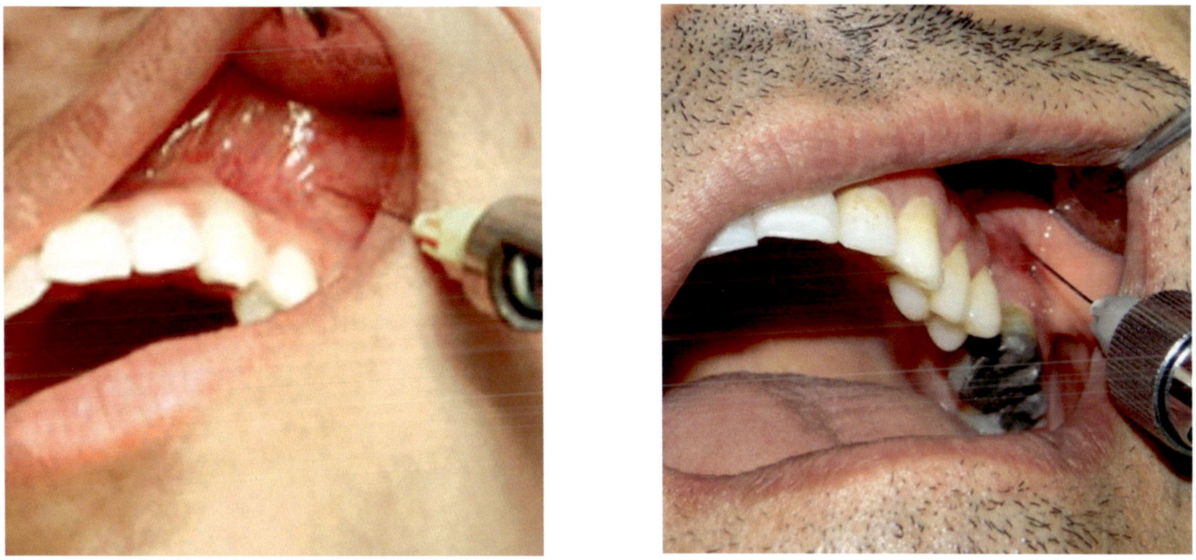

Figure 3.12 Infraorbital nerve block: intraoral approach.

Video 3.7 Infraorbital nerve block

3.5.3.6 Mental Nerve Block

- Disinfect.
- Palpate at the mid-pupillary line in the middle of the mandible, just lateral to the third tooth.
- Soft touch with needle to the periosteum.
- Aspirate and inject 0.2–0.5 mL.
- Consider injecting multiple smaller boluses.

See Figure 3.13 to visualize the mental nerve block and Figure 3.14 targeting the same nerve but intraorally.

3.5.3.7 Mucosal Nerve Block

- Identify landmarks: first and second premolars of upper and lower teeth.
- Apply topical local anesthetic (e.g. cetacaine spray to these injection sites).
- Cleanse area and have patient rinse with disinfectant (e.g. chlorhexidine oral rinse).

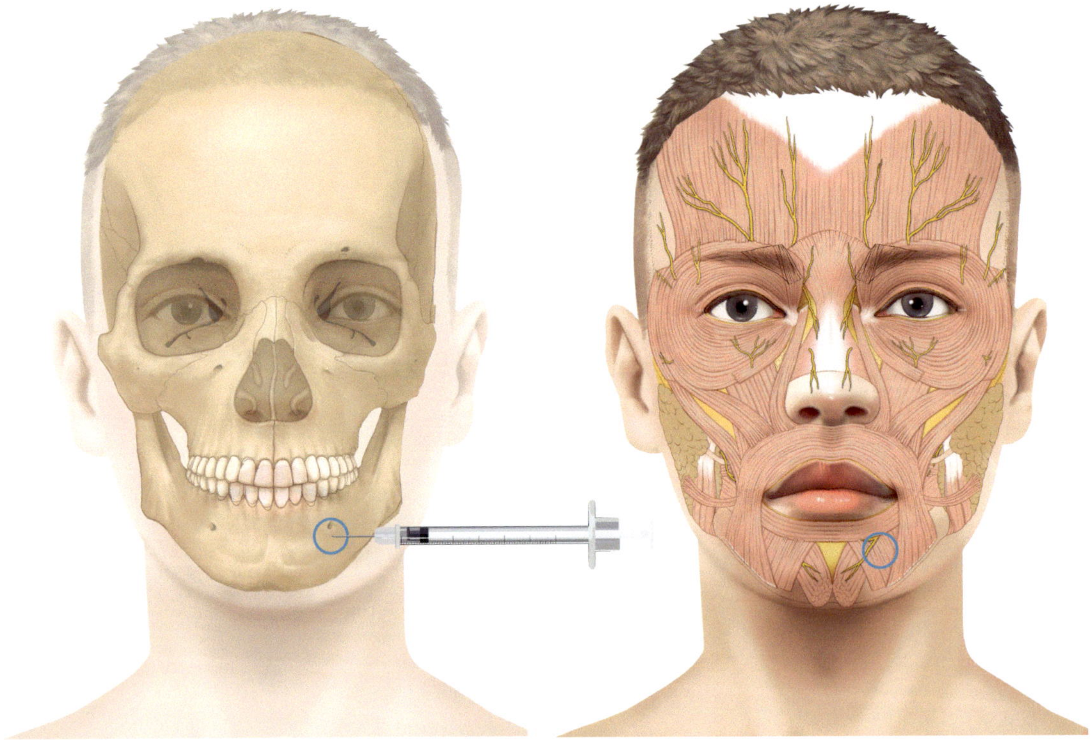

Figure 3.13 Mental nerve block.

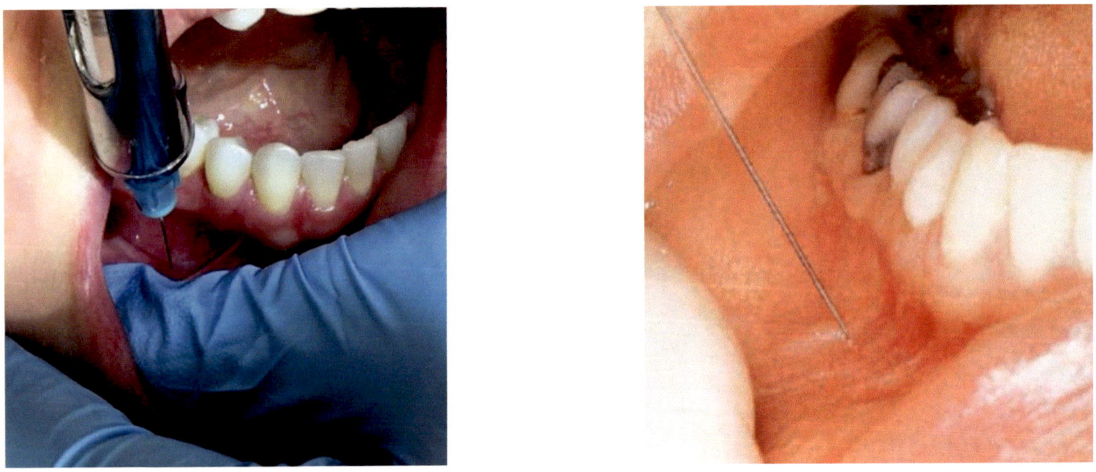

Figure 3.14 Mental nerve block: intraoral approach.

- Identify superficial landmarks by palpating the infraorbital and mental foramina. Maintain location with finger of non-dominant hand when performing each block.
- Introduce the needle transmucosally and direct lateromedially to the supraorbital foramen superiorly and to the mental foramen inferiorly through proprioception, i.e., direct needle tip underneath finger of non-dominant hand placed above either foramen by sensing the location.
- Aspirate and inject 0.5–1.0 mL.

See Video 3.8 on how to perform a mucosal nerve block from the oral mucosa.

Video 3.8 Mucosal nerve block.

3.5.3.8 Superior Labial Block

- As the largest of the three terminal infraorbital nerve branches, the superior labial branches descend beneath the levator labii superioris muscle to supply innervation to the skin and mucous membrane of the upper lip and buccal vestibule [7].
- Targeting the pyriform aperture is a great alternative to the intraoral approach.
- Disinfect the area.

- Soft touch with needle to the periosteum just lateral to the nose ala.
- Aspirate and inject 0.2–0.5 mL.

See Video 3.9 on how to perform a superior labial block.

Video 3.9 Superior labial block.

3.5.3.9 Mandibular Nerve Block

- Target branches of the mandibular nerve, i.e., auriculotemporal (AT) nerve within the temporomandibular joint (TMJ).
- Identify the tragus of the ear. Identify the joint space by having the patient open and close the mouth, leaving it slightly ajar. The joint is anterior to the tragus and behind the lateral pole of the condyle. The mental nerve branches can be found on the lateral surface of the condyle.
- Disinfect.
- Introduce the needle inferiorly to the zygomatic arch within the joint space with the needle slightly upward and slightly forward so that it slides beneath the zygoma, along the back of the condyle towards the posterior uppermost slope of the articular eminence if the joint space allows.
- Aspirate and inject 0.2–0.5 mL. This volume should be sufficient to fill the joint space.

See Video 3.10 on how to perform a mandibular nerve block.

Video 3.10 Mandibular nerve block.

3.5.3.10 Auriculotemporal Nerve Block

- The auriculotemporal (AT) nerve may be blocked anywhere along its course; the more proximal the location, the wider the area of distribution, and the more distal, the more specific. To anesthetize the lateral temple area, the area anterior or superior to the tragus of the ear immediately posterior to the superficial temporal artery is acceptable.
- Identify the landmarks and palpate the pulse of the superficial temporal artery.
- Disinfect.
- Soft touch with needle to the periosteum.
- Aspirate and inject 0.2–0.5 mL.

See Video 3.11 on how to perform an AT nerve block.

Video 3.11 Auriculotemporal nerve block.

3.5.3.11 Greater Occipital and Lesser Occipital Nerve Blocks

- Identify the greater occipital protuberance and the mastoid process. Divide this imaginary line connecting these two landmarks into thirds.
- Palpate for the greater occipital artery pulse at the medial third and aim medial to the pulse.

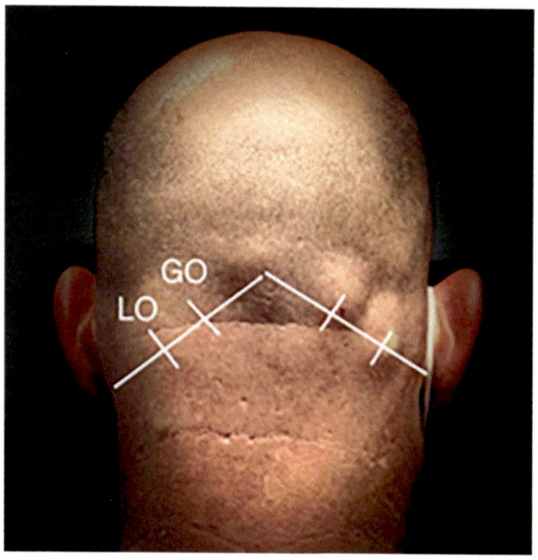

Figure 3.15 Landmarks to conduct blocks on the greater occipital and lesser occipital nerves.

- Disinfect the area.
- Soft touch with needle to the periosteum.
- Aspirate and inject 0.2–0.5 mL.
- Target the lateral third of the line connecting the greater occipital protuberance and the mastoid process for the lesser occipital (LO) block.

See Figure 3.15 to visualize the landmarks of the greater occipital (GO) and LO nerves and Video 3.12 on how to perform a GO and LO nerve blocks.

Video 3.12 Greater and lesser occipital nerve block.

3.5.3.12 Superficial Cervical Plexus Nerve Block

- With the patient sitting upright, identify the midpoint of the sternocleidomastoid (SCM) muscle.
- Disinfect the area.
- Gently pull the SCM away from the neck and introduce the needle deep to the muscle within the parasagittal plane.
- Aspirate and inject 0.2–0.5 mL.

See Video 3.13 on how to perform a superficial cervical plexus nerve block.

Video 3.13 Superficial cervical plexus nerve block.

3.6 ADVERSE EFFECTS

Local anesthetics can sometimes lead to side effects. Some individuals may experience ringing in the ears or dizziness. Others might report numbness beyond the intended area or involuntary muscle twitching. A metallic taste in the mouth can also be an indicator of a reaction to the anesthetic. In more severe cases, a person may experience seizures. Cardiovascular effects can include a drop in blood pressure (hypotension) and a slower heart rate (bradycardia). Additionally, some people may encounter difficulties in breathing after receiving a local anesthetic. It's crucial to monitor for these side effects, especially after administration, to ensure patient safety.

3.7 CONTRAINDICATIONS

- Known allergic or hypersensitivity reactions.
- Infection in skin at or near injection sites.
- Severe ischemic heart disease or cardiac failure.
- Do not use adrenaline in peripheries/adnexa.

3.8 SAFETY CONCERNS

- Not every facility or clinic may have the necessary credentials, equipment, or expertise to perform all types of nerve blocks. While most facilities may be authorized to do simpler procedures like trigger point injections or field blocks, more advanced nerve blocks (e.g. brachial plexus block, sciatic nerve block) may require specialized training and facilities.
- A well-stocked crash cart is crucial in case of any emergencies.
- Key items include:
    - Oxygen with a functioning delivery system
    - Oximetry
    - Essential medications such as adrenaline, which can be crucial during an emergency
    - Other medications for allergic reactions, cardiac events, or respiratory distress
- Most airway concerns are related to nerve blocks in the neck. For example, a brachial plexus block may inadvertently target recurrent laryngeal nerve or phrenic nerve. To avoid such risks, the professional performing the block should have deep knowledge of anatomy and the specific region being targeted.

REFERENCES

[1] M. Goerig et al., "Carl Koller, cocaine, and local anesthesia: Some less known and forgotten facts," *Reg Anesth Pain Med*, vol. 37, no. 3, pp. 318–324, 2012.
[2] S. Zhou et al., "Synthesis and biological activities of local anesthetics," *RSC Adv*, vol. 9, no. 70, p. 41173, 2019.
[3] C. M. Brummett, B. A. Williams, "Additives to local anesthetics for peripheral nerve blockade," *Int Anesthesiol Clin*, vol. 49, no. 4, pp. 104–116, 2011.
[4] A. Rękas-Dudziak et al., "The use of local anaesthetics in dermatology, aesthetic medicine and plastic surgery: Review of the literature," *Adv Dermatol Allergol/Postępy Dermatologii i Alergologii*, vol. 40, no. 1, p. 22, 2023.
[5] A. Hadzic, J. Vloka, *Peripheral Nerve Blocks: Principles and Practice*. New York: McGraw Hill, 2004.
[6] S. Waldman, *Comprehensive Atlas of Ultrasound-Guided Pain Management Injection Techniques*, 2nd edn. Wolters Klubers Health, 2020.
[7] W. E. Shankland, "The trigeminal nerve. Part III: The maxillary division," *Cranio*, vol. 19, no. 2, pp. 78–83, 2001.

The Upper Third of the Face

Forehead Lift

4

JANI VAN LOGHEM

4.1 INTRODUCTION

Bone resorption plays an important role in the aging process and contributes significantly to sagging of soft tissue. The skull becomes smaller in diameter and the soft tissue becomes relatively wide, resulting in a downward migration of the forehead skin and of the brows. Due to reduced origin to insertion distance, the frontalis muscle may become hyperdynamic: the origin in the galea aponeurotica and insertion in the skin of the brows. CaHA can be used to correct volume loss of the skull and can be placed in the subgaleal space, which is a potential space, a glide plane between the galea aponeurotica and the periosteum (Figures 4.1–4.2) [1]. The ideal instrument is a nontraumatic cannula of 25G or thicker to reduce the chance of intra-arterial injection of especially the supraorbital and supratrochlear arteries and their branches.

4.2 CANNULA TECHNIQUE (THREE OR FIVE ENTRY POINTS)

For injection placement, see Figure 4.3.

4.2.1 Step-by-Step Technique

A cannula will provide more precision with respect to product placement in the subgaleal layer compared to sharp needle injection [3].

1. Disinfect both the skin and the hair.
2. Supratrochlear, supraorbital, and zygomaticotemporal nerve blocks may be considered. Inject approx. 0.1–0.2 mL of 1% lidocaine with adrenaline (1:200000) close to the exit location of the nerve (supraorbital and supratrochlear notch/foramen. Also consider a zygomaticotemporal nerve block with approximately 0.5 mL adrenalized lidocaine (please see block anesthesia in Chapter 3).
3. Check for pulsation and mark one entry point per side, just inferior to the hairline at the temporal crest and anaesthetize with adrenalized 1% lidocaine (Figure 4.4).
4. Make a pre-hole in the skin with a 23G needle (Figure 4.5).

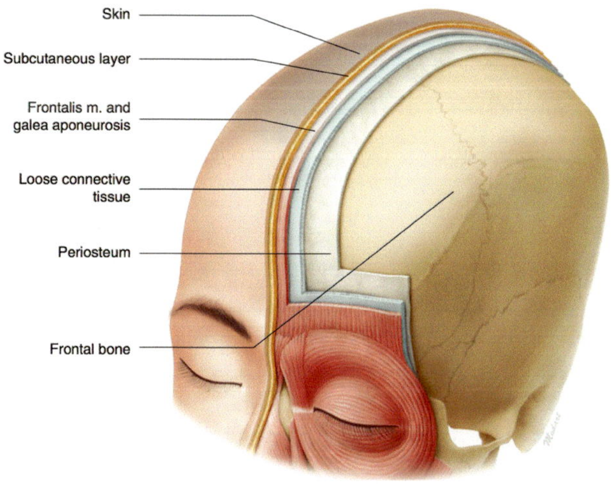

Figure 4.1 Layers of the head. The safest injection plane of the filler is in the loose connective tissue on the periosteum, in the subgaleal space [2]. (Reproduced from Kim HJ *et al. Clinical Anatomy of the Face for Filler and Botulinum Toxin Injection*, Springer Science+Business: Singapore, 2016; with permission).

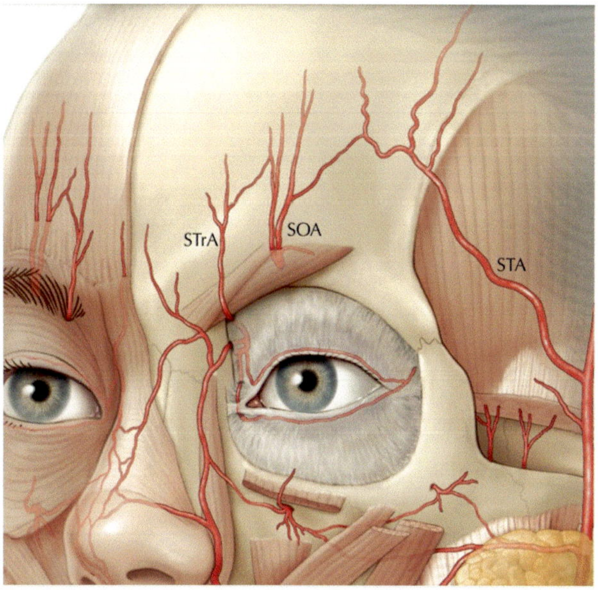

Figure 4.2 Arterial danger zones for the treatment of the forehead are: supraorbital artery (SOA) branches, supratrochlear artery (STrA) branches, and superficial temporal artery branches (STA) [4].

DOI: 10.1201/9781003617129-4

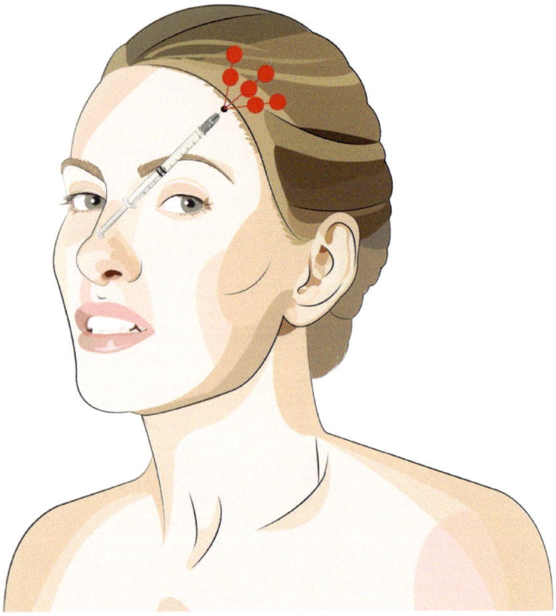

Figure 4.3 Product injection for the forehead lift. The black dot indicates the entry point on the left side. The red dots mark subgaleal boluses of CaHA. For symmetry, the same should also be done on the other side.

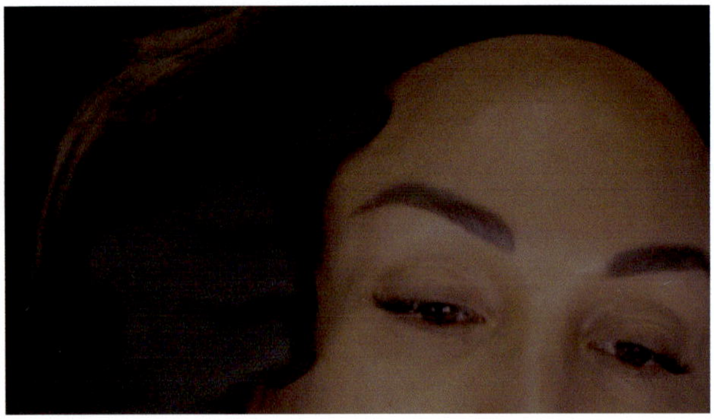

Figure 4.4 Checking for pulsation prior to anesthesia.

5. With a nontraumatic cannula (suggested 25G, 38 mm, or 50 mm cannula), advance through the skin until the subcutaneous fat is reached.
6. With thumb and index finger of the nondominant hand, pinch the skin just in front of the cannula so that the galea aponeurotica is lifted from the periosteum. In this way, a path of least resistance toward the deep level has been created (Figure 4.6).
7. Maneuver the cannula through the resistance of the galea aponeurotica. Usually, a pencil-rolling technique can be of value, where the syringe is rotated between the fingers in order to let the tip of the cannula can find the path of least resistance.
8. Advance the cannula in the subgaleal space while lifting the muscle in front of the cannula.
9. Place multiple boluses and retrogrades of maximum 0.1 mL of undiluted or minimally diluted CaHA (Figure 4.7).

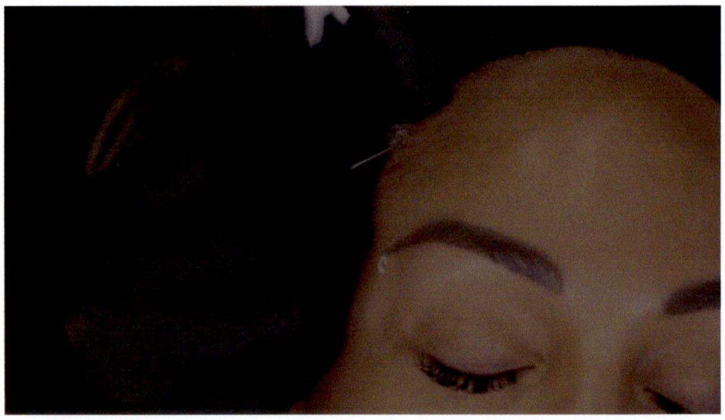

Figure 4.5 Pre-hole at the entry point with a 23G sharp needle.

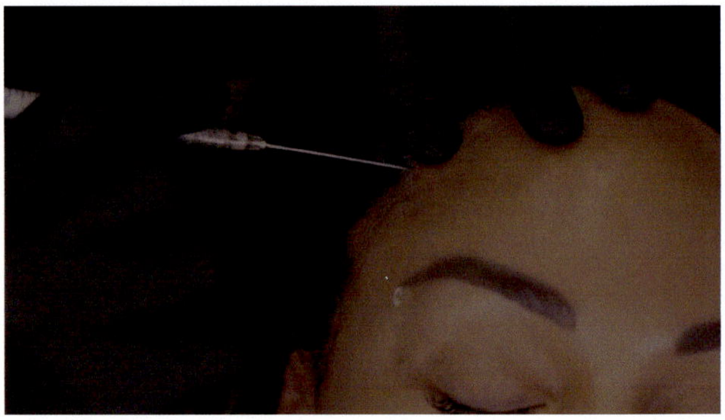

Figure 4.6 Advancing the cannula to the periosteal level while rotating the syringe with the fingers to pass any resistance.

10. A total of at least 1.5 mL of product is recommended per side.
11. Check for visible irregularities and massage gently to correct them if needed.
12. Check the amount of forehead lift and consider adding more product. Take into consideration that the frontalis muscle might be relaxed due to the anesthesia and that a temporary brow ptosis might occur due to the anesthesia.

4.3 AFTERCARE

After injection, the frontalis muscle might be temporarily relaxed due to the lidocaine in the anesthesia and the product. Also, transient distension of the veins can be observed due to increased pressure in the area. Swelling might be uneven in the forehead, so the patient should be advised that any swelling is to be expected and is temporary but can last up to five days. Swelling might also descend into the eyelids.

4.4 ADDITIONAL TREATMENTS FOR OPTIMAL RESULTS

Additional treatments to raise the position of the brows may be:

- Frontal concavity (Chapter 5)
- Temporal hollows (Chapter 6)
- Lateral brow lift (Chapter 7)

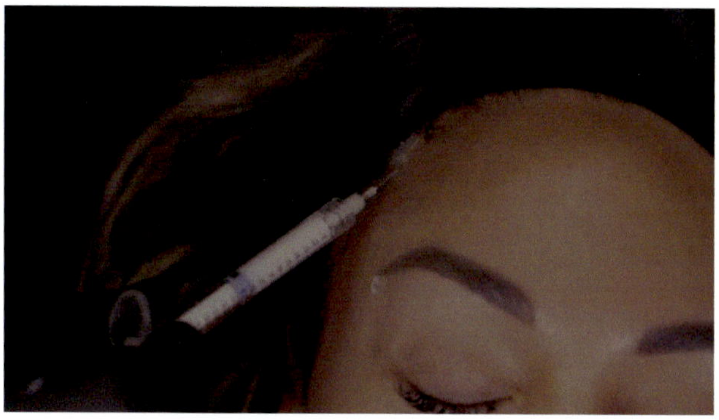

Figure 4.7 Subgaleal injection of CaHA.

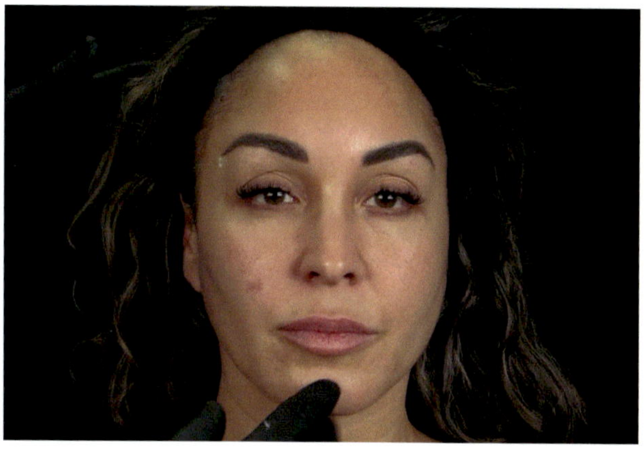

Figure 4.8 Example of a patient treated with 1.5 mL of CaHA at the subgaleal level on her right side only, resulting in an elevated lateral brow.

- C-angle (Chapter 9)
- Botulinum toxin of the depressor muscles of the brows
- Focused ultrasound
- Thread
- Surgical lift

As a filler placed in the subgaleal region, it will stretch the frontalis muscle; hence the horizontal forehead wrinkles can be expected to reduce [5,6].

See also Figure 4.8 and Video 4.1 to visualize end results and product application technique, respectively.

Video 4.1 Forehead lift: Cannula technique.

REFERENCES

[1] R. J. Warren et al., "Face lift," *Plast Reconstr Surg*, vol. 128, no. 6, 2011.

[2] J. A. J. van Loghem et al., "Cannula versus sharp needle for placement of soft tissue fillers: An observational cadaver study," *Aesthet Surg J*, vol. 38, no. 1, pp. 73–88, 2017.

[3] R. B. Shaw et al., "Aging of the facial skeleton: Aesthetic implications and rejuvenation strategies," *Plast Reconstr Surg*, vol. 127, no. 1, pp. 374–383, 2011.

[4] C. Faris et al., "The midline central artery forehead flap: A valid alternative to supratrochlear-based forehead flaps," *JAMA Facial Plast Surg*, vol. 17, no. 1, pp. 16–22, 2015.

[5] H.-J. Kim et al., "Clinical anatomy of the face for filler and botulinum toxin injection," in: *Clinical Anatomy of the Face for Filler and Botulinum Toxin Injection*. Springer, 2016.

[6] J. A. J. van Loghem, "Use of calcium hydroxylapatite in the upper third of the face: Retrospective analysis of techniques, dilutions and adverse events," *J Cosmet Dermatol*, vol. 17, no. 6, pp. 1025–1030, 2018.

The Upper Third of the Face

Frontal Concavity

5

YATES YEN-YU CHAO, NIAMH CORDUFF, AND JANI VAN LOGHEM

5.1 INTRODUCTION

The forehead, when measured in size, is almost one third of our face. When talking about either facial contouring or facial rejuvenation, the forehead shape is definitely an important part of the whole face and must be addressed as well. An ideal forehead shape should be full, with optimum convexity, smoothly continuous with the brow, glabella, temples, and then the cheekbones. Complete treatment of the upper face should cover the forehead, glabella, brow, and temples.

However, most doctors hesitate to go into the forehead and glabella mainly because of the concern with many vulnerable vessels in this area. Supratrochlear/supraorbital arteries and veins penetrate via the superior margin of the orbital rim, piercing the corrugator muscles, and then distribute in the surface of frontalis muscle. The superficial temporal artery transverses from the superficial aponeurotic system to the subcutaneous plane from the lateral hairline to the lateral forehead. In the temporal area, most of the other vascular structures run deep to the deep temporal fascia. Filler injection of the upper face is certainly feasible when taking these anatomical geographies into good consideration.

Temple volume augmentation can be performed either in the supraperiosteal space or the interfascial layer. When fillers are intended for the supraperiosteal space, sharp needles are more convenient and can easily penetrate the deep temporal fascia and temporalis muscle to the bone. Bolus injection with malleable substance can easily fill the space with reasonable spread. While volumizing fillers are planned for the interfascial space, thinner fillers are ideal for a more even distribution in this rather superficial layer. When filler material is used in the interfascial layer, the author prefers using cannulas to ensure a safer and more precise treatment process. An entry hole created to the position of zygomatic prominence is the usual technique employed by the author, because of the easier access to full extent of the temporal hollow. The author suggests using a 23G or thicker cannula for less bending of the cannula and better precision of filler delivery. Thinner cannulas behave more like needles and can heighten the risks for vascular damage.

The interfascial space of the temporal fossa ends in the temporal ridge, where the temporalis muscle inserts into the frontal bone. The continuous curve of the temples to forehead should be considered when both the augmentation of the forehead and of the temples must be performed.

For the forehead region, the subgaleal space is the most suitable level for placing the exogenous filling material. For most candidates, their forehead bone is full of curves, with prominent and depressed areas, and the subgaleal space is actually a space occupied by thin fibrous tissue, not as loose as described in some textbooks, but rather dense. Our frontal area has a unique anatomy, with our frontal bone responsible for most of the forehead shape and then, when going upward, the periosteum, glide space, frontalis aponeurosis (galea aponeurotica), frontalis muscle, subcutaneous fat, and skin. The periosteum is tightly bound to the frontal bone. The frontalis muscle and the forehead superficial fat compartment are both quite thin in structure—playing minor roles for the shape—only softening the contour. Skin thickness varies in different patients, with males having thicker skin, while women, Caucasians, or the aged have thinner skin. Even for patients with thick skin, forehead filling jobs can be very unforgiving. Any uneven distribution of the filler, or unnatural curve, can be easily visible through the overlying thin, soft tissue.

Dissection of tissue itself is a little uncomfortable and may be painful when approaching the vital structures of nerves and vessels. The pain sensation of our own body is itself an innate protective system. Therefore, local infiltration of anesthetics, or nerve blocks, numbs the patient and blocks this alarm system. During the injection process, we should avoid aggressive and rude punching of the cannula and listen to how patients respond. If patients complain of pain, then we should be cautious in that area, do it more slowly, or turn to a different route. But if the patient has been totally blocked off from his or her pain sensation, then it becomes more difficult to detect the occurrence of vessel disruption.

Because of the pain and concerns about intravascular injection, the contouring work of the forehead usually is really disturbing to the patient and difficult for the injector. However, with the help of the novel technique of saline hydrodissection, the whole process becomes much easier and safer [1,2].

5.2 ARTERIAL DANGER ZONES

Arterial danger zones must be considered, and care should be taken that the needle tip does not proceed

DOI: 10.1201/9781003617129-5

through the dermis but rather remains intradermal [3]. The important arteries present in this area are similar to the ones described in Chapter 4, which include the medial branch from the supraorbital artery, the supratrochlear artery, and the frontal branches from the superficial temporal artery (Figure 5.1).

5.3 SAFETY CONSIDERATIONS

For safety concerns, when performing contouring of the forehead, cannulas are preferred to needles—using cannulas in the forehead region is still very challenging. The cannula must be inserted through the limited subgaleal space. The process of a cannula traveling in the subgaleal space is a dissection of tissue. If we want thorough and even distribution of filler but do not dissect the space enough, the thin fibrotic tissue still can limit the spreading and distribution of the filler. This can result in an uneven surface and suboptimal contour.

5.4 THOROUGH UPPER FACE CONTOURING WITH THE AID OF SALINE HYDRODISSECTION

For injection placement, see Figure 5.2.

5.4.1 Step-by-Step Technique

1. Disinfect the forehead, mark the frontal concavity, determine the entry points at the temporal crests just above the brows, and estimate the amount of product needed for augmentation.
2. Puncture the skin with a 20G needle (consider numbing the skin first with local anesthesia).
3. Prepare a 3 mL syringe filled with normal saline and attach it to a 22G cannula.
4. Introduce the cannula through the skin and advance it to the subgaleal space.
5. When sure that the cannula is on the periosteum, start infiltrating normal saline (without lidocaine) in the pre-marked area.
6. Use a bolus pattern of injection of saline (Figure 5.3). The saline itself will not block nerve sensation and leave the treatment areas staying alert for the subsequent filling process.

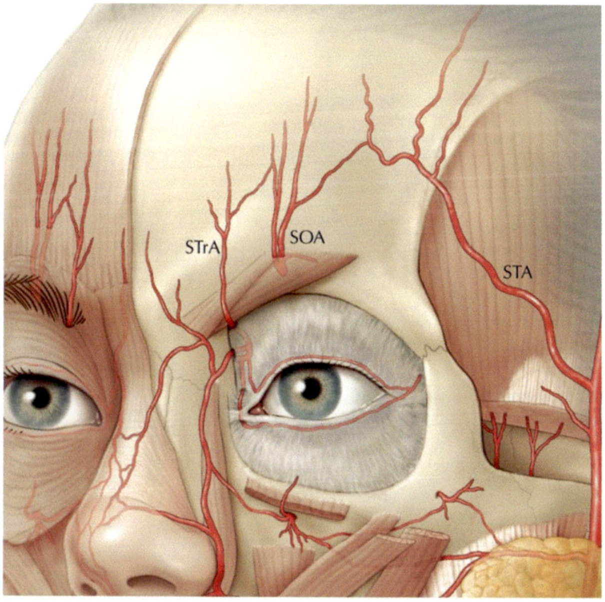

Figure 5.1 Arterial danger zones for the treatment of the frontal concavity are: supraorbital artery (SOA) branches, supratrochlear artery (STrA) branches, and superficial temporal artery (STA) and its frontal branches.

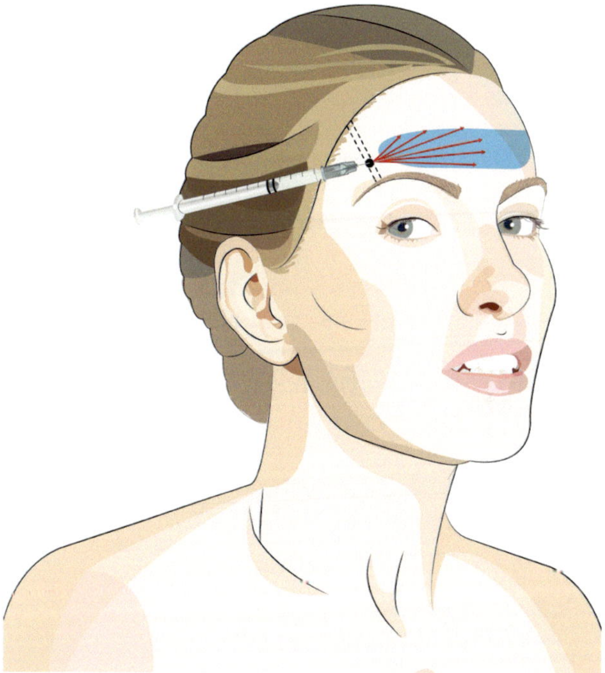

Figure 5.2 Schematic drawing of product injection at the frontal concavity. The straight dotted lines mark the temporal crest. The black dot indicates the entry point. The blue color marks adjuvant infiltration of saline in the subgaleal space. The red lines mark subgaleal retrograde linear threads of CaHA injected from one side (for symmetry, the same should be done from the other side).

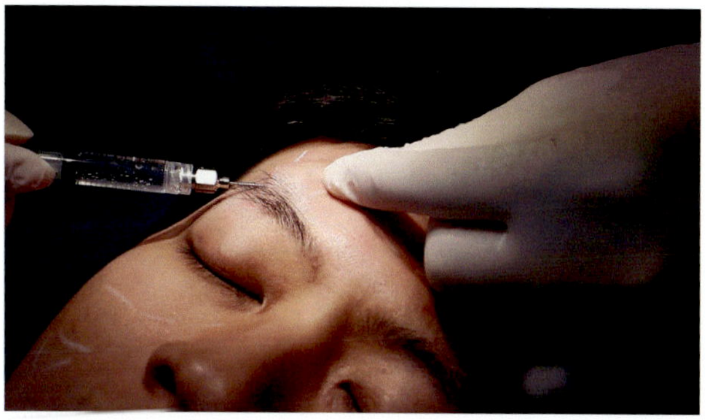

Figure 5.3 Saline infiltration at the subgaleal space with blunt cannula in a bolus hydrodissection technique.

7. Use a hand pressing/pushing maneuver to direct the hydrostatic pressure to dissect the peripheral subgaleal space around the injected boluses. The hydrodissected area then becomes confluent together after the multifocal deployment of the saline.
8. The physician can wait for a couple of minutes before injecting the filling material (Figure 5.4).
9. Even though the subgaleal space has been well prepared by the saline dissection, the second step of filler infusion must be done very carefully. Nevertheless, according to the author's experience, the second step is usually not painful at all and would encounter very limited resistance.
10. The glabella area is also covered by the aponeurosis of procerus muscle, with only the most lateral border attached by the corrugator muscle. Contouring of this area can be achieved more easily using a similar hydrodissection technique, but the cannula must pass through a more critical area near the medial brow. Thus, injectors must be much more careful in this area.
11. After enough filler has been infiltrated and satisfactory distribution of the filler has been achieved, we can use our hands to mold the subgaleal filler into the desired shape, curve, and projective magnitude.

5.5 CANNULA TECHNIQUE (THREE OR FIVE ENTRY POINTS)

For injection placement, see Figure 5.5.

5.5.1 Step-by-Step Technique

1. As an alternative to Dr. Chao's advice of avoiding anesthesia, a supraorbital and supratrochlear nerve block may be considered. Inject approximately 0.1–0.5 mL of 1% lidocaine with adrenaline close to the exit location of the supraorbital, supratrochlear, and zygomaticotemporal nerves; see block anesthesia in Chapter 3.
2. Mark the frontal concavity and the lateral border of the temporal crest, and mark the entry points. If necessary, also mark two additional entry points at the temporal crest close to the hairline, depending on the shape of the frontal concavity.

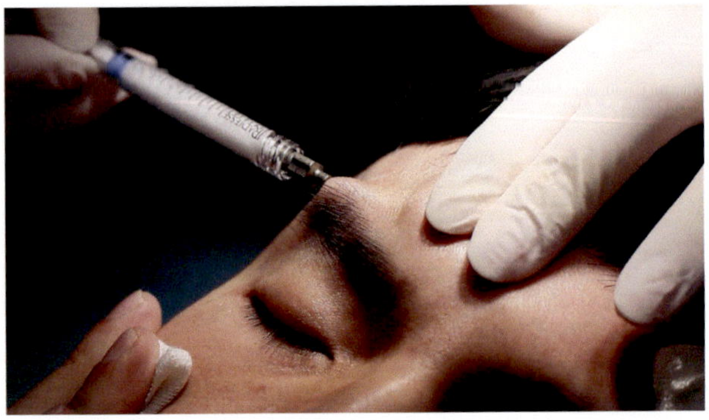

Figure 5.4 Careful injection of CaHA at the pre-hydrodissected subgaleal space with blunt cannula.

3. On the line of the lateral border of the temporal crest, approximately 1 cm above the orbital rim, a low-risk access point can be marked (Figure 5.6), although the superficial temporal artery is known for its high anatomic variability. The temporal branch of the facial nerve divides into many branches, while the main branch normally passes the temporal crest more cranially to this entry point.
4. If needed, anaesthetize this point with adrenalized lidocaine 1% before using a 21G needle to make a pre-hole in the skin.
5. With a rigid cannula (suggested 25G, 38 mm cannula, or 22G, 50 mm cannula), advance through the skin until the subcutaneous fat is reached.

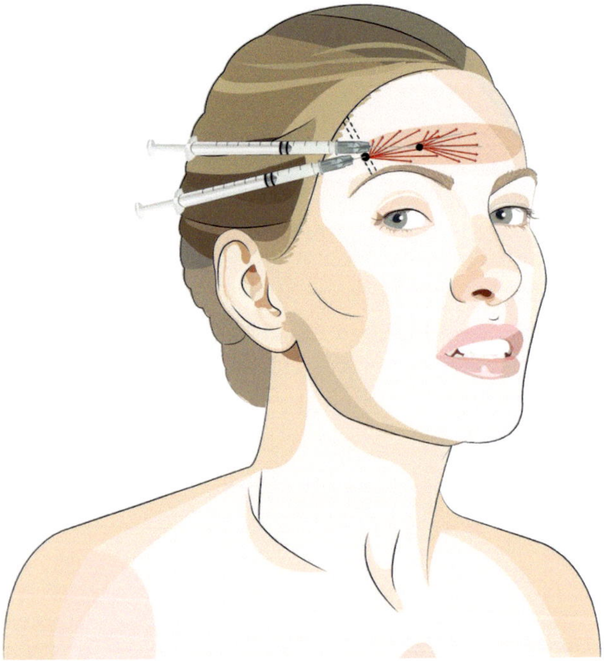

Figure 5.5 Schematic drawing of product injection at the frontal concavity. The black dots indicate the entry points and the red lines mark subgaleal retrograde linear threads of CaHA injected from one side (for symmetry, the same should be done from the other side).

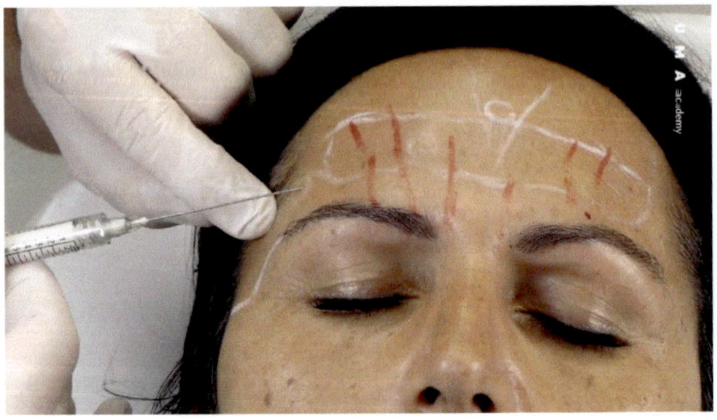

Figure 5.6 Entry of the cannula.

6. With thumb and index finger of the nondominant hand, pinch the skin just in front of the cannula so that the muscle is lifted from the periosteum. In this way, a horizontal path of least resistance toward the deep level has been created (Figure 5.7).
7. Maneuver the cannula through the resistance of the galea aponeurotica. This requires a well-dosed amount of force, as the galea can be quite tough here. Usually, a pencil-rolling technique can be of value, where the syringe is rotated between the fingers in order to let the tip of the cannula find the path of least resistance.

   Advance the cannula in the subgaleal space while lifting the muscle in front of the cannula and start at the most caudal part of the frontal concavity. As many products contain lidocaine that will anaesthetize the supraorbital nerve, beginning at the lower part will subsequently numb the higher parts of the frontal area when no nerve bock is used.
8. Place multiple retrograde linear threads using a fanning pattern (Figure 5.8)
9. The second entry point is in between the midline and the lateral entry point.

   The possible third entry point is the midline entry point. It can be found immediately cranial to the marked frontal concavity in the midline.

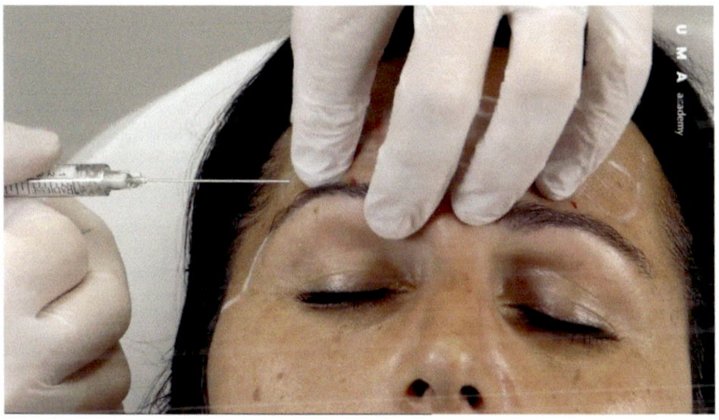

Figure 5.7 Creating a path below the galea aponeurotica in front of the cannula.

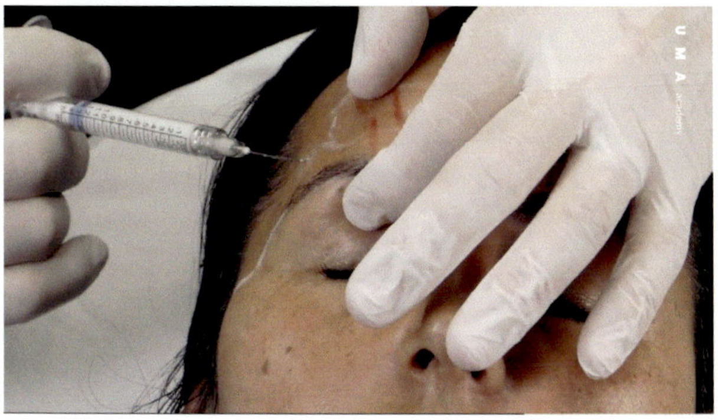

Figure 5.8 Compressing supraorbital artery with finger and injecting retrograde linear threads.

10. Anesthetize if necessary and also place some lidocaine at the periosteal level in order to hydrodissect.
11. Create an opening with a sharp needle and advance the cannula in lateral direction underneath the galea aponeurotica.
13. Place multiple retrograde linear threads in a fanning pattern. To reduce chance of serious vascular complications, maximize the size of the retrograde threads to 0.025 mL per thread and keep pressure on the supraorbital or supratrochlear arteries with the thumb and index finger of the nondominant hand (Figure 5.8).
14. Even out the product with direct massage.

5.6 SUBGALEAL SHARP NEEDLE BOLUS TECHNIQUE

For injection placement, see Figure 5.9.

Cautionary message: sharp needles in the frontal/glabellar area are associated with an increased risk of vascular complications. The cannula technique is considered safer in this area. Only if the injector does not inject with cannulas, needles may be considered, taking this extra safety advice into consideration: Use small-gauge needles (27–28 G); place the bevel down using an angled approach; lift the vessels up, away from the needle bevel, by pulling on the skin around the needle; use small volume boluses on periosteum with low pressure on the plunger; and compress the supratrochlear arteries when injecting. Aspiration can be performed when the needle is not primed.

5.6.1 Step-by-Step Technique

1. A supraorbital and supratrochlear nerve block may be considered. Inject approx. 0.1–0.2 mL of 1% lidocaine with adrenaline close to the exit location of the nerve (supraorbital and supratrochlear notch/foramen). See Chapter 3 for nerve blocks.
2. Mark the frontal concavity and the lateral border of the temporal crest and the location of the supraorbital and corrugator creases (indicate approximate location of the arteries) (Figure 5.11).

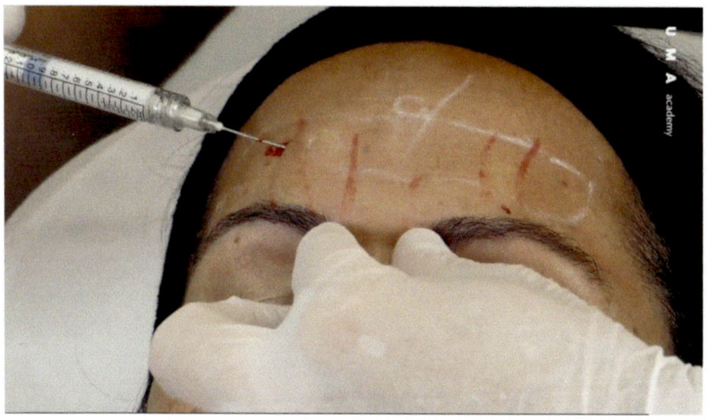

Figure 5.9 Subgaleal injection through midline entry point while giving pressure on supratrochlear arteries with the fingers.

3. Choose a short 27G needle.
4. Use a standard dilution of CaHA.
5. Tent the forehead skin in front of the needle with the nondominant thumb and index finger by lifting up the brow (Figure 5.12).
7. Advance the needle to the periosteum with an angled approach of approximately 45° with the bevel down (Figure 5.13).
8. Aspiration with a primed needle will always give negative results, so aspiration should be avoided and negative aspiration (no blood in the hub) should never be regarded as proof of being extravascular.
9. Change position of nondominant fingers to give pressure on supratrochlear arteries.
10. Softly touching the periosteum, inject a maximum 0.025 mL of periosteal bolus.
11. Partially retract, without exiting the skin, reorient, and readvance the needle to the periosteum.
12. Inject an additional bolus of max 0.025 mL.
13. Repeat as needed.
14. Exit the needle and repeat every 0.5 cm until full correction.
15. Even out the product with purposeful molding.

See Videos 5.1–5.5 for product placement using different application techniques.

Video 5.1 Forehead hydrodissection (courtesy of Niamh Corduff).

Video 5.2 Frontal concavity cannula anesthesia.

Video 5.3 Frontal concavity cannula technique 1: 3-point technique.

Video 5.4 Frontal concavity cannula technique 2: 5-point technique.

Video 5.5 Subgaleal sharp needle bolus technique.

5.7 AFTERCARE

After injection, the frontalis muscle might be temporarily relaxed due to the lidocaine in the product. Also, transient distension of the veins can be observed due to increased pressure in the area. Swelling might be uneven in the forehead, so the patient should be advised that any swelling is to be expected and should be temporary but can last up to five days. Swelling might also descend into the eyelids.

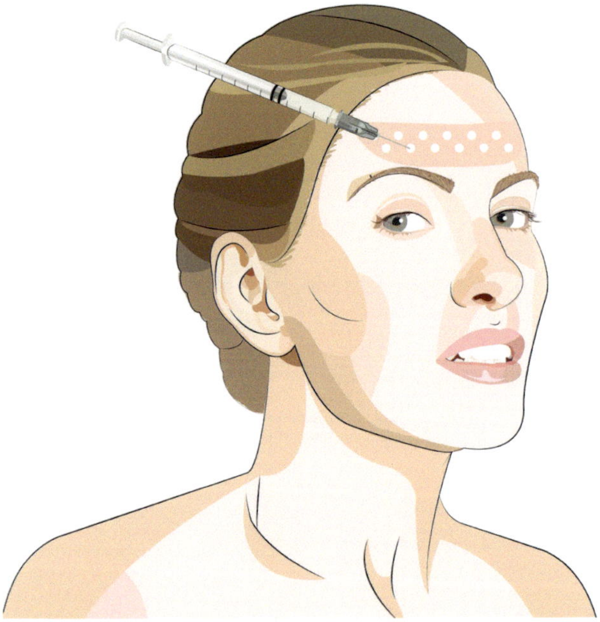

Figure 5.10 Schematic drawing of product injection at the frontal concavity with a sharp needle. All periosteal boluses should be maximized to 0.025 mL each.

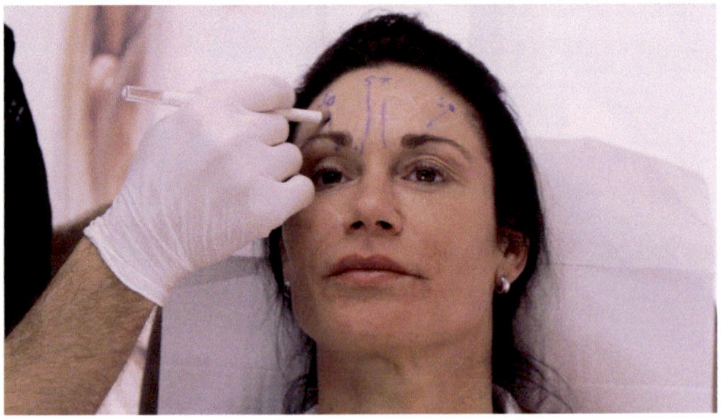

Figure 5.11 Marking of the area.

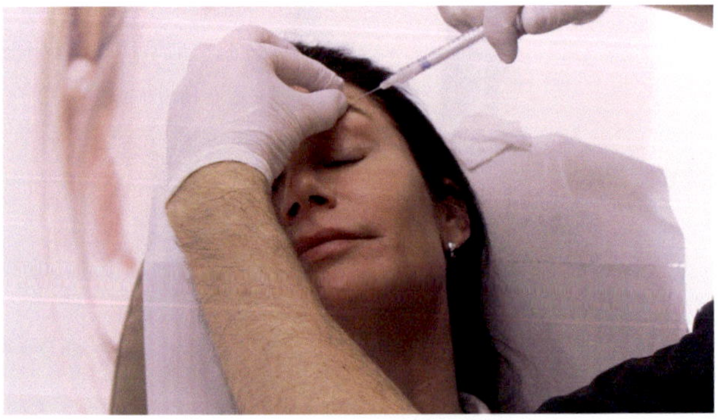

Figure 5.12 Tenting the skin, bevel down.

5.8 ADDITIONAL TREATMENTS FOR OPTIMAL RESULTS

Thin to medium thickness soft tissue fillers can be used for dermal treatment of wrinkles, while keeping

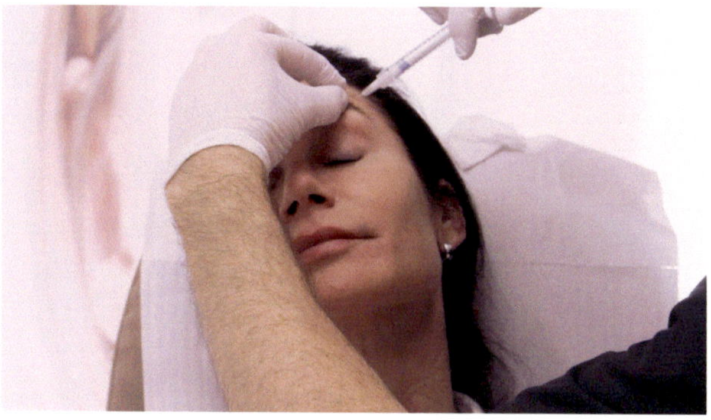

Figure 5.13 Syringe placement at 45° to the periosteum; injection of 0.025 mL bolus.

in mind that the wrinkles here are dynamic and will also benefit from pretreatment with botulinum toxin. Ideally, a hyaluronic acid filler with a low viscoelasticity but high cohesivity should be used, preferably in an intradermal (blanching) technique, indicating papillary dermis placement, to correct forehead wrinkles. For intradermal injections, a sharp needle should be used, as nontraumatic cannulas do not penetrate the dermis readily.

Intra-arterial injection into any of these arteries can potentially lead to permanent blindness, so injection with a nontraumatic cannula should be considered, ideally horizontally, perpendicular to the (vertical) direction of the arteries. Superficially placed product can potentially be seen during movement of the brows, as the position of the filler will change relative to the concavity. This will result in a visible convexity just above the concavity when the patient raises the brows, which aesthetically might be a suboptimal result [4].

Soft tissue fillers are generally not injected intramuscularly, as muscular contractions can displace the product and cause visible nodules. Both intramuscular injection and intragaleal injection will result in the same aesthetic problem as with a subcutaneous injection: the position of the product will change on animation.

As a subgaleal placed filler may stretch the frontalis muscle, horizontal forehead wrinkles can be expected to be reduced (Figure 5.14) [5].

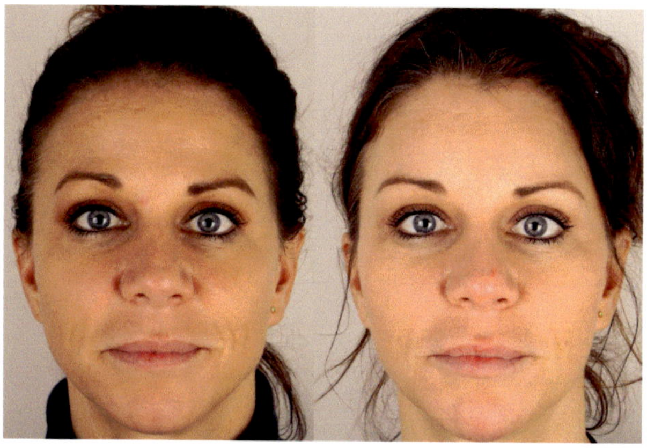

Figure 5.14 Before (left) and after (right) pictures of a patient treated with 1.5 mL of CaHA at the subgaleal level, resulting in a more optimal light reflection and contour of the forehead [6]. (Reproduced with permission from ref 6.)

REFERENCES

[1] J. Sykes, "Applied anatomy of the temporal region and forehead for injectable fillers," *J Drugs Dermatol*, vol. 8, no. Suppl 10, pp. 24–27, 2009.

[2] Y. Y. Y. Chao, "Saline hydrodissection: A novel technique for the injection of calcium hydroxylapatite fillers in the forehead," *Dermatol Surg*, vol. 44, no. 1, pp. 133–136, Jan. 2018.

[3] W. Prager, P. Micheels, "A prospective, comparative survey to investigate practitioners' satisfaction with a cohesive, polydensified matrix(®), hyaluronic acid-based filler gel with and without lidocaine for the treatment of facial wrinkles," *J Cosmet Dermatol*, vol. 14, no. 2, pp. 124–129, Jun. 2015.

[4] X. Li et al., "A novel hypothesis of visual loss secondary to cosmetic facial filler injection," *Ann Plast Surg*, vol. 75, no. 3, pp. 258–260, Sep. 2015.

[5] R. B. Shaw et al., "Aging of the facial skeleton: Aesthetic implications and rejuvenation strategies," *Plast Reconstr Surg*, vol. 127, no. 1, pp. 374–383, 2011.

[6] J. A. J. van Loghem, "Use of calcium hydroxylapatite in the upper third of the face: Retrospective analysis of techniques, dilutions and adverse events," *J Cosmet Dermatol*, vol. 17, no. 6, pp. 1025–1030, Dec. 2018.

The Upper Third of the Face

Temporal Hollows

6

POLINA HOLOVINA, AINA CERVERA-BAREA, AND JANI VAN LOGHEM

6.1 INTRODUCTION

During the aging process, the temples become hollow and the orbital rim more apparent, leading to a skeletonized appearance, due to resorption of bone and fat. This region contains the *temporal retaining ligament* which consists of an adhesion area (*temporal ligamentous adhesion*; TLA) located along the superior temporal fusion line. This structure is a low-density fibrous tissue connecting the deep and superficial fascias and restricting mobility in all directions. Two branches sprout from the TLA: the *superior* and the *inferior temporal septa* (Figure 6.1) [1]. As far as the septa go, some authors do not categorize them as true ligaments, since the STS only passes between the deep fascia and the superficial temporal fascia, albeit being fibrous walls [1]. Replacing lost volume on the periosteum and lifting the temporal region (by targeting the TLA), like Amaral and others suggest [2], may therefore create a natural rejuvenated appearance. In this chapter, we describe different treatment techniques of the temporal hollows with both sharp needles and nontraumatic cannulas. Cannulas will provide more precision with respect to product placement in the subcutaneous, interfacial, or supraperiosteal level compared to sharp needle injection [3]. Sharp needles are generally easier to control. Due to the high level of anatomic variation in this area, the exact location of the arteries cannot be exactly predicted, and therefore, safe techniques must be used to avoid intraarterial injection (Figure 6.2) [4]. More information on ligament liftings can be found in Chapter 11.

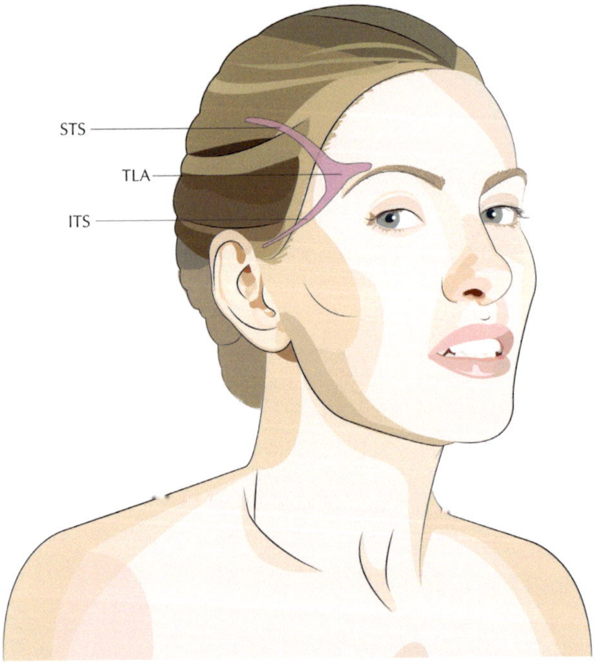

Figure 6.1 Schematic drawing of the temporal (pink) retaining ligament from the upper and middle thirds of the face. In the upper third, the temporal ligamentous adhesion (TLA), the superior temporal septum (STS), and the inferior temporal septum (ITS) can be found.

6.2 TEMPORAL HOLLOWS (SHARP NEEDLE PERIOSTEAL BOLUS TECHNIQUE)

For injection placement, see Figure 6.3.

6.2.1 Step-by-Step Technique

1. Disinfect and mark the temporal crest, the lateral orbital rim, and the zygomatic arch. Determine the area of maximum depression (Figure 6.4).

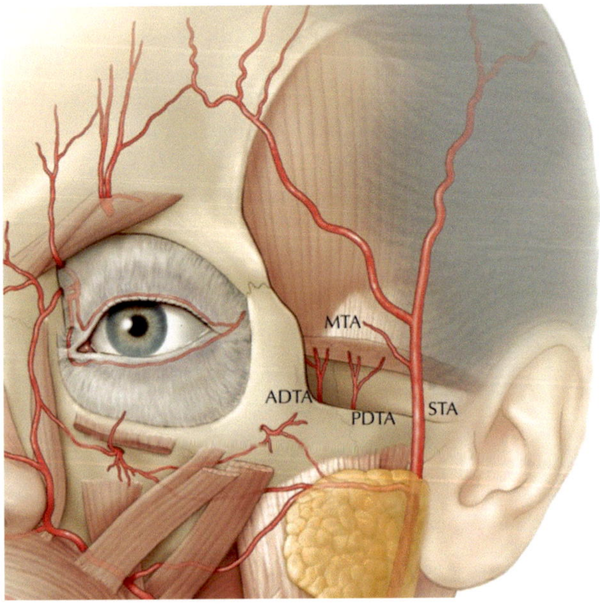

Figure 6.2 Arterial danger zones for the treatment of the temporal hollows are: superficial temporal artery (STA), medial temporal artery (MTA), anterior (ADTA) and posterior (PDTA) deep temporal artery.

DOI: 10.1201/9781003617129-6

2. A zygomaticotemporal nerve block may be considered. Inject approx. 0.5–1 mL of 2% lidocaine deep to the lateral orbital rim at the fusion point of the zygomatic arch; please see block anesthesia in Chapter 3.
3. Use full viscosity (undiluted) CaHA.
4. Check for pulsations and avoid hitting the superficial temporal artery and veins.
5. Advance the 27G, 19 mm cannula perpendicular to the skin, slowly to the periosteum (Figure 6.5). The needle should have a soft touch to the periosteum, and the patient might feel some pressure.
6. Aspiration is not necessarily indicated, as it yields false-negative results, and physicians should not solely rely on this technique to avoid intravascular injection [5].
7. Inject approximately 0.05–0.1 mL of nondiluted CaHA slowly, with low pressure in a bolus on the periosteum (Figure 6.6).
8. Partially retract, reorient, and readvance the needle back to the periosteum, about 5 mm away from the first bolus.
9. Inject another bolus of approximately 0.05–0.1 mL of non-diluted CaHA with the bevel down.
10. Repeat these steps until the hollow is satisfactorily corrected.
11. Even out with light massage (Figure 6.7).

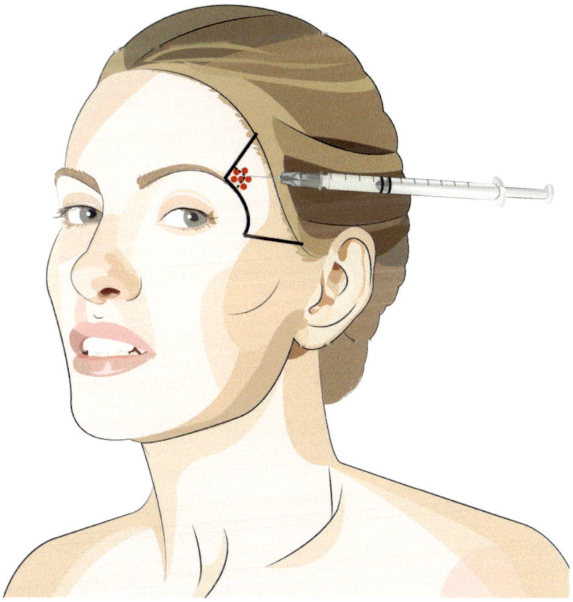

Figure 6.3 Sharp needle injection at the temporal hollow. The black lines mark the temporal crest, lateral orbital rim, and upper border of the zygomatic arch. The black dotted lines lateral to the temporal crest indicate the low-risk zone of 1 cm by 1 cm. The red dots indicate sharp needle bolus injection of CaHA on the periosteum.

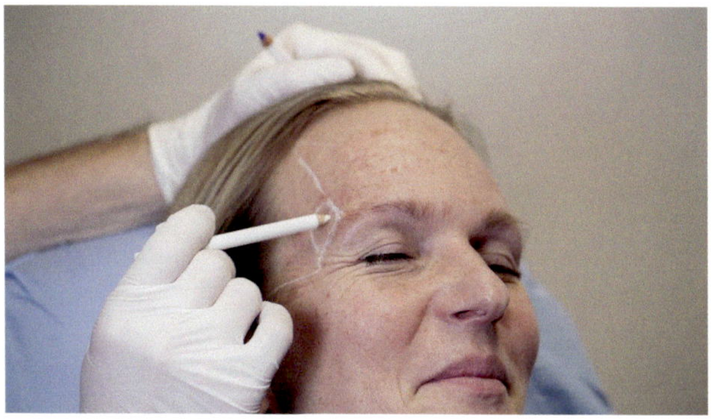

Figure 6.4 Marking of the temporal area and area of maximum depression.

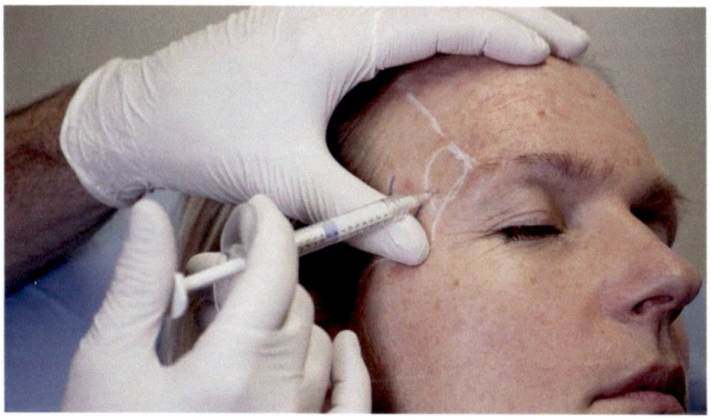

Figure 6.5 Perpendicular to 45° to the skin, advance the needle to the periosteum.

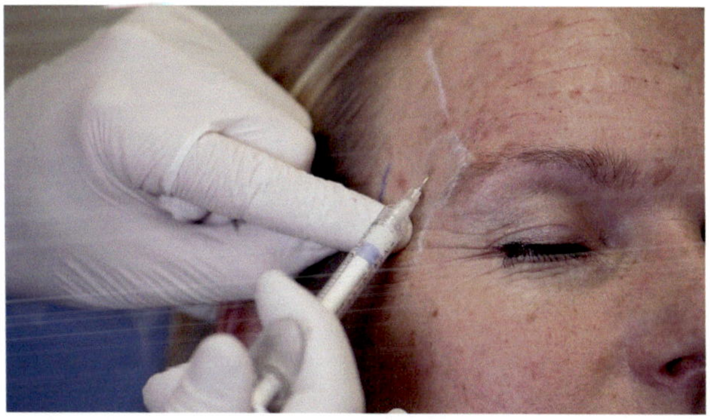

Figure 6.6 Using the same entry point, without exiting the needle from the skin, retract, reorient, readvance, and inject multiple boluses on the periosteum of approximately 0.05–0.1 mL per bolus with bevel down.

6.3 TEMPORAL HOLLOWS (INTERFASCIAL CANNULA TECHNIQUE; ZYGOMATIC ARCH ENTRY POINT)

For injection placement, see Figure 6.8.

6.3.1 Step-by-Step Technique

1. Disinfect and mark the temporal crest, the lateral orbital rim, and the zygomatic arch. Determine the

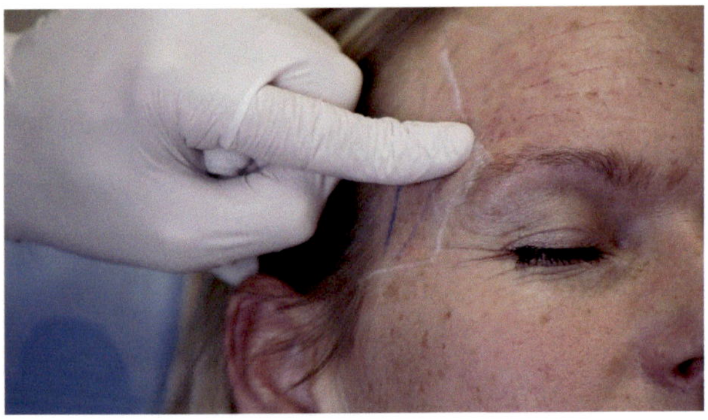

Figure 6.7 Even out with mild pressure.

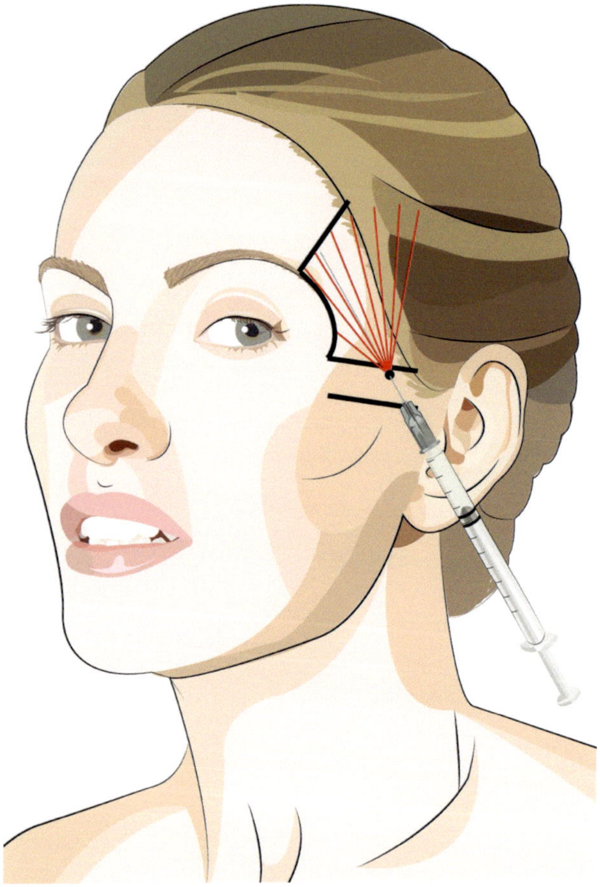

Figure 6.8 CaHA injection with blunt cannula in the interfascial space of the temporal hollow. The black lines mark the temporal crest, lateral orbital rim, and upper border of the zygomatic arch. The red lines indicate retrograde linear threads injection of CaHA.

area of maximum depression. Palpate and mark the superficial temporal artery and determine the entry point so that the trajectory of the cannula is not parallel to this artery.

2. A zygomaticotemporal nerve block may be considered. Inject approx. 0.5–1 mL of 2% lidocaine deep to the lateral orbital rim at the fusion point of the zygomatic arch; see block anesthesia in Chapter 3.
3. At the zygomatic arch, anterior to the hairline, mark the entry point and anesthetize.
4. Use a 23G needle for the pre-hole.
5. Maneuver the cannula through the skin to the subcutaneous fat. As a test, advance the cannula and pull it up to see the thickness of the skin over the cannula (Figure 6.9).
6. Retract the tip back to the entry point and now orient it 45° down until resistance is felt (Figure 6.10).
7. Rotate the cannula and press through that resistance (the temporoparietal fascia).
8. To test whether the cannula is indeed one layer down, check if the tissue over the cannula is thicker by pulling up the cannula again (Figure 6.11).
9. Advance to the temporal crest and start fanning.

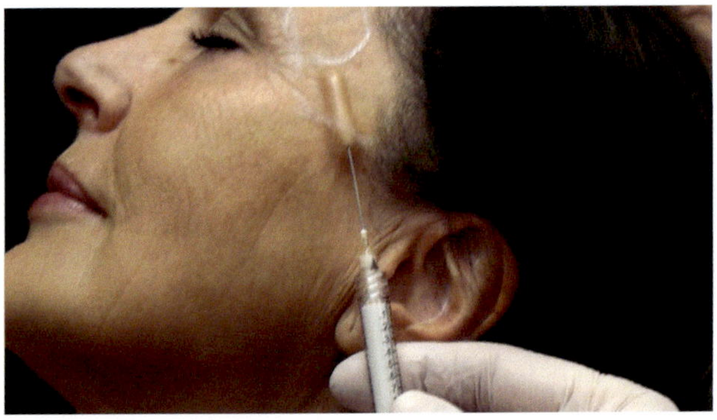

Figure 6.9 Cannula is subcutaneous.

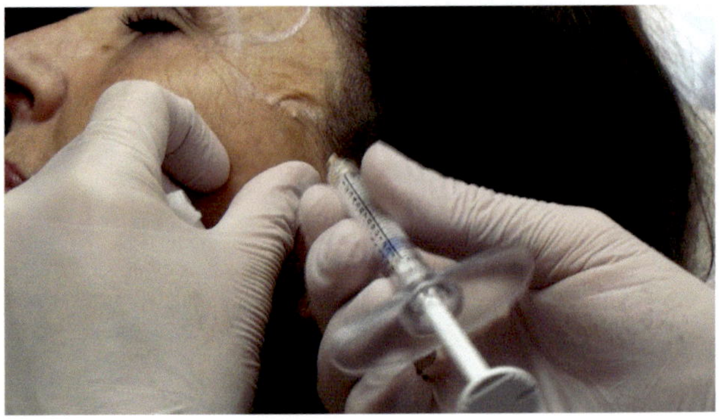

Figure 6.10 Cannula passes the resistance of the temporoparietal fascia.

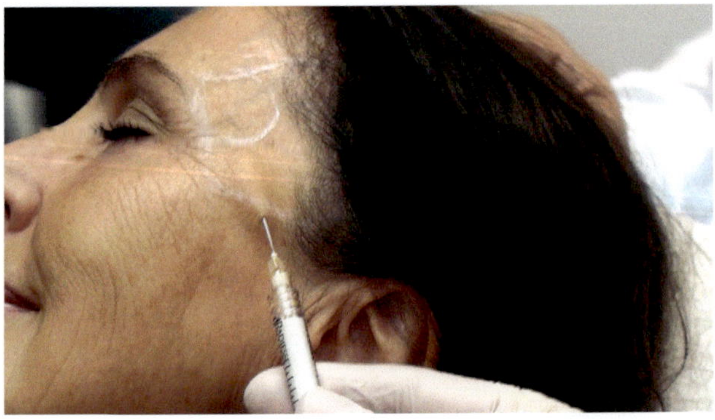

Figure 6.11 Cannula is now positioned between the two fascias.

10. Consider also advancing to the area below the hair to improve hair thickness and lifting of the lateral cheek.
11. Even out with light massage.

6.4 TEMPORAL HOLLOWS (SUBCUTANEOUS CANNULA TECHNIQUE; ZYGOMATIC ARCH ENTRY POINT)

For injection placement, see Figure 6.8.

6.4.1 Step-by-Step Technique

1. Disinfect and mark the temporal crest, the lateral orbital rim, and the zygomatic arch. Determine the area of maximum depression.
2. Palpate and mark the superficial temporal artery and determine the entry point so that the trajectory of the cannula is perpendicular to this artery.
3. Use CaHA standard dilution (adding 0.3 mL of 2% lidocaine to 1.5 mL of CaHA) or CaHA in 1:1 dilution depending on the thickness of the tissue.
4. Mark the entry point from the zygomatic arch, anterior to the hairline, and anesthetize the region (Figure 6.12). You can use a 23G needle for the pre-hole.
5. Maneuver the tip of the 25G, 50 mm cannula from the skin to the subcutaneous fat. Place the syringe almost parallel to the surface of the treated area and advance the cannula while slowly rotating the syringe. Check the depth by pulling the cannula up.
6. Advance the cannula all the way in while lifting the lateral part of the temple with the non-dominant hand (Figure 6.13).
7. Start fanning; place tiny retrograde lines of up to 0.05 mL per line (Figure 6.14).
8. Make sure to create a new tunnel for each retrograde linear thread to distribute the product evenly.
9. If resistance is encountered, most likely it is due to the inferior temporal septum. Rotate the syringe, and that will help the cannula to slide through the tissue.
10. Consider also advancing to the area beyond the hairline to improve hair thickness and lifting of the lateral cheek.
11. Even out the product with a light massage (Figure 6.15).

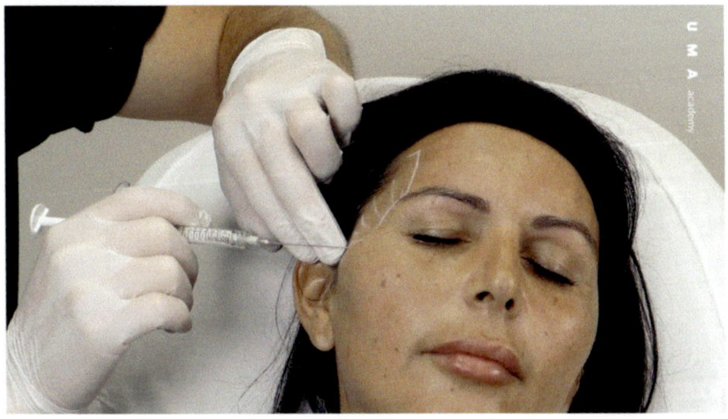

Figure 6.12 Creation of the entry hole for the cannula.

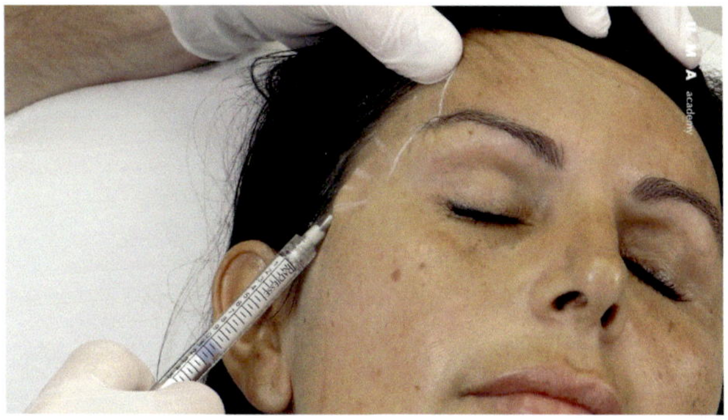

Figure 6.13 Advancement of the cannula through the temporal crest prior initiating a retrograde deposition technique.

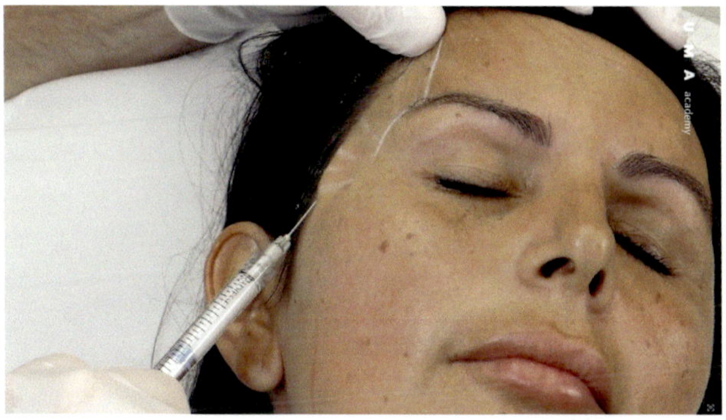

Figure 6.14 Product deposition using a retrograde, fanning technique.

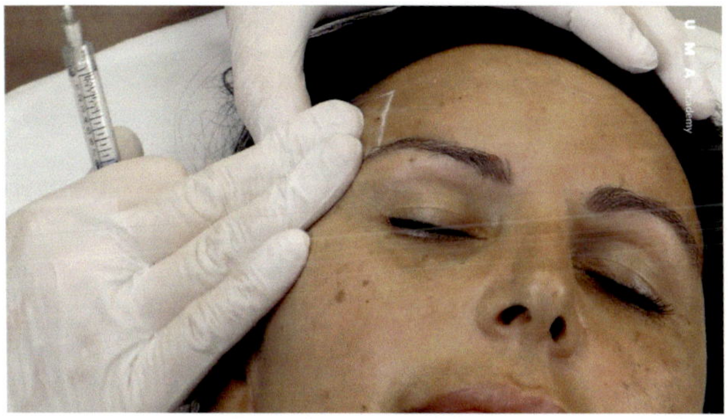

Figure 6.15 Molding the product to ensure desired volumizing effects.

6.5 TEMPORAL HOLLOWS (PERIOSTEAL CANNULA TECHNIQUE; TEMPORAL CREST ENTRY POINT)

For injection placement, see Figure 6.16.

6.5.1 Step-by-Step Technique

1. Disinfect and mark the temporal crest, the lateral orbital rim, and the zygomatic arch. Determine the area of maximum depression.
2. A zygomaticotemporal nerve block may be considered. Inject approx. 0.5–1 mL of 2% lidocaine

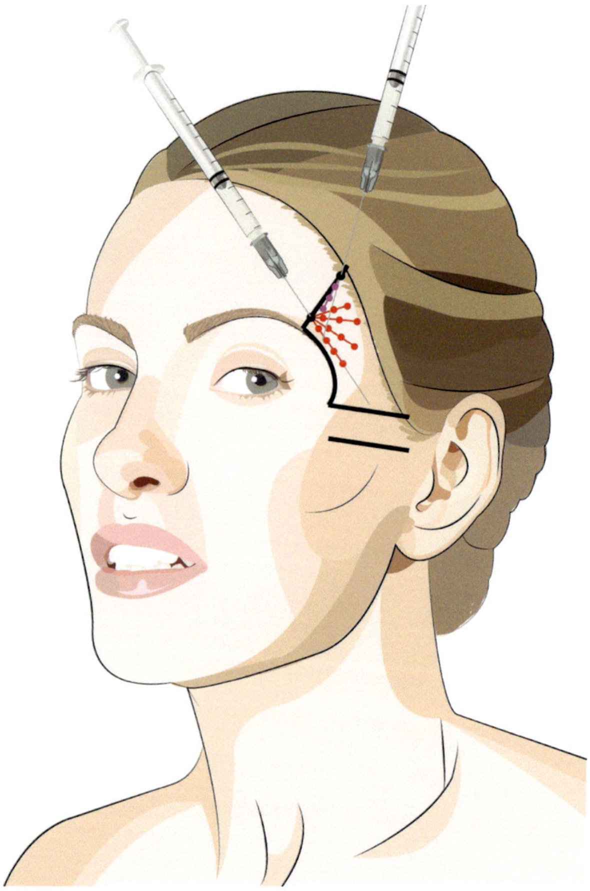

Figure 6.16 CaHA injection with blunt cannula on the periosteum of the temporal hollow. The black lines mark the lateral temporal crest, lateral orbital rim, and upper border of the zygomatic arch. The red dots indicate small bolus injections of CaHA.

deep to the lateral orbital rim at the fusion point of the zygomatic arch; please see block anesthesia in Chapter 3.

3. Check for pulsations and avoid hitting the superficial temporal artery and veins.
4. Approximately 1 cm superior to the orbital rim, mark the entry point just lateral to the lateral border of the temporal crest.
5. Anesthetize subcutaneously with 1% lidocaine with adrenaline and advance the needle further to the periosteum of the temporal hollow. The resistance of the deep temporal fascia may be felt (Figure 6.17).
6. With the needle touching the periosteum, inject approximately 0.2 mL of local anesthesia for patient comfort.
7. The needle should not be too deep. Reposition if needed until the most cranial trajectory to the periosteum is found.
8. Remember the direction of the needle of the anesthesia.
9. Use a thicker gauge needle (18–23G) for making the entry point in the skin.
10. Without manipulating the position of the skin, advance the needle further (in the direction of the periosteum; Figure 6.18).
11. While softly touching the periosteum, rotate the needle once and retract.
12. Switch to undiluted CaHA with a 25G rigid cannula.
13. In the same direction as the entry needle and without manipulating the position of the skin, advance the cannula through the skin and through the deep temporal fascia (Figure 6.19).

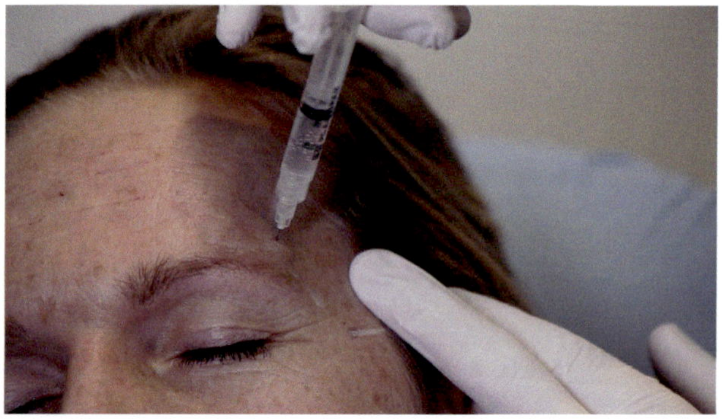

Figure 6.17 Determine the direction to the periosteum with the needle of the anesthesia.

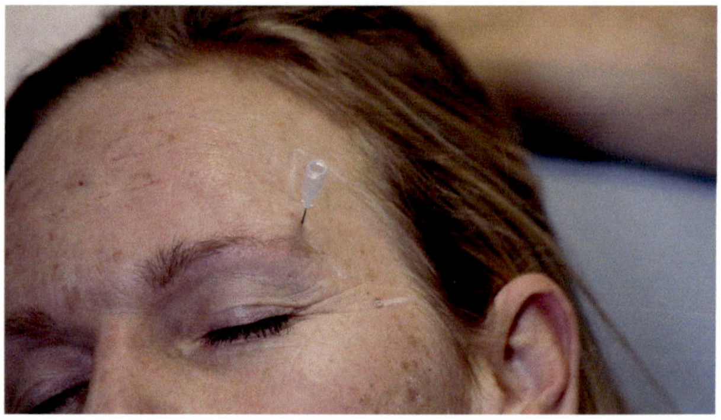

Figure 6.18 Advance the needle through the skin and the deep temporal fascia until the periosteum.

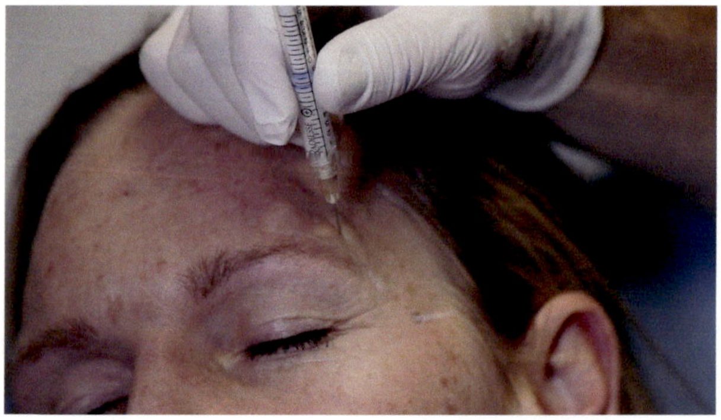

Figure 6.19 Advance the cannula through the deep temporal fascia until it is at the periosteal level.

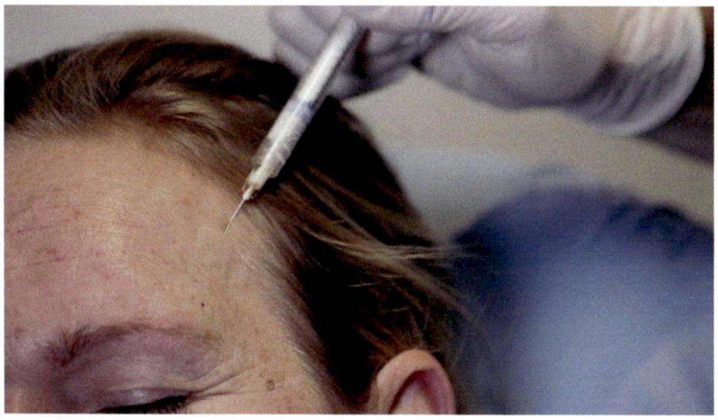

Figure 6.20 Place multiple boluses of maximum 0.1 mL.

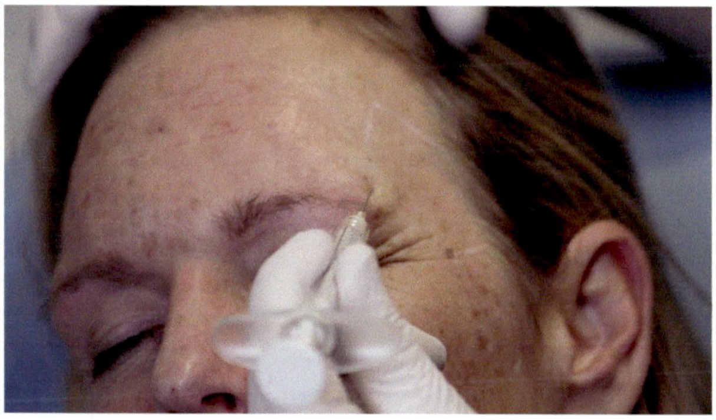

Figure 6.21 Creation of a second entry point.

14. When the cannula is on the periosteum, the typical scraping of the cannula over the periosteum can be felt.
15. Advance the cannula and give multiple boluses of approximately 0.05–0.1 mL until the desired result. Maximize the boluses to 0.1 mL per bolus (Figure 6.20).
16. If necessary, an additional entry point can be made close to the hairline (Figure 6.21). Disinfect and repeat from step 5.
17. Even out with a light massage.

6.6 TEMPORAL HOLLOWS (INTERFASCIAL CANNULA TECHNIQUE; TEMPORAL CREST ENTRY POINT)

For injection placement, see Figure 6.22.

6.6.1 Step-by-Step Technique

1. Disinfect and mark the temporal crest, the lateral orbital rim, and the zygomatic arch. Determine the area of maximum depression.
2. A zygomaticotemporal nerve block may be considered. Inject approx. 0.5–1 mL of 2% lidocaine deep to the lateral orbital rim at the fusion point of the zygomatic arch; please see block anesthesia in Chapter 3.

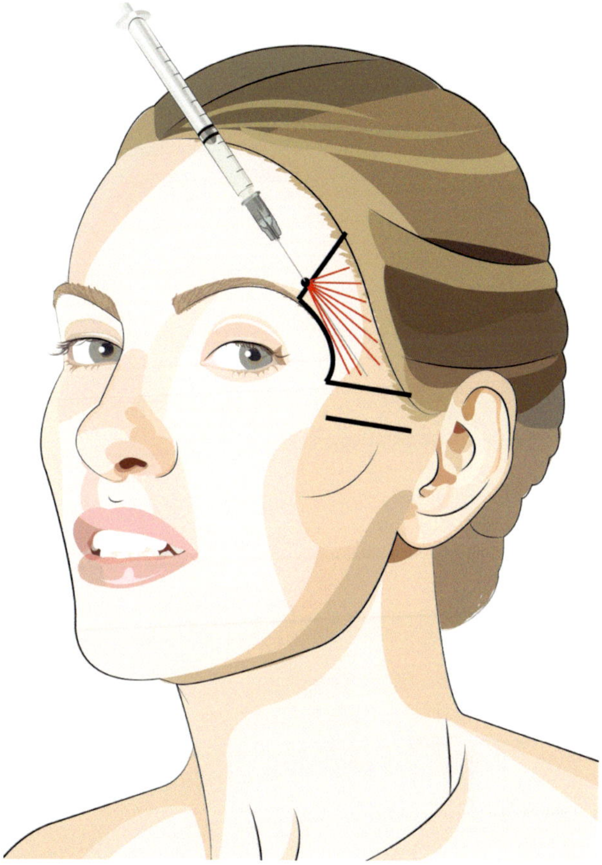

Figure 6.22 CaHA injection with a blunt cannula in the interfascial space, temporal crest entry point. The black lines mark the temporal crest, lateral orbital.

3. Check for pulsations and avoid hitting the superficial temporal artery and veins.
4. Approximately 1 cm superior to the orbital rim, mark the entry point just medial to or at the medial border of the temporal crest.
5. Anesthetize subcutaneous with 1% lidocaine with adrenaline and advance the needle further to the periosteum of the frontal bone at the temporal crest to anesthetize deeper.
6. Create a pre-hole with a 23G needle.
7. Use CaHA product with slightly reduced viscosity to reduce the risk of lumpiness (e.g. 0.3 mL lidocaine per 1.5 mL CaHA syringe).
8. Introduce the cannula and advance it to the periosteum of the frontal bone (Figure 6.23).
9. Advance it over the periosteum through the temporal crest. As the anatomical layer of the periosteum and the deep temporal fascia are continuous, the cannula will now be positioned between the deep temporal fascia and the temporoparietal fascia (Figure 6.24).
10. Place multiple retrograde linear threads of approximately 0.1 mL per thread or consider injecting multiple boluses of approximately 0.05–0.1 mL per bolus and then manually distributing the diluted product between the fascias.

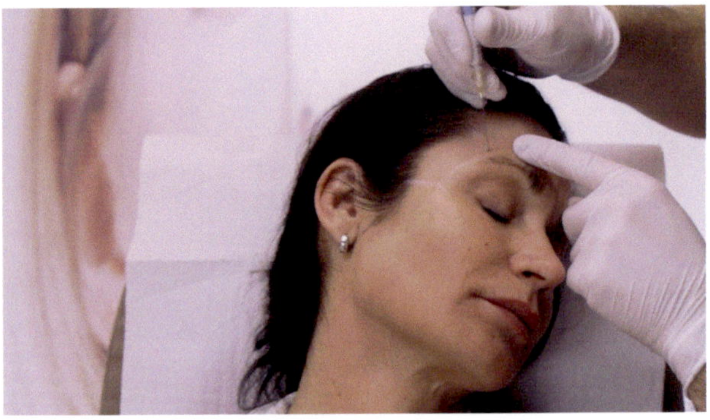

Figure 6.23 Entry point just medial to the temporal crest: advance to frontal bone.

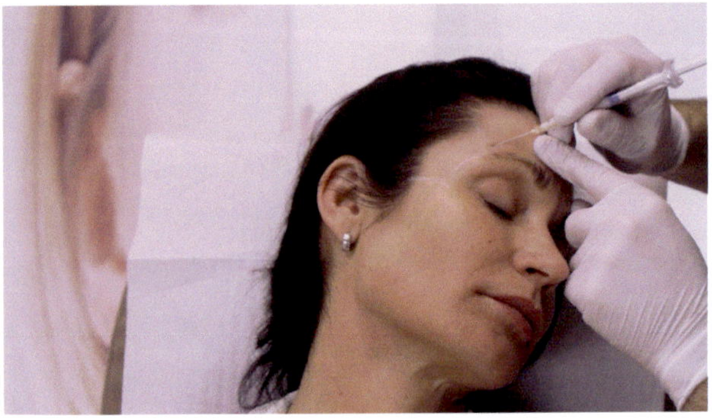

Figure 6.24 Advance lateral passing the temporal crest and inject in the interfascial space.

6.7 AFTERCARE

If necessary, the area can be manually massaged to even out the product. After injection, distension of the veins and superficial temporal artery can be observed due to increased pressure in the area. Swelling might be uneven in the temples, so the patient should be advised that any swelling is to be expected and is temporary, lasting usually one day, but can last up to five days. When injecting in the subcutaneous layer, swelling is more severe than injecting in deeper layers. When injecting periosteally with a sharp needle, pain on mastication can be expected, as the product is mostly injected intramuscularly using this technique.

6.8 ADDITIONAL TREATMENTS FOR OPTIMAL RESULTS

To further improve the aesthetics of the temporal area, brow reshaping with botulinum toxin and fillers can be considered. Also, skin improvement with topical creams, peels, and lasers might be advisable depending on the patients and their needs.

See Figure 6.25 and Videos 6.1–6.5 for before and after results and distinct product placement techniques. Additionally, in Video 44.1 from Chapter 44, an example of temporal ligament lifting can also be found.

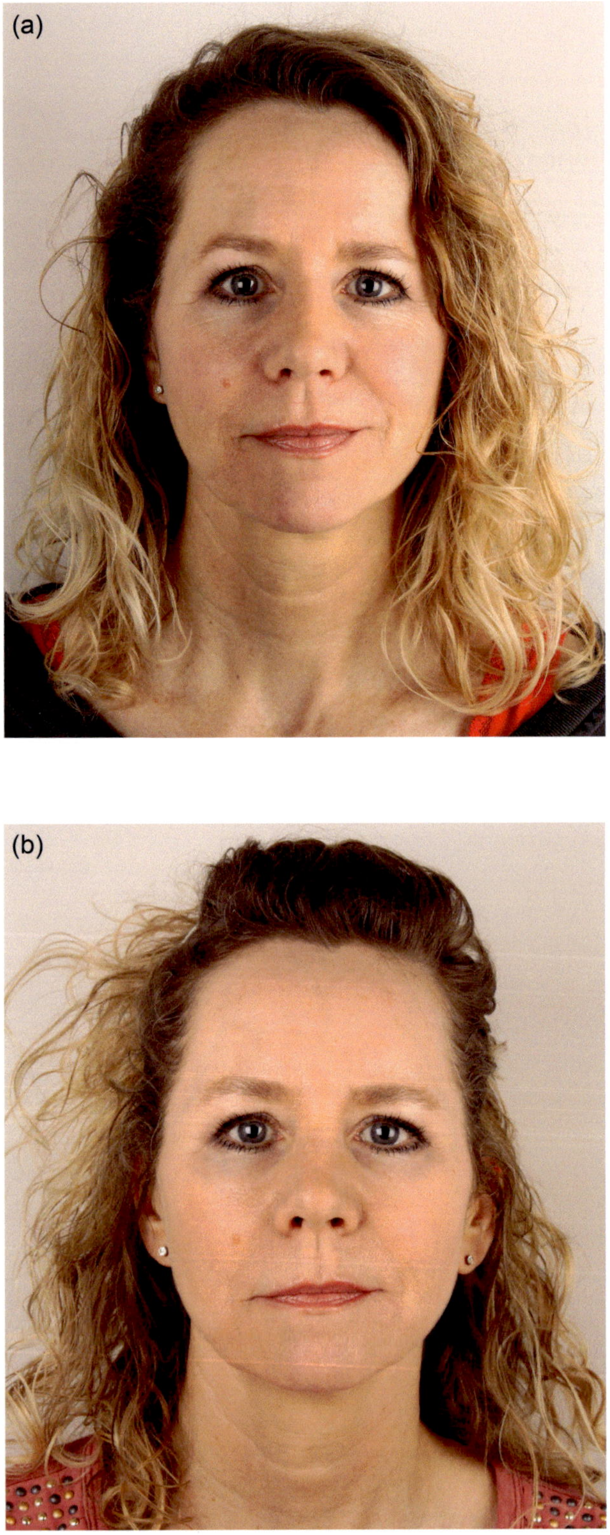

Figure 6.25 Example of a patient (a) before and (b) three months after treatment with CaHA.

Video 6.1 Temporal hollows: interfascial cannula technique 1 (including frontal concavity).

Video 6.2 Temporal hollows: interfascial cannula technique 2.

Video 6.3 Temporal hollows: supraperiosteal cannula technique.

Video 6.4 Temporal hollows: supraperiosteal needle technique.

Video 6.5 Temporal hollows: interfascial cannula technique (zygomatic entry point).

REFERENCES

[1] C. J. Moss et al., "Surgical anatomy of the ligamentous attachments in the temple and periorbital regions," *Plast Reconstr Surg*, vol. 105, no. 4, pp. 1491–1498, 2000.
[2] V. M. Amaral et al., "An innovative treatment using calcium hydroxyapatite for non-surgical facial rejuvenation: The vectorial-lift technique," *Aesthet Plast Surg*, vol. 48, no. 17, pp. 3206–3215, 2024.
[3] J. A. J. van Loghem et al., "Cannula versus sharp needle for placement of soft tissue fillers: An observational cadaver study," *Aesthet Surg J*, vol. 38, no. 1, pp. 73–88, 2017.
[4] J. A. J. van Loghem et al., "Calcium hydroxylapatite: Over a decade of clinical experience," *J Clin Aesthet Dermatol*, vol. 8, no. 1, p. 38, 2015.
[5] J. A. J. van Loghem et al., "Sensitivity of aspiration as a safety test before injection of soft tissue fillers," *J Cosmet Dermatol*, vol. 17, no. 1, pp. 39–46, 2018.

The Upper Third of the Face

Lateral Brow Lift

7

JANI VAN LOGHEM

Lateral brow lift can improve the look of the patient by giving a sense of a more open and awake eye. This can make the patient look more youthful and attractive. Even though small quantities are used, one should realize that the arteries are variable in position and are not always exactly as drawn in Figure 7.1. They can run in all anatomical levels here, from deep to superficial, and as they are connected to the supraorbital artery, a terminal branch of the ophthalmic artery, there is the risk of blindness. Therefore, we advise injecting small amounts per bolus or retrograde linear thread.

7.1 LATERAL BROW LIFT (SHARP NEEDLE MULTILEVEL TECHNIQUE 1)

For injection placement, see Figure 7.2 [1].

7.1.1 Step-by-Step Technique

1. Disinfect and mark the ideal position of the tail and the peak of the brow.
2. Use full viscosity (undiluted) CaHA or CaHA with up to standard dilution (0.3 mL lidocaine per 1.5 mL syringe).
3. Check for pulsations and avoid hitting the superficial veins.
4. Enter through the skin at the tail of the brow at a 45° angle. Advance the 27G needle, 19 mm cannula through the skin and keep the dermal–subdermal junction as target depth.
5. The position of the needle should be just below the hairline of the brow and should be advanced along the lower hairline to the peak of the brow.
6. With two retrogrades, inject a total of 0.05 mL (Figure 7.3).
7. Remove the needle from the skin.
8. Apply direct pressure to the injected area to prevent bruising of this well-vascularized area (Figure 7.4).
9. Move the brow upward with the nondominant fingers. Place the thumb at the lower border of the supraorbital rim to prevent the needle from entering the orbit.

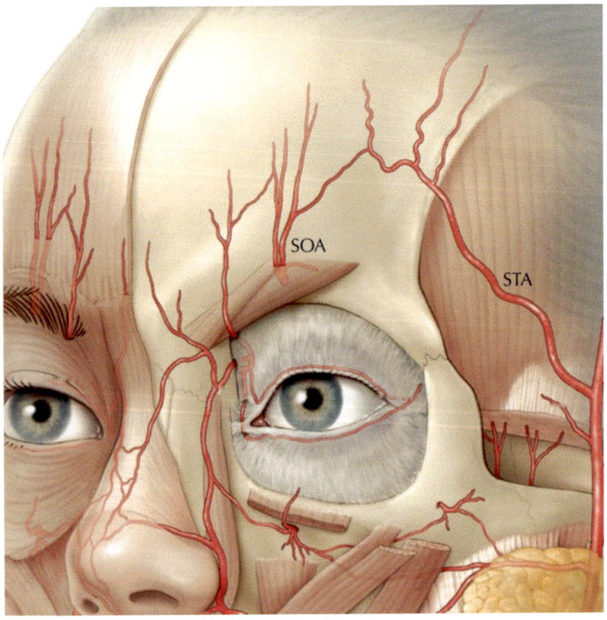

Figure 7.1 Arterial danger zones for the treatment of the brows are: supraorbital artery (SOA) and superficial temporal artery (STA).

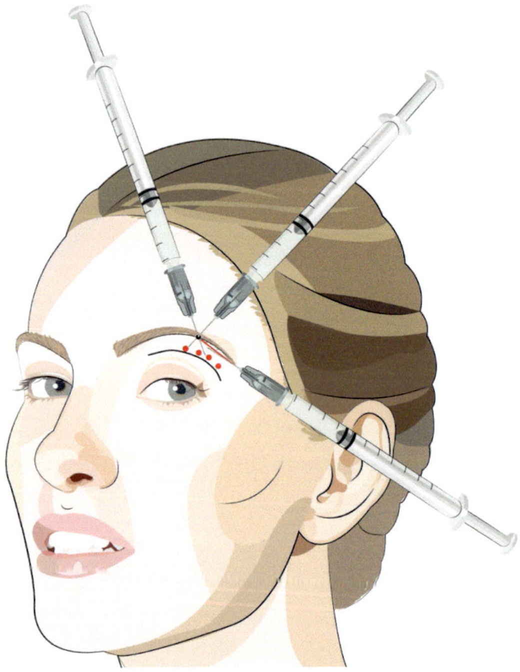

Figure 7.2 Sharp needle multilevel injection technique of the lateral brow lift using subcutaneous retrograde linear threads and periosteal boluses. The black line represents the supraorbital rim. The red line represents a subcutaneous retrograde linear thread, and the red circles represent supraperiosteal boluses.

DOI: 10.1201/9781003617129-7

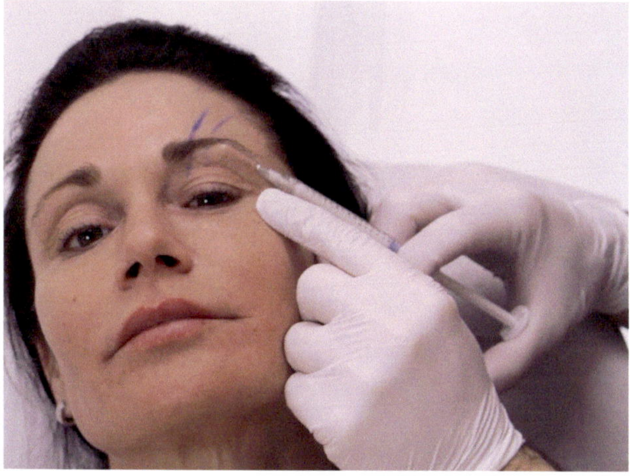

Figure 7.3 Subcutaneous retrograde linear thread.

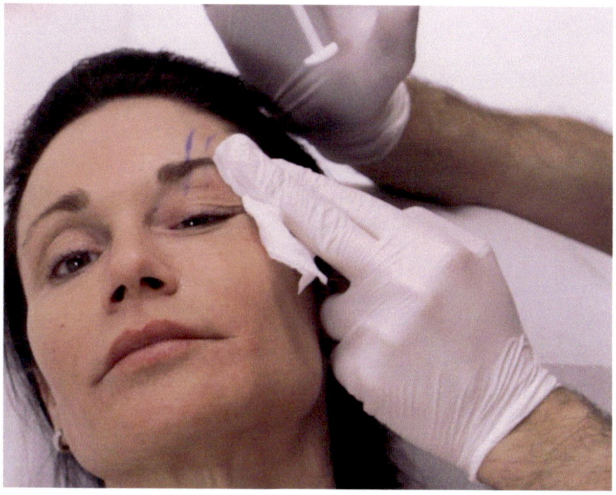

Figure 7.4 Applying direct pressure to avoid ecchymosis.

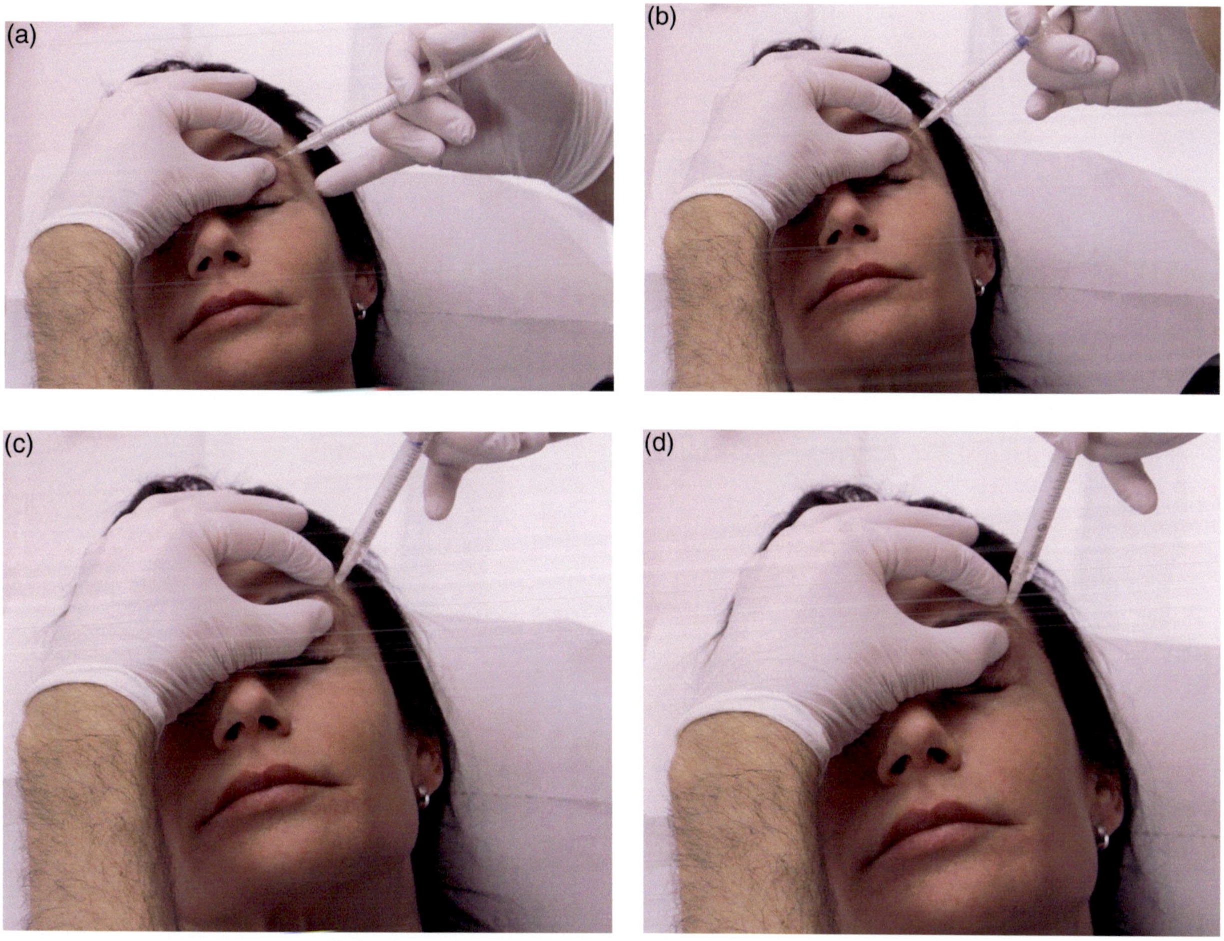

Figure 7.5 (a–d) Administration of supraperiosteal boluses.

10. Below the hairline, at the peak of the brow, advance the needle straight to the periosteum of the orbital rim, just medial to the peak of the brow.
11. Without taking out the needle completely, inject four or five small boluses of 0.025 mL each with the needle in constant contact with the periosteum, "walking" over the periosteum towards the tail of the brow (Figure 5.5).
12. Keeping the brow pulled up with the nondominant hand, remove the needle and even out the product (Figure 5.6).

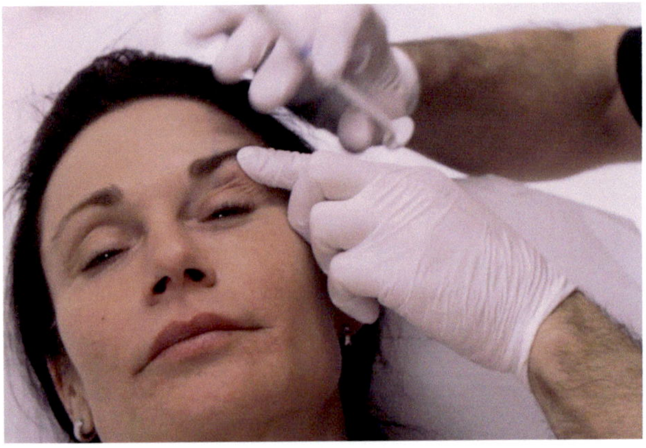

Figure 7.6 Evening out the product.

7.2 LATERAL BROW LIFT (SHARP NEEDLE MULTILEVEL TECHNIQUE 2)

For injection placement, see Figure 7.7.

7.2.1 Step-by-Step Technique

1. Disinfect and mark the ideal position of the tail and the peak of the brow (Figure 7.8).
2. Use full viscosity (undiluted) CaHA or CaHA with up to standard dilution (0.3 mL lidocaine per 1.5 mL syringe).
3. Check for pulsations and avoid hitting the superficial veins.
4. Enter through the skin at the tail of the brow at a 45° angle. Advance the 27–28G needle, 19 mm cannula through the skin and keep the dermal–subdermal junction as target depth.
5. The position of the needle should be just below the hairline of the brow and should be advanced along the hairline to the peak of the brow.
6. With two retrogrades, inject a total of 0.05 mL (Figure 7.9).
7. Without taking out the needle completely, lift the brow with the nondominant hand and advance the needle to the periosteum (Figure 7.10).
8. Advance the needle over the periosteum of the orbital rim and inject a total of 0.1 mL in about four retrograde linear threads (Figure 7.11).
9. Make sure the needle is always moving on injection.
10. Keeping the brow pulled up with the nondominant hand, remove the needle and even out the product.

7.3 LATERAL BROW LIFT (MULTILEVEL CANNULA TECHNIQUE)

For injection placement, see Figure 7.12.

7.3.1 Step-by-Step Technique

1. Disinfect and if needed inject a very small amount of anesthesia (0.05 mL of lidocaine with adrenaline) just lateral to the lateral tip of the brow (Figure 7.13).

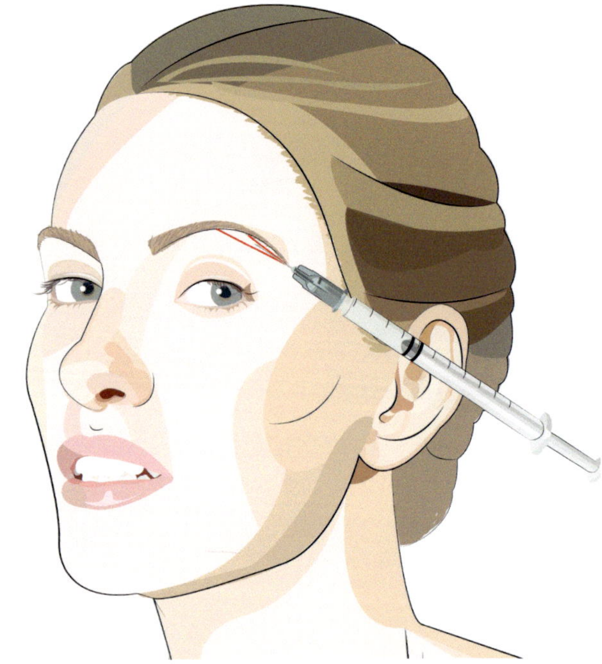

Figure 7.7 Sharp needle multilevel injection technique of the lateral brow lift using subcutaneous and periosteal retrograde linear threads (red lines).

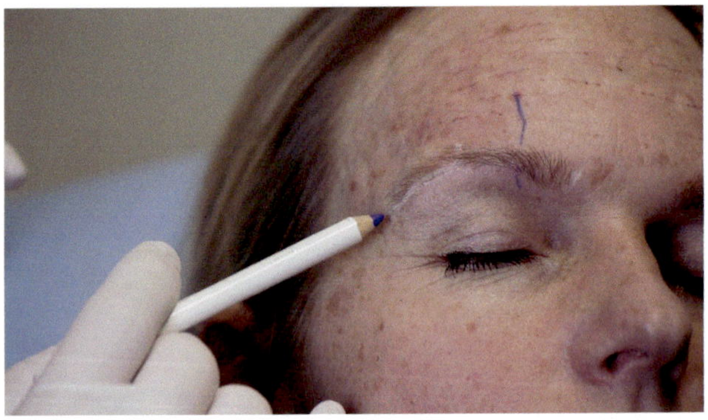

Figure 7.8 Marking according to ideal proportions.

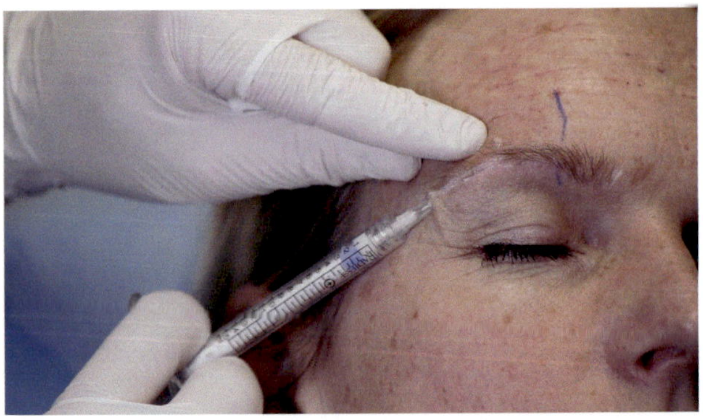

Figure 7.9 Subcutaneous retrograde linear thread.

2. Use full viscosity (undiluted) CaHA or CaHA with up to standard dilution (0.3 mL lidocaine per 1.5 mL syringe).
3. Check for pulsations and avoid hitting the superficial veins.

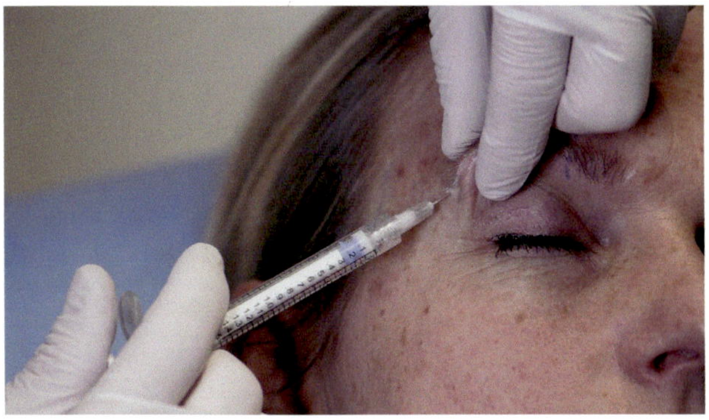

Figure 7.10 Lifting the brow to advance the needle to the orbital rim.

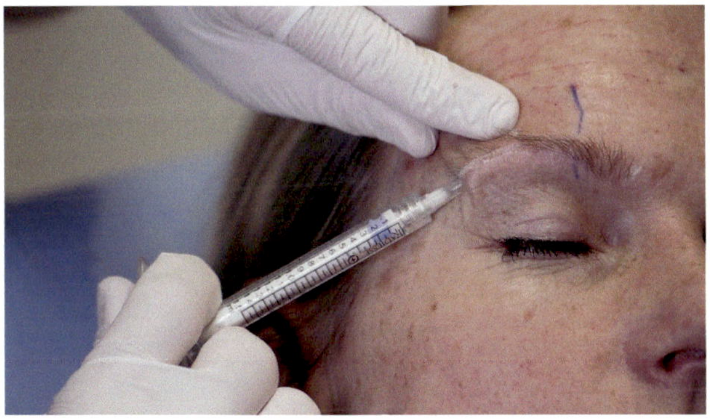

Figure 7.11 Periosteal retrograde linear thread.

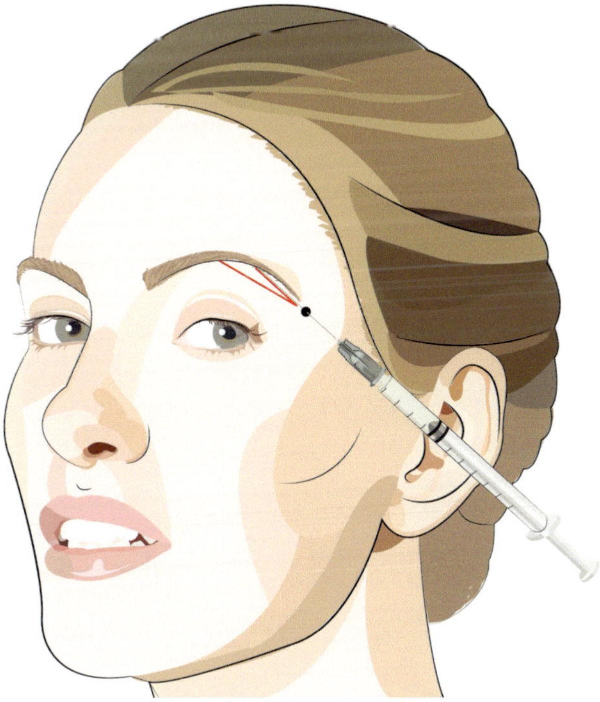

Figure 7.12 Multilevel cannula technique of the lateral brow lift.

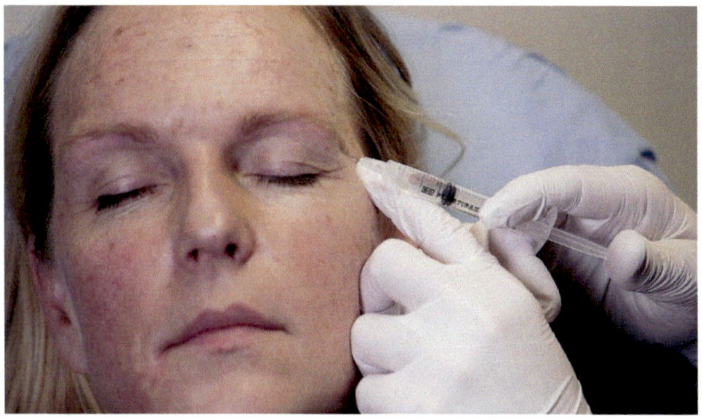

Figure 7.13 Lifting the brow to maneuver the cannula to the supraperiosteal plane

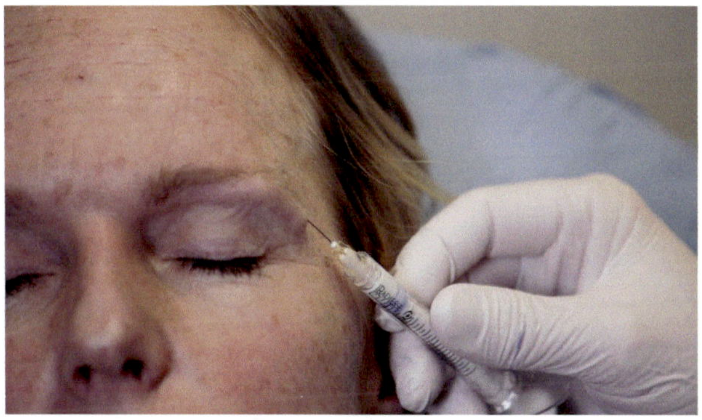

Figure 7.14 Subcutaneous retrograde linear thread.

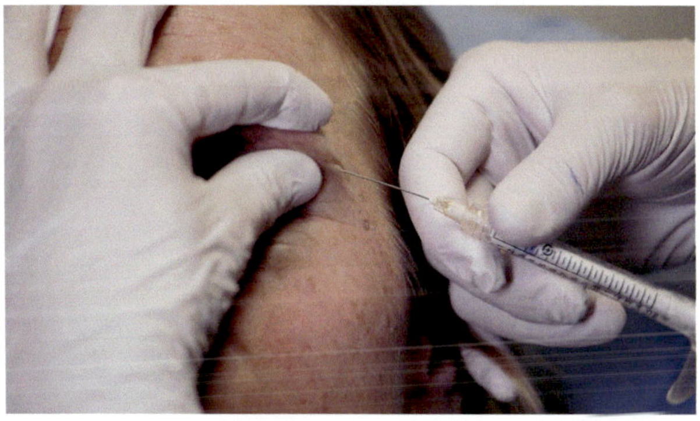

Figure 7.15 Lifting the brow to maneuver the cannula to the supraperiosteal plane.

4. Enter through the skin at the tail of the brow at a 45° angle. Advance the 25G, 38 mm cannula through the skin and keep the dermal-subdermal junction as target depth.
5. The position of the cannula should be just below the lower hairline of the brow and should be advanced along the hairline to the peak of the brow.
6. With one or two retrogrades, inject a total of 0.05 mL (Figure 7.14).
7. Without having to completely remove the cannula, lift the brow away from the orbital rim. Advance the cannula through the resistance of the muscle

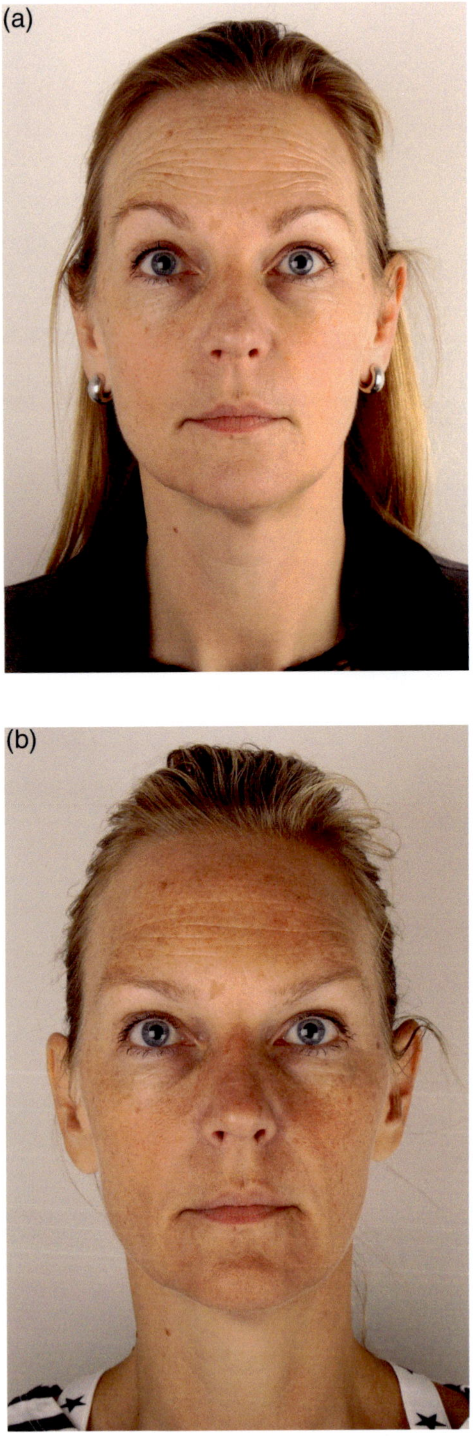

Figure 7.16 Example of a patient treated with CaHA (a) before and (b) two months after the treatment (patient received treatment in other areas as well).

toward the periosteum of the orbital rim. A typical "click" can be heard when passing the resistance.

8. While keeping the brow lifted, advance the cannula over the supraorbital rim to lateral of the supraorbital foramen (Figure 7.15).
9. Inject slow retrograde linear threads totaling about 0.1 mL in total over the orbital rim toward the lateral tip of the brow.
10. Even out as needed.

See also Videos 7.1–7.4 to visualize different application techniques.

7.3.2 Aftercare

If necessary, the area can be manually massaged to even out the product. After injection, edema can be observed and can typically last for one day. Due to the abundant vascular structures in the brow, ecchymosis can be expected, especially when injecting with a sharp needle. Prophylactic compression after injection can be advised to prevent hematoma.

7.3.3 Additional Treatments for Optimal Results

To further improve the aesthetics of the brow, reshaping with botulinum toxin and fillers in the adjacent areas (temples, forehead) can be considered. Also, advice can be given on plucking or not plucking of the brow. See also Figure 7.16.

Video 7.1 Lateral brow lift, needle 1: periosteal bolus.

Video 7.2 Lateral brow lift, needle 2: periosteal retrograde technique.

Video 7.3 Lateral brow lift: multilevel cannula technique.

Video 7.4 Lateral brow lift: cannula workshop.

REFERENCE

[1] J. A. J. van Loghem et al., "Calcium hydroxylapatite: Over a decade of clinical experience," *J Clin Aesthet Dermatol*, vol. 8, no. 1, p. 38, 2015.

The Upper Third of the Face

Frontal Bossing in Men

8

JANI VAN LOGHEM

Frontal bossing is typically a male facial characteristic, and its enhancement will create a masculine look in the patient. The frontal bone in males has a more prominent ridge parallel to the orbital rim than in females. Therefore, the ideal depth of placement of CaHA is the periosteal level. Here, the subgaleal cannula technique will be explained. The major danger cone in this area is the neurovascular bundle ascending from the supraorbital foramen/notch. As the supraorbital artery is in tight tissue, close to the periosteum, possible intravascular events should be avoided. To minimize risk, do not force the cannula through any resistances in this area. See also Figure 8.1 to be aware of the arterial danger zones when treating the frontal bossing.

8.1 FRONTAL BOSSING IN MALES (CANNULA TECHNIQUE)

For injection placement, see Figure 8.2.

8.1.1 Step-by-Step Technique

1. Mark the area and disinfect. Consider anesthesia of the entry points, supratrochlear, and supraorbital nerve blocks.

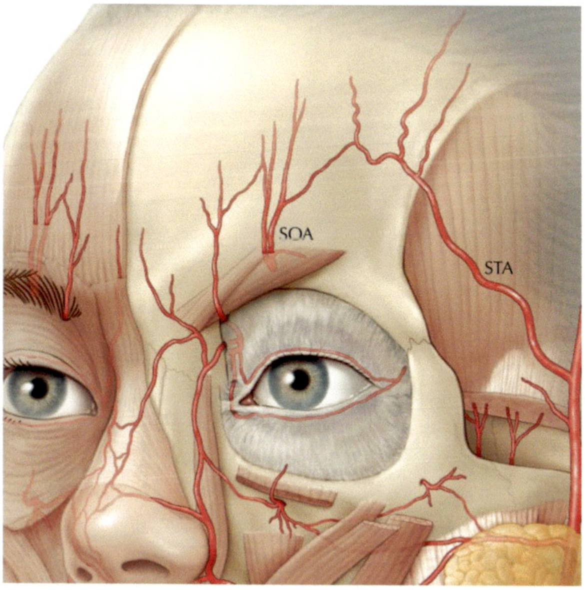

Figure 8.1 Arterial danger zones for the treatment of the forehead are: supraorbital artery (SOA) and superficial temporal artery (STA).

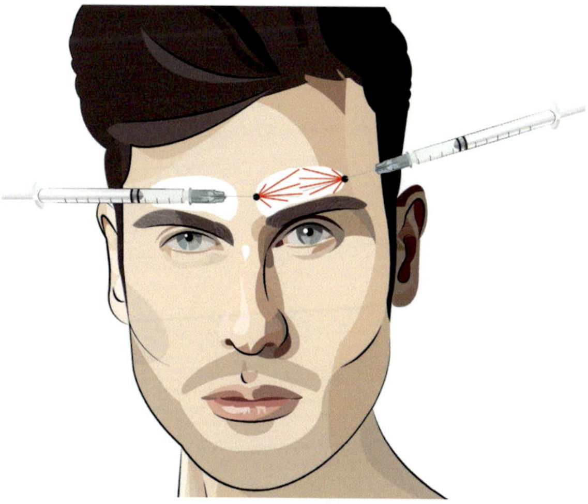

Figure 8.2 Schematic drawing of subgaleal cannula technique for enhancing frontal bossing in males.

2. Use a 23G needle to make entry points for the 25G cannula (preferred is the 22G cannula for reducing vascular complications even more) (Figure 8.3).
3. Use full viscosity (undiluted) CaHA or CaHA with up to standard dilution (0.3 mL lidocaine in a 1.5 mL syringe).
4. Stretch the skin to get the cannula through the dermis to pass resistance; rolling the syringe between thumb and index finger could be considered.
5. Lift the tissue in front of the cannula to make a path of least resistance to the periosteum.
6. Gently advance the cannula over the periosteum without using force. When injecting, use a finger of your nondominant hand to press against the supraorbital notch.
7. Place multiple retrograde linear threads over the periosteum of maximum 0.05 mL per retrograde (Figure 8.4). Do not force the cannula through resistance, as the area around the supraorbital foramen contains the neurovascular bundle.
8. Inject a slow retrograde linear thread of 0.1 mL in total over the orbital rim toward the lateral tip of the brow.
9. From the medial entry point, approximately 2–3 cm above the orbital rim (Figures 8.5 and 8.6), horizontally advance the cannula to the periosteum. Keep a finger of the nondominant hand on the orbital rim to apply pressure.

DOI: 10.1201/9781003617129-8

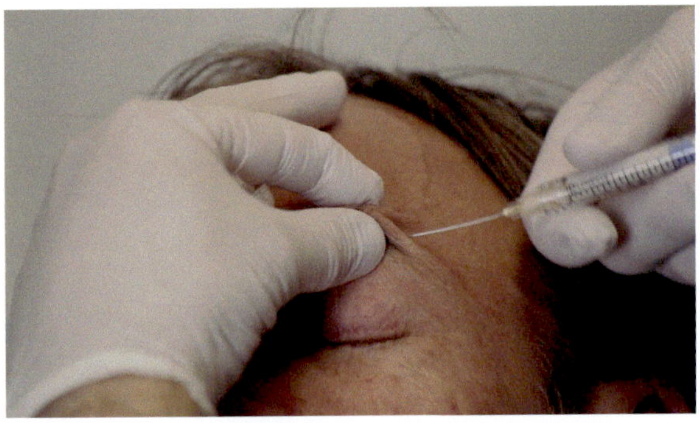

Figure 8.3 Lateral entry point.

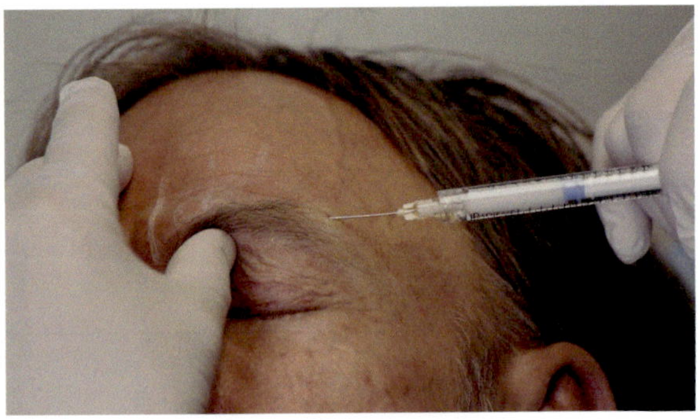

Figure 8.4 Periosteal injection.

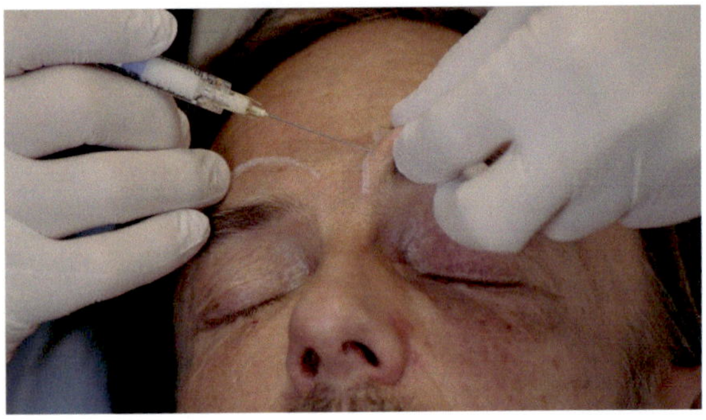

Figure 8.5 Medial entry point.

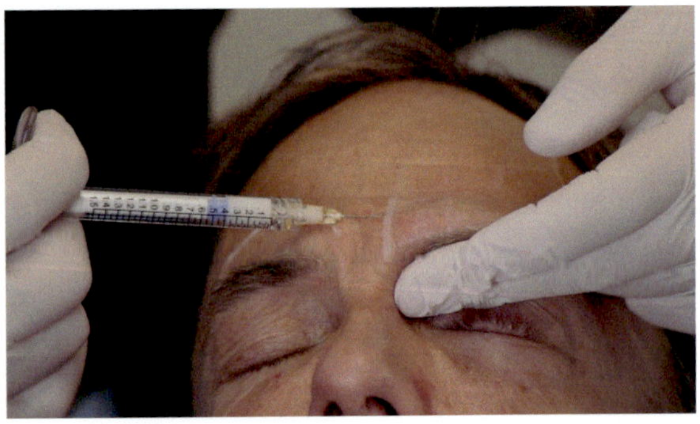

Figure 8.6 Keep pressure on arteries with non-dominant finger.

10. Advance the cannula over the periosteum and inject retrograde linear threads of approximately 0.025 mL per thread to keep within the maximum limit of 0.04 mL [1].
11. Even out as needed.

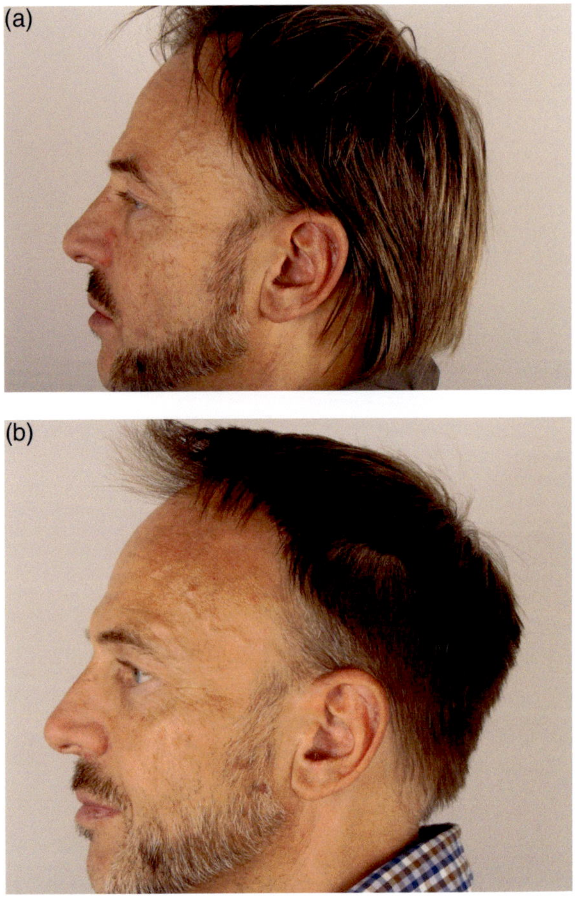

Figure 8.7 Example of a male patient before (a) and after (b) treatment with 0.75 mL of CaHA per side to increase frontal bossing.

See also Figure 8.7 and Video 8.1 to visualize before and after results and application technique, respectively.

8.2 AFTERCARE

If necessary, the area can be manually massaged to even out the product. After injection, edema can be observed, typically lasting for one day. As edema is close to the supraorbital foramen, the swelling may descend into the eyelids. When this occurs, the swelling typically stays for a few days.

8.3 ADDITIONAL TREATMENTS FOR OPTIMAL RESULTS

To further improve the aesthetics of the frontal male area, botulinum toxin injection in the frontalis muscle can be used to lower the brows and relax the mimic muscles. Fillers in the adjacent areas (temples, frontal concavity) can be considered.

Video 8.1 Frontal bossing: cannula technique.

REFERENCE

[1] T. T. Khan et al., "An anatomical analysis of the supratrochlear artery: Considerations in facial filler injections and preventing vision loss," *Aesthet Surg J*, vol. 37, no. 2, pp. 203–208, 2017.

The Upper Third of the Face

9

Horizontal Forehead Lines and C-Angle

JANI VAN LOGHEM

9.1 HORIZONTAL FOREHEAD LINES

Horizontal forehead lines are not generally treated with CaHA. This is due to the fact that these lines are essentially dynamic wrinkles, and so botulinum toxin is often chosen to treat them. CaHA in its original form is too viscous, and thus superficial injection can result in both lumpiness and whitish discoloration visible through the skin. Soft hyaluronic acid fillers are the first choice for treating horizontal forehead lines when selecting fillers to treat these lines intradermally. Diluted CaHA can aid in improving the quality of the forehead skin and thereby contribute to reducing the horizontal forehead lines.

See also Figure 9.1 to be aware of the danger zones of for the forehead.

9.2 HORIZONTAL FOREHEAD LINES: HYPER DILUTION, SHARP NEEDLE TECHNIQUE

For injection placement, see Figure 9.2.

9.2.1 Step-by-Step Technique

1. Consider pretreatment with botulinum toxin and volumizing the subgaleal space to relax the frontalis muscle.

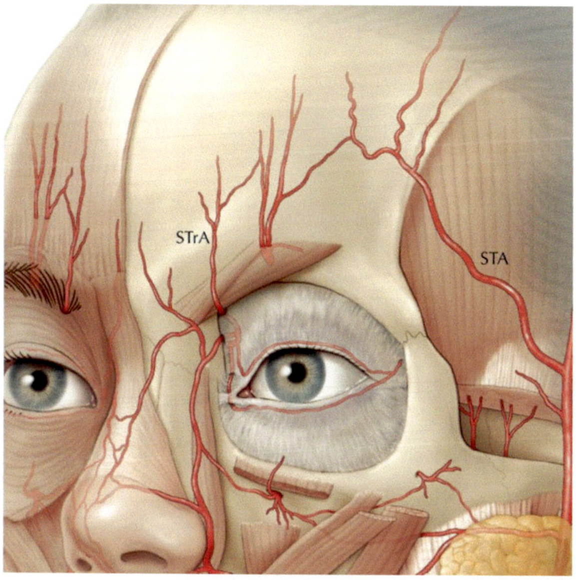

Figure 9.1 Arterial danger zones for the treatment of the forehead are: superficial temporal artery (STA) and supratrochlear artery (STrA).

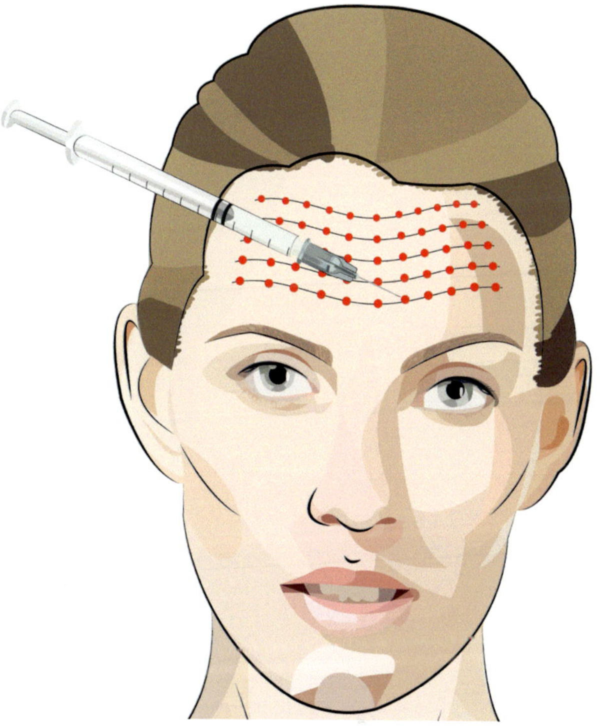

Figure 9.2 Injection technique using a sharp needle, intradermal retrograde linear threads (black lines), and serial punctures (red dots) in the wrinkles.

2. Disinfect the skin of the forehead. Consider supratrochlear and supraorbital nerve blocks.
3. Use hyper diluted CaHA of 1–1.5 mL lidocaine with adrenaline (1:200000) per 1.5 mL syringe.
4. Advance the 27G or 28G needle with bevel up into the dermis with an angle of approximately 10–20° to prevent the needle from advancing through the dermis.
5. Inject in the deep dermis with the bevel up; not too superficial (the grey of the needle should not be visible) and not too deep; the danger zones run mostly in the subcutaneous fat here. Inject along the horizontal wrinkles, either retrograde or small aliquots of maximum 0.025 mL (Figure 9.3).
6. Use low pressure on injection; use low volume (stay well below 0.04 mL per retrograde) [1].
7. Even out as needed.

DOI: 10.1201/9781003617129-9

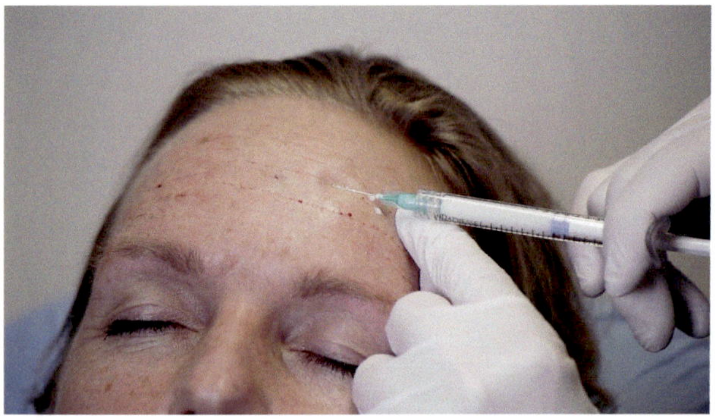

Figure 9.3 Injecting retrograde linear threads, and small aliquots of max. 0.025 mL, intradermally in the wrinkles.

9.3 AFTERCARE

If necessary, the area can be manually massaged to even out the product. After injection, edema can be observed and can typically last for one day. Advise the patient that the skin rejuvenation shall be a slow process over the next few months, even though immediate results may be observed.

9.4 ADDITIONAL TREATMENTS FOR OPTIMAL RESULTS

To further reduce the horizontal forehead lines, botulinum toxin can be used to relax the frontalis muscle, ideally one to two weeks prior to the CaHA treatment. Fillers placed deep to the frontalis muscle (frontal concavity) can be considered to induce myomodulation, whereby stretching the muscle will have a lower basic tonus and muscular activity.

See further Figure 9.4 and Video 9.1 for before and after results and application technique, respectively.

9.5 C-ANGLE

The C-angle is a C-shaped area around the eyes, spanning from the retro orbicularis oculi fat pad (ROOF) in the supraorbital area along the temple, the lateral orbital rim, and the palpebromalar groove to the V-frame deformity and the tear trough in the infraorbital area. The C-angle is, therefore, a key anatomic subunit in the perception of eye attractiveness [2], and one must be careful when treating it, as it constitutes one of the topographical areas of the face with high risk of vascular complications due to the ample number of arteries traversing the periorbital region (supraorbital artery, angular artery, infraorbital artery, zygomaticofacial artery, zygomaticotemporal artery, and their respective branches) (Figure 9.5).

During the aging process, significant bone resorption impacts the position of soft tissues. The aged appearance is characterized by the apparent descent of the brow, which could be due to the upward movement of the supraorbital rim due to bone resorption. The temple and the temporal crest show skeletonization due to volume loss. The infraorbital area shows volume loss of the infraorbital rim, resulting in deepening of the palpebromalar groove, the V-frame deformity, and the tear trough. Replacing lost volume on the periosteum and lifting the temporal region (by targeting the TLA), like Amaral and others suggest [3], may therefore create a natural rejuvenated appearance. In this section we share an injection technique with a combination of needle and cannula and an injection technique

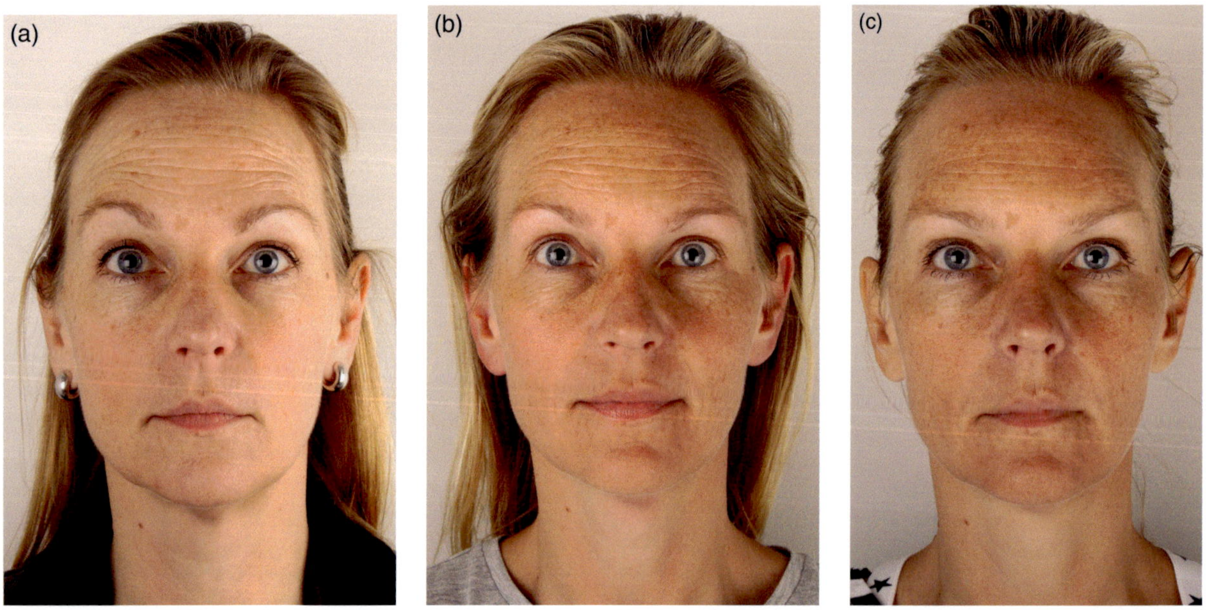

Figure 9.4 Example of a patient treated with 0.5 mL of diluted CaHA per side (patient was also treated in other areas). (a) Before (one month after only CaHA); (b) one month after Botulinum toxin; and (c) two months after CaHA.

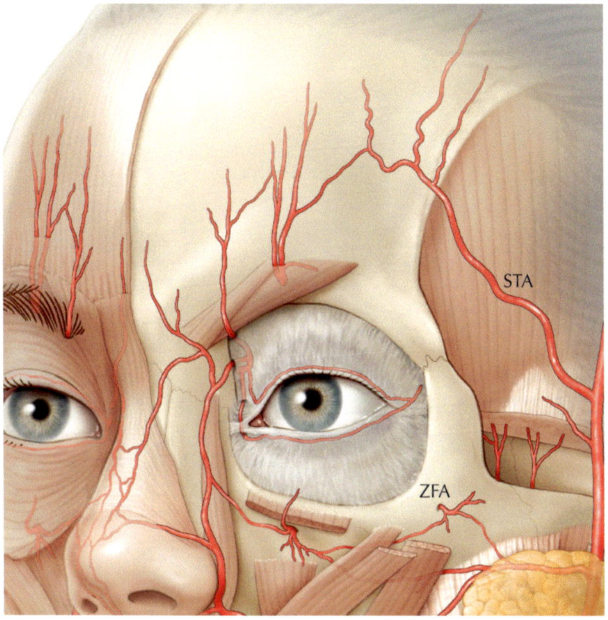

Figure 9.5 Arterial danger zones of the C-angle include the superficial temporal artery (STA) and the zygomaticofacial artery (ZFA).

using only cannulas. It is of the utmost importance to place the product on the periosteum, especially in the infraorbital area, to avoid malar edema.

9.5.1 C-Angle Needle and Cannula Technique

For injection placement, see Figure 9.6 and video 9.2.

9.5.2 Step-by-Step Technique

1. Disinfect and mark the lateral brow, temporal crest, temporal hollow, palpebromalar groove, V frame deformity, and tear trough (Figure 9.7).
2. Local anesthesia may be considered for the entry points at the lateral brow and the tear trough.
3. Check for blood vessels and make an entry point at the tail of the brow.
4. Use full viscosity (undiluted) CaHA with a 25G, 38 mm cannula or thicker.
5. Advance the cannula through the skin.
6. Prop up the brow with the non-dominant hand in order to pass the cannula through the orbicularis oculi muscle into the ROOF.
7. Make sure the cannula is on the periosteum and gently advance it medially along the supraorbital rim until approximately 1–2 cm lateral from the supraorbital notch.
8. When the cannula is at the maximum distance, keep the brow elevated with the non-dominant hand and inject a retrograde linear thread of max 0.025 mL (Figure 9.8).
9. Repeat until approximately 0.1–0.2 mL has been injected.
10. Remove the cannula and attach a 27G, 19 mm needle.

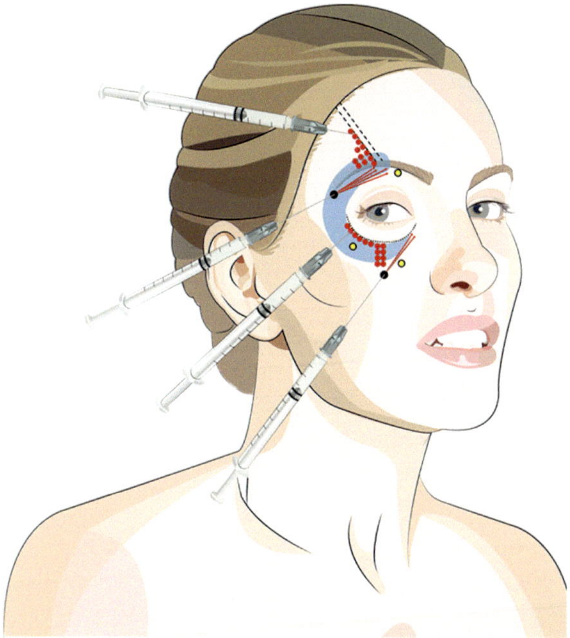

Figure 9.6 Schematic drawing of cannula and sharp needle injection at the C-angle. The blue area indicates the C-shaped target area. The black dashed lines mark the temporal crest; the dotted black line marks the infraorbital rim. The yellow circles mark the supraorbital notch, zygomaticofacial foramen, and infraorbital foramen. The red dots indicate sharp needle bolus injection of CaHA on the periosteum. The red lines indicate periosteal retrograde linear threads.

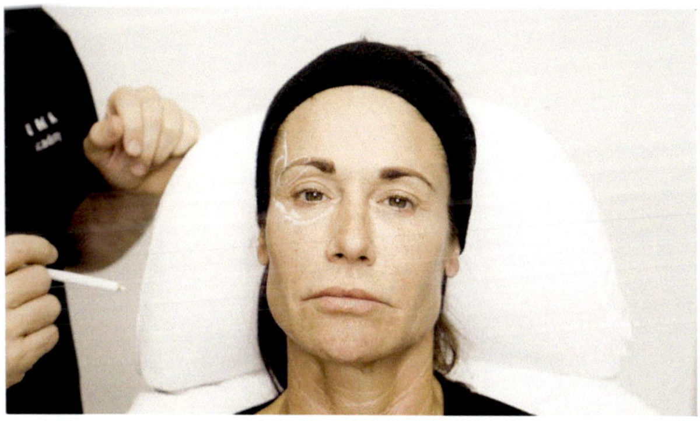

Figure 9.7 Marking of the C-angle: lateral brow, temporal crest, temporal hollow, palpebromalar groove, V-frame deformity, and tear trough.

11. Feel for pulsations in the temporal area and mark these in order to avoid injecting into the superficial temporal artery (Figure 9.9).
12. With the brow lifted, advance the needle with the bevel down to the periosteum of the area where the temporal crest and the lateral orbital rim meet and inject 0.05 mL.
13. Retract partially and readvance the needle to the periosteum of the lateral temporal crest to inject multiple additional boluses of 0.05 mL while keeping the brow lifted.

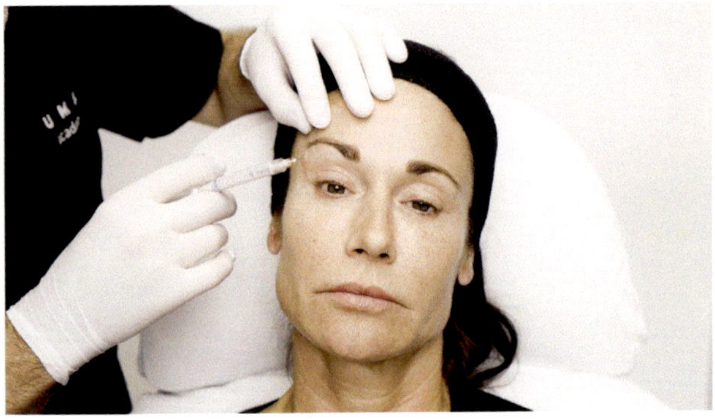

Figure 9.8 The cannula is positioned under the orbicularis oculi muscle at the periosteal level. Retrograde linear threads of 0.025 mL CaHA are injected with the brow lifted upward.

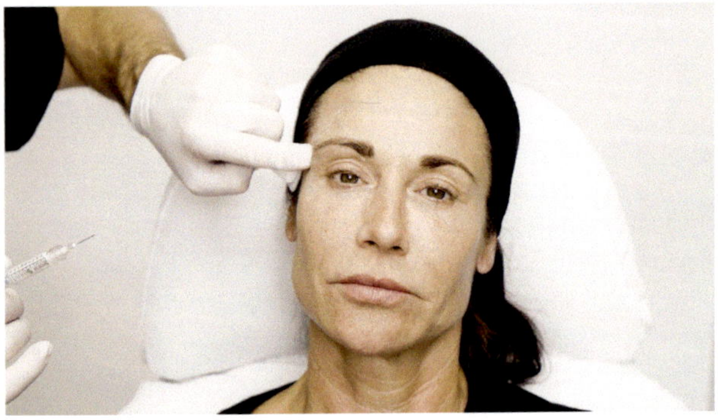

Figure 9.9 Check and mark areas where pulsations of the superficial temporal artery can be felt.

14. If needed, continue injecting multiple boluses along the temporal crest to lift the lateral brow and in the temporal hollow to volumize the temple (Figure 9.10).
15. Even out and mold the product upward along the temporal crest.
16. Determine a needle entry point for the palpebromalar groove. Re-check the possible position of the zygomaticofacial foramen. Advance the needle to the periosteum of the inferolateral rim, just beneath the orbicularis retaining ligament (ORL) (Figure 9.11).
17. Inject a bolus of approximately 0.025 mL.
18. Partially retract, reorient, and readvance 1–2 mm away from the first bolus and inject another bolus of 0.025 mL.
19. If needed, the apex of the cheek may be included.
20. Repeat until approximately 0.1–0.3 mL has been injected.
21. Determine the area of the V-frame deformity, just lateral to the infraorbital foramen (Figure 9.12).
22. Advance the needle to the periosteum of the infraorbital rim, just below the ORL.
23. At the periosteum with the bevel down, inject multiple boluses of approximately 0.05 mL each.

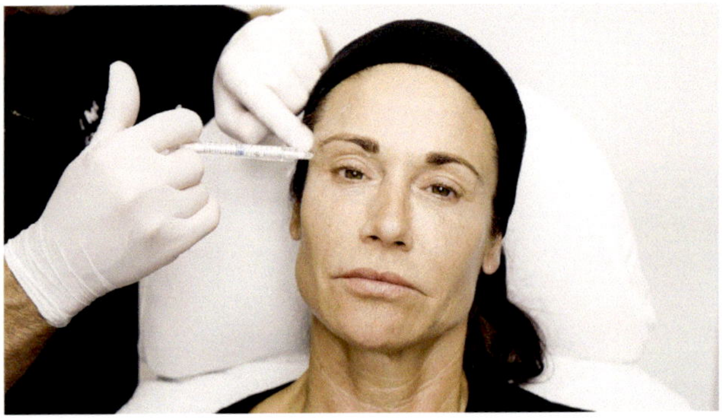

Figure 9.10 The needle is advanced to the temporal crest in Layer 4 and temporal hollow in Layer 5. Then small aliquots (0.05 mL) at the superior temporal septum and temporal hollow are injected.

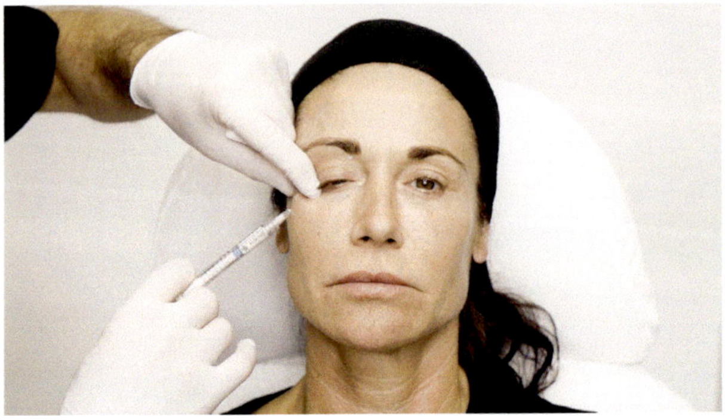

Figure 9.11 At the palpebromalar groove, the needle is advanced to the periosteum of the orbital rim. Small retrogrades (0.05 mL) just below the orbicularis retaining ligament are injected. The non-dominant hand controls the needle to stay extraorbitally.

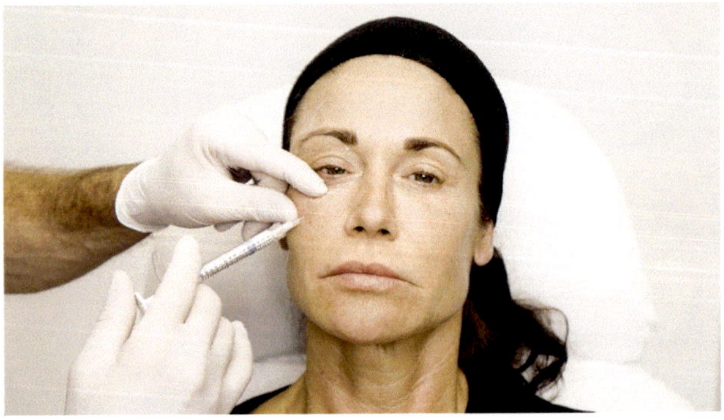

Figure 9.12 The needle is advanced to the periosteum. Small boluses (0.05 mL) just below the orbicularis retaining ligament are injected. Additional aliquots of 0.05 mL are injected to support the zygomatic cutaneous ligament.

24. While lifting the cheek with the non-dominant hand, also inject multiple periosteal boluses just below the zygomatic cutaneous ligament (ZCL).
25. Remove the 27G needle and replace it with a 25G, 38 mm cannula.

26. Determine the entry point in such a way that it is lateral to the insertion of the ZCL and the cannula can reach the medial tear trough (Figure 9.13).
27. Make the pre-hole and advance the cannula through the orbicularis oculi (and the superficial musculo-aponeurotic system; SMAS) and the premaxillary glide space (malar septum) to the periosteum.
28. Advance the cannula over the periosteum to the medial tear trough.
29. With the bevel down, inject retrograde linear threads of approximately 0.05 mL each, totaling about 0.1–0.2 mL.
30. Even out with a light massage.

9.5.3 C-Angle Cannula-Only Technique

For injection placement, see Figure 9.14 and Video 9.3.

9.5.4 Step-by-Step Technique

1. Disinfect and mark the lateral brow, temporal crest, temporal hollow, palpebromalar groove, V-frame deformity, and tear trough (Figure 9.15).
2. Mark and anesthetize the pre-holes.
3. Check for blood vessels and make an entry point at the tail of the brow.
4. Use full viscosity (undiluted) CaHA with a 25G, 38mm cannula or thicker.
5. Advance the cannula through the skin.
6. Prop up the brow with the non-dominant hand in order to pass the cannula through the orbicularis oculi muscle into the ROOF (Figure 9.16).
7. Make sure the cannula is on the periosteum and gently advance the cannula medially along the supraorbital rim until approximately 1–2 cm lateral from the supraorbital notch.
8. When the cannula is at the maximum distance, keep the brow elevated with the non-dominant hand and inject a retrograde linear thread of max 0.025 mL.
9. Repeat until approximately 0.1–0.2 mL has been injected.

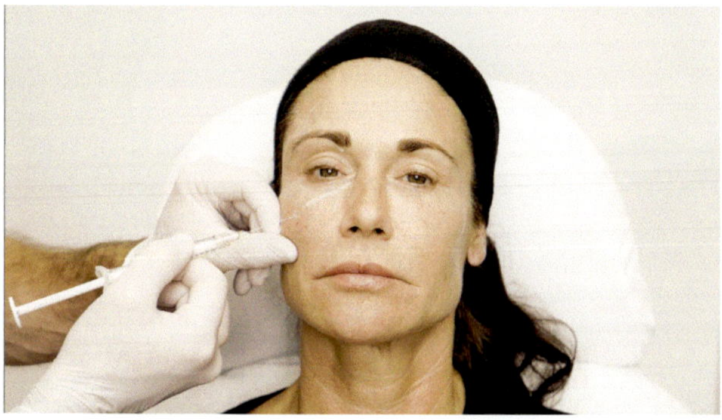

Figure 9.13 The cannula is advanced through the orbicularis oculi and the malar septum to the periosteum. Small retrogrades (0.05 mL) are injected between the orbicularis retaining ligament and the zygomatic cutaneous ligament.

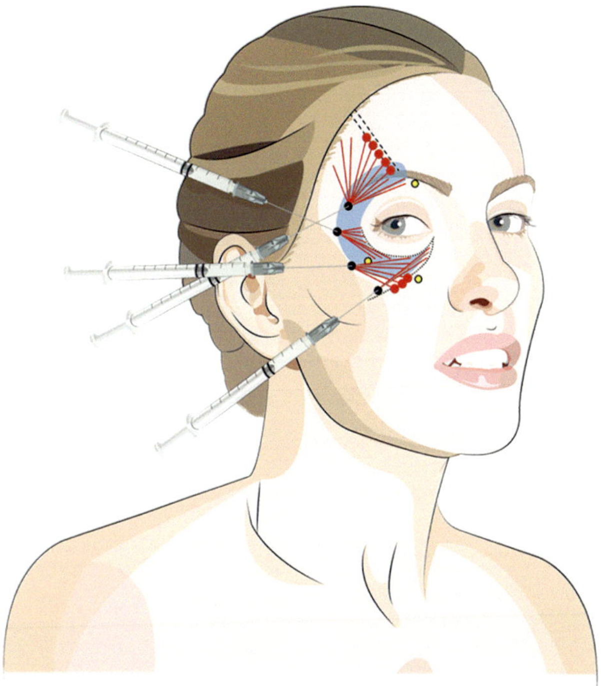

Figure 9.14 Schematic drawing of cannula-only injection technique at the C-angle. The blue area indicates the C-shaped target area. The black dashed lines mark the temporal crest; the dotted black lines mark the infraorbital rim and the zygomatic cutaneous ligament. The yellow circles mark the supraorbital notch, zygomaticofacial foramen, and infraorbital foramen. The red dots indicate bolus deposits of CaHA on the periosteum. The red lines indicate retrograde linear threads.

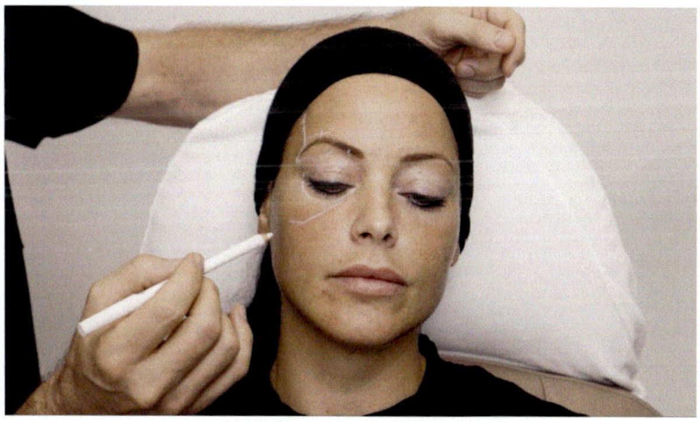

Figure 9.15 Marking the temporal crest, tail of the brow, temporal hollow, lateral and infraorbital rims, tear trough, palpebromalar groove, and tear trough that conform to the C-angle area.

10. After the brow has been injected, advance the cannula in anatomical Layer 4 (under the orbicularis oculi muscle, under the temporoparietal fascia) to the temporal crest.
11. With the non-injecting hand, the brow is being propped up while the cannula is advanced along the temporal crest (Figure 9.17).

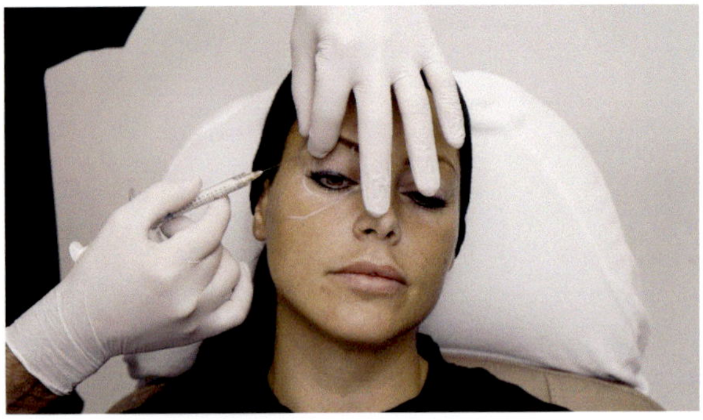

Figure 9.16 The cannula is advanced through the orbicularis oculi muscle to reach the supraorbital rim and elevate the eyebrow. Retrograde linear threads of 0.025 mL CaHA are injected with the brow lifted upward.

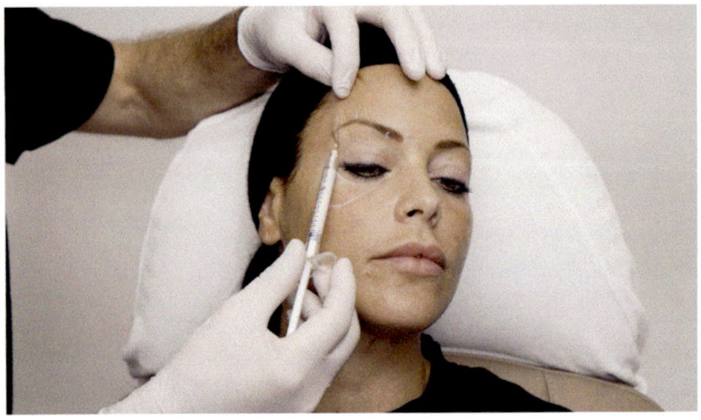

Figure 9.17 Through the orbicularis oculi muscle, the cannula is advanced laterally to the temporal crest. While lifting the skin, retrograde linear threads of CaHA are deposited.

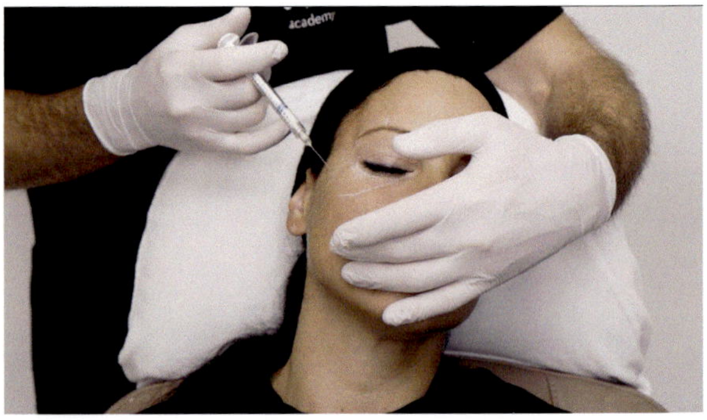

Figure 9.18 CaHA is deposited on top of the orbicularis and zygomatic retaining ligaments to facilitate the ligament lifting and give volume and projection to the cheek.

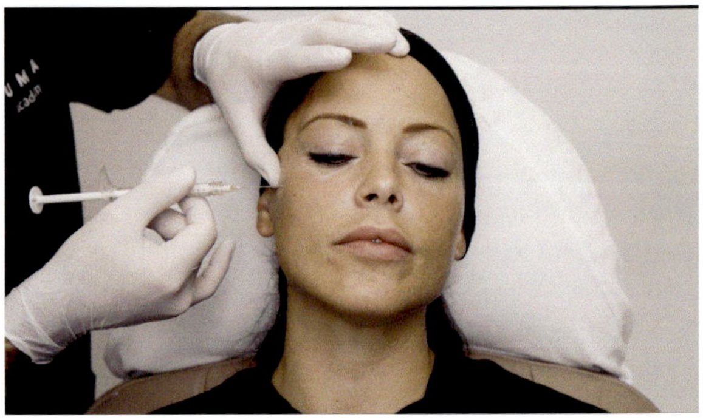

Figure 9.19 The cannula is advanced below the sub-orbicularis oculi fat (SOOF) and above the periosteum to treat the V-frame deformity with 0.05 mL boluses of CaHA.

12. Multiple passes may be used while product is injected in boluses of approximately 0.05 mL along the temporal crest.
13. A purposeful molding technique may be used, where the product is massaged upward to support the superior temporal septum.
14. From a second entry hole, additional retrograde linear threads may be injected in the temporal hollows in the interfascial space.
15. Taking advantage of this second entry point, we can conduct a ligament lifting of the ORL and the zygomatic retaining ligament (Figure 9.18).
16. Advance the cannula to the periosteum. Some force may be necessary to advance the cannula through the lateral orbital thickening.
17. Inject small retrograde linear threads of approximately 0.025–0.05 mL just below the ORL on the periosteum.
18. A third entry point can also be used to treat the palpebromalar groove beside the V-frame deformity.
19. Advance the cannula into the periosteum between the ORL and the ZCL toward the mid pupillary line (Figure 9.19).
20. Inject small retrogrades of approximately 0.05 mL.
21. Advance the cannula through the ZCL.

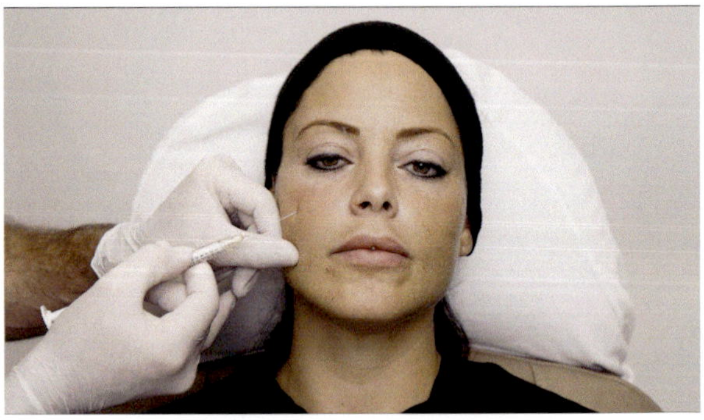

Figure 9.20 Retrograde linear threads of 0.05–0.1 mL CaHA are administered to treat the tear trough.

22. Inject small boluses of 0.05 mL below the ligament and retrogrades of 0.05 mL, moving back to the entry point.
23. The fourth entry point is used to treat the tear trough (Figure 9.20).
24. Make the pre-hole and advance the cannula through the orbicularis oculi (SMAS) and the premaxillary glide space (malar septum) to the periosteum.
25. Advance the cannula over the periosteum to the medial tear trough.

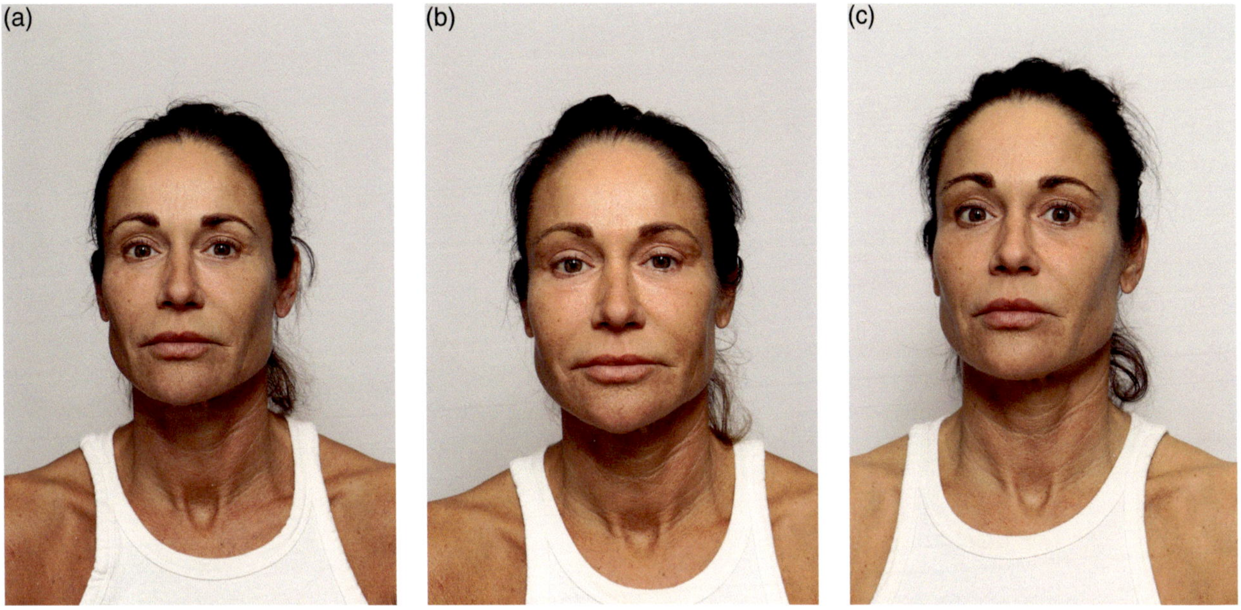

Figure 9.21 Before (a), 1-month (b), and 2-month (c) after results of a 45-year-old woman who underwent a C-angle rejuvenation with CaHA.

26. With the bevel down, inject retrograde linear threads of approximately 0.05 mL each, totaling about 0.1–0.2 mL.
27. Even out with a light massage.

9.6 AFTERCARE

If necessary, the area can be manually massaged to even out the product. When doing so, use a purposeful molding ("rock and roll") technique where the tissue is lifted upward and then the product is massaged into its desired shape, especially around the retaining ligaments along the temporal crest (the superior temporal septum), the temple (the inferior temporal septum, palpebromalar groove, orbicularis retaining ligament, canthal ligament), V-frame deformity (ZCL), and tear trough (tear trough ligament). After injection, distension of the veins and superficial temporal artery can be observed due to increased pressure in the area. Swelling might be uneven in the injected area, so the patient should be advised that any swelling is to be expected and is temporary, lasting usually one day, but can last up to five days. When injecting periosteally with a sharp needle in the temple, pain on mastication can be expected, as the product is mostly injected intramuscularly using this technique.

9.7 ADDITIONAL TREATMENTS FOR OPTIMAL RESULTS

To further improve the aesthetics of the C-angle, brow reshaping and wrinkle reduction with botulinum toxin can be considered. Also, skin improvement with topical creams, peels, and lasers might be advisable depending on the patients and their needs.

Video 9.1 Horizontal forehead lines: needle technique.

Video 9.2 C-Angle: needle technique.

Video 9.3 C-Angle: cannula-only technique.

REFERENCES

[1] T. T. Khan et al., "An anatomical analysis of the supratrochlear artery: Considerations in facial filler injections and preventing vision loss," *Aesthet Surg J*, vol. 37, no. 2, pp. 203–208, Feb. 2017.
[2] M. S. Alghoul et al., "Enhancing the lateral orbital 'C-Angle' with calcium hydroxylapatite: An anatomic and clinical study," *Aesthet Surg J*, vol. 41, no. 8, pp. 952–966, Aug. 2021.
[3] V. M. Amaral et al., "An innovative treatment using calcium hydroxyapatite for non-surgical facial rejuvenation: The vectorial-lift technique," *Aesthetic Plast Surg*, vol. 48, no. 17, pp. 3206–3215, Sep. 2024.

The Upper Third of the Face

10

Temporal Crest Smoothing

JANI VAN LOGHEM

Here, we describe treatment techniques for reducing the sharpness of the temporal crest with both sharp needles and nontraumatic cannulas. Smoothing the temporal crest will reduce the skeletonized appearance and therefore has a subtle rejuvenating power. Often, the frontalis muscle extends laterally beyond the temporal crest. The preferred depth of injection is therefore in the subgaleal plane that extends to the interfascial plane in the temporal area (Figure 10.1).

10.1 TEMPORAL CREST SMOOTHING (SHARP NEEDLE MULTIPLE BOLUS TECHNIQUE)

For injection placement, see Figure 10.2 [1].

10.1.1 Step-by-Step Technique

1. Disinfect and mark the temporal crest (Figure 10.3).
2. Use full viscosity (undiluted) CaHA or standard dilution of CaHA.
3. Check for pulsations and avoid hitting the superficial temporal artery and veins.
4. Advance the 27G, 19 mm needle 45–90° to the skin, slowly to the periosteum just lateral to the temporal crest (Figure 10.4). The patient may note a cracking noise as the needle passes through the fascias and is placed at the periosteum.
5. The beveled down needle should have a soft touch to the periosteum, and the patient might feel some pressure.

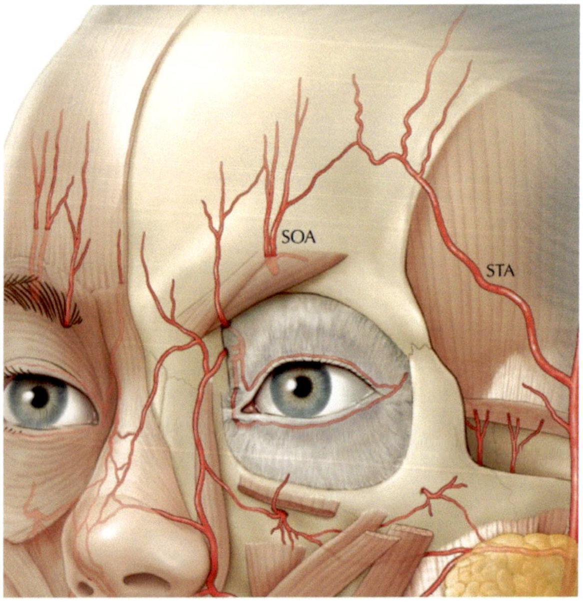

Figure 10.1 Arterial danger zones to consider during temporal crest smoothing are: frontal branch of the superficial temporal artery (STA) and the supraorbital artery (SOA).

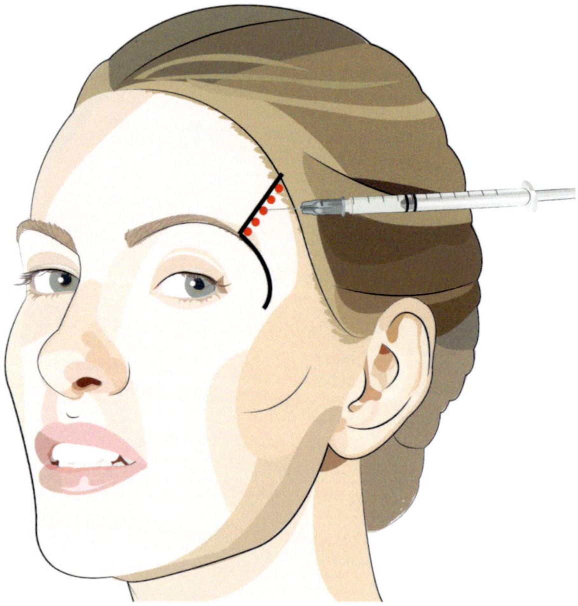

Figure 10.2 Sharp needle injection at the lateral temporal crest. The black lines mark the temporal crest and lateral orbital rim. The red dots indicate sharp needle bolus injection of CaHA on the periosteum.

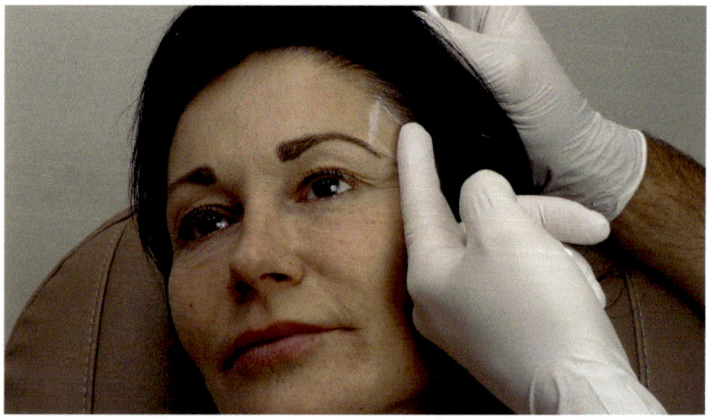

Figure 10.3 Marking the temporal crest. The frontalis muscle usually extends laterally beyond the temporal crest.

DOI: 10.1201/9781003617129-10

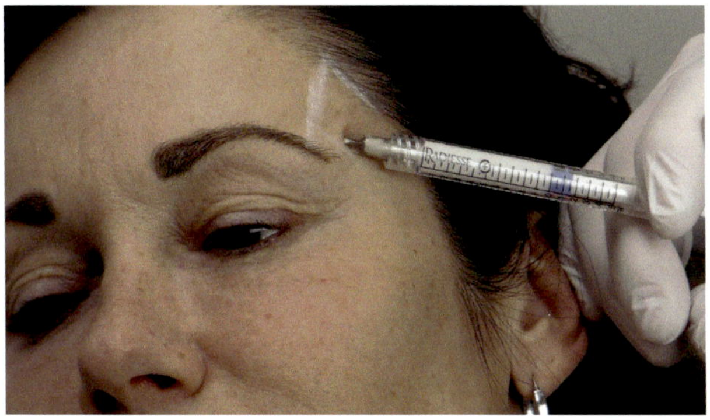

Figure 10.4 Perpendicular to 45° to the skin, advance the needle to the periosteum of the lateral temporal crest, bevel down.

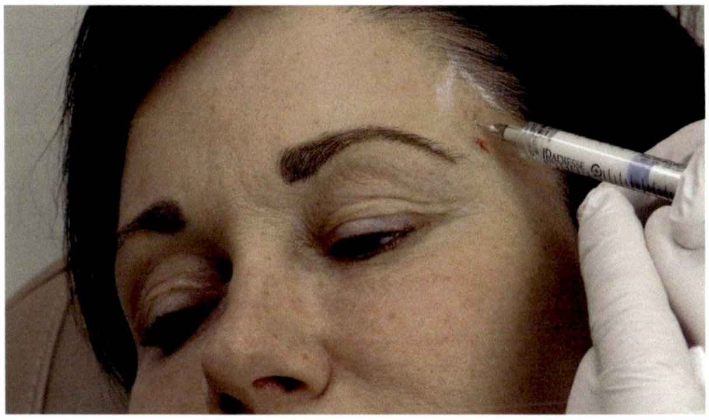

Figure 10.5 Using the same entry point, without exiting the needle from the skin, retract, reorient, readvance, and inject one or two more boluses on the periosteum of the lateral temporal crest of approximately 0.05–0.1 mL per bolus with bevel down. Use a second and optionally a third entry point and repeat.

6. Aspiration is not necessary, as it is not reliable [2].
7. Inject approximately 0.05 mL of CaHA slowly, with low pressure in a bolus on the periosteum (Figure 10.5).
8. Partially retract, reorient, and readvance the needle back to the periosteum, about 5 mm away from the first bolus.
9. Inject another bolus of approximately 0.05 mL of CaHA with the bevel down.
10. Repeat these steps until the crest is satisfactorily corrected.
11. Repeat with additional entry points.
12. Even out with purposeful molding: from lateral to medial.

10.2 TEMPORAL CREST SMOOTHING (SUBMUSCULAR CANNULA TECHNIQUE 1)

See Figure 10.6 for injection placement.

10.2.1 Step-by-Step Technique

1. Disinfect and mark the temporal crest.
2. At the lateral brow, mark the entry point and anesthetize.

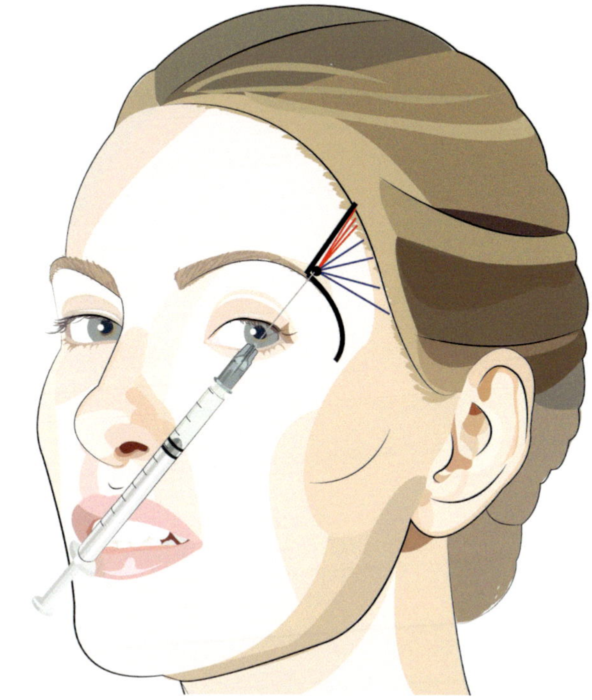

Figure 10.6 CaHA injection with blunt cannula in the submuscular layer of the lateral temporal crest. The black lines mark the temporal crest and lateral orbital rim. The red lines indicate retrograde linear thread injections of CaHA, and the blue lines indicate possible additional retrogrades in the temporal hollows (interfascial technique).

3. Use a 23G needle for the pre-hole.
4. Use standard dilution of CaHA or undiluted product.
5. Maneuver the cannula through the skin to the subcutaneous fat and through the frontalis muscle plus the galea aponeurotica (Figure 10.7).
6. Advance along the lateral temporal crest and inject one or more retrograde linear threads (Figure 10.8).
7. Continue fanning in the interfascial space (Figure 10.9).
8. Even out with light massage.

10.3 TEMPORAL CREST SMOOTHING (INTERFASCIAL AND SUBGALEAL CANNULA TECHNIQUE 2)

See Figure 10.10 for injection placement.

10.3.1 Step-by-Step Technique

1. Disinfect and mark the temporal crest, the supraorbital rim, the lateral orbital rim, and the zygomatic arch (Figure 10.11). Mark the C-shaped area to augment and take note of the trajectory of the superficial temporal artery.
2. A zygomaticotemporal and supraorbital nerve block may be considered; please see block anesthesia in Chapter 3.
3. Use full viscosity (undiluted) CaHA or standard dilution.

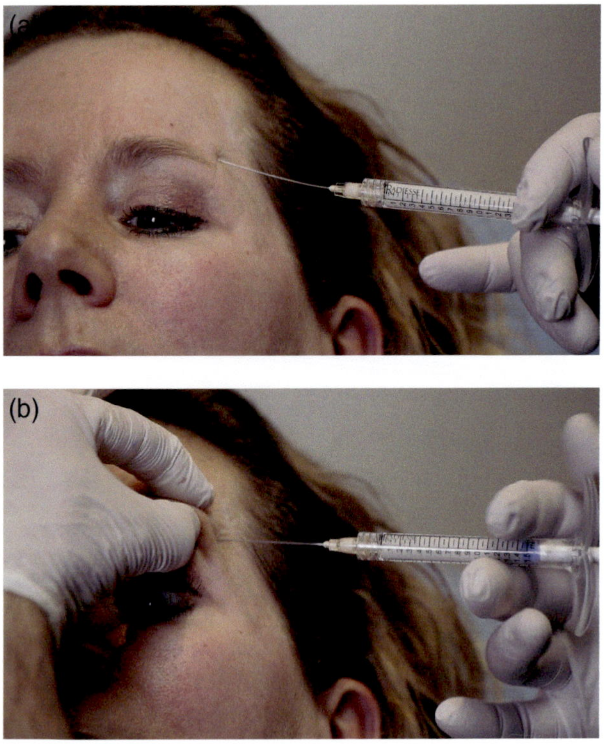

Figure 10.7 Cannula is entered through the pre-hole in the dermis (a) and advanced through the galea aponeurotica while lifting up the tissue with the non-dominant hand (b).

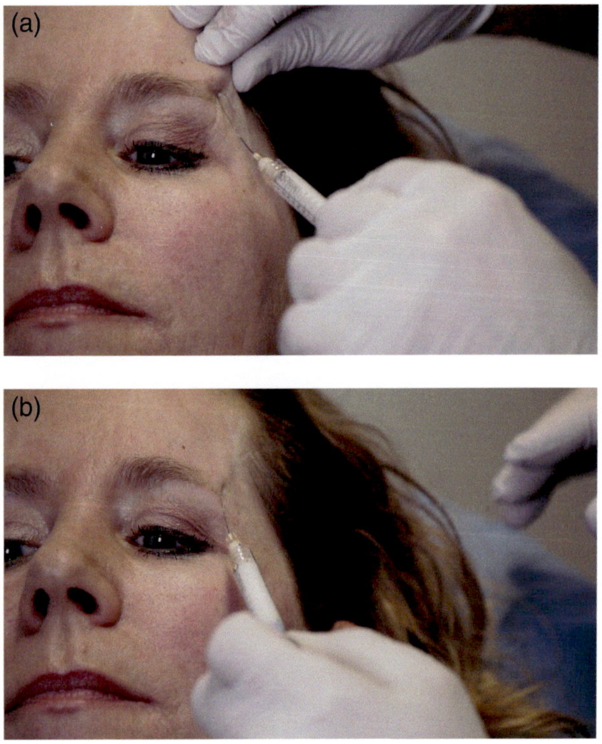

Figure 10.8 Cannula is advanced deep to the galea aponeurotica (a) and advanced just lateral to the temporal crest (b).

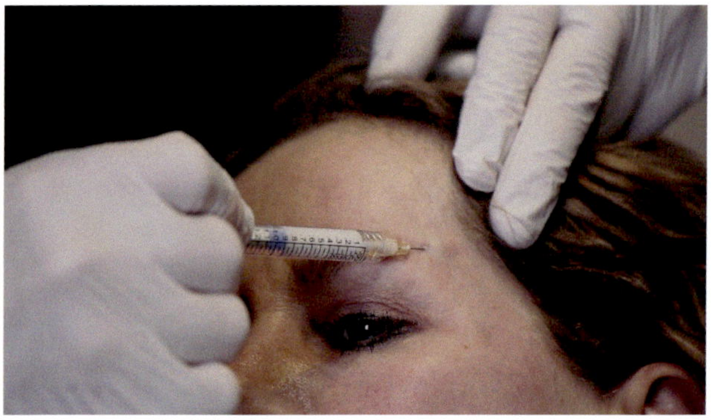

Figure 10.9 Cannula is advanced in the interfascial space in the temporal area.

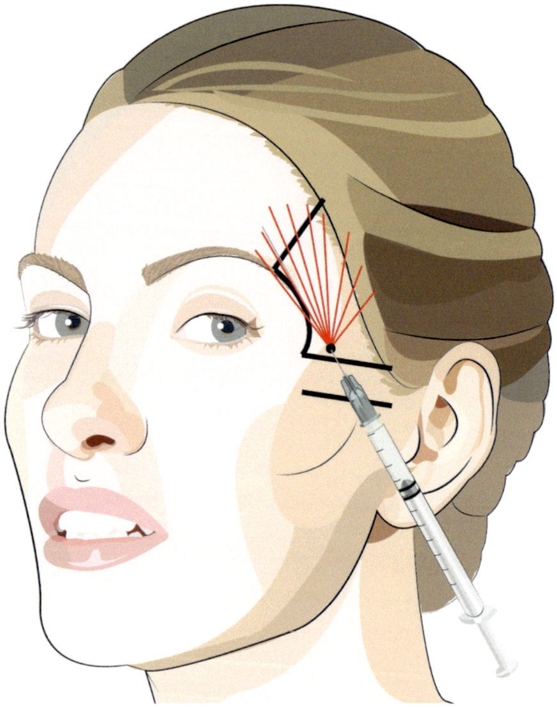

Figure 10.10 Cannula injection at the temporofrontal concavity. The black lines mark the temporal crest, supra-orbital rim, lateral orbital rim, and upper border of the zygomatic arch. The red lines indicate retrograde linear thread injection of CaHA on the periosteum of the frontal bone and interfascial placement in the temporal area.

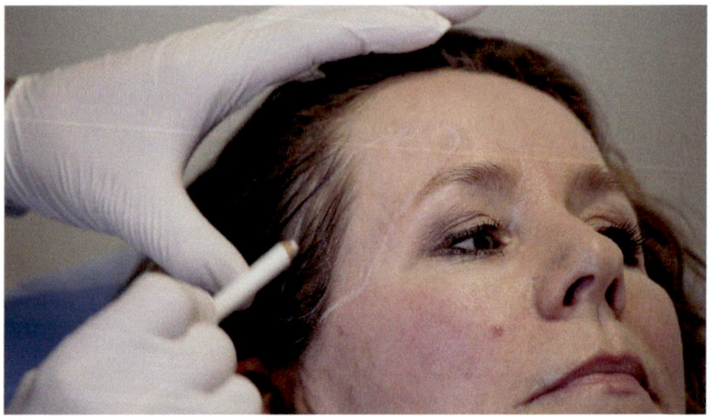

Figure 10.11 Marking of the temporofrontal area.

4. At the upper border of the zygomatic arch approximately midway between the helix of the ear and the lateral canthus, mark the entry point and anesthetize.
5. Use a 23G needle for the pre-hole.
6. Maneuver the cannula through the skin to the subcutaneous fat.
7. Rotate the cannula and press through the resistance of the temporoparietal fascia (Figure 10.12).
8. At the temporal crest, lift up the frontalis muscle in order to advance the cannula beyond the temporal crest (Figure 10.13).
9. Use the flexibility of the skin to advance the cannula into the frontal area and inject product in the subgaleal space (Figure 10.14).
10. As the anatomical layer of the deep temporal fascia is continuous with the periosteum of the frontal bone, advancing from the interfascial space through the temporal crest will position the cannula in the subgaleal space.
11. Consider also advancing to the area beyond the hairline to reduce temporal hollowing.
12. Repeat these steps until the area is satisfactorily corrected.
13. Even out with light massage.

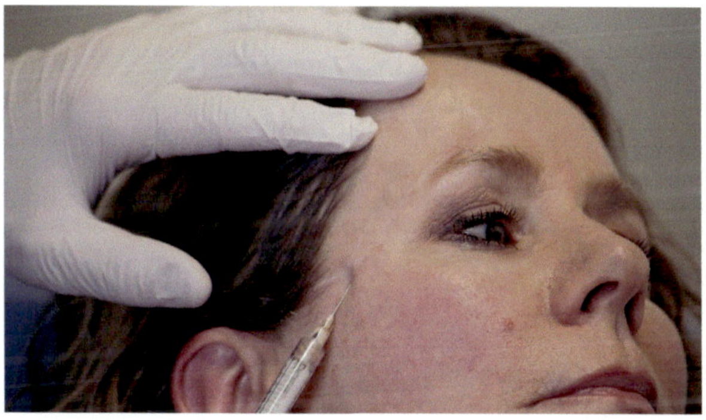

Figure 10.12 Fanning in the interfascial space.

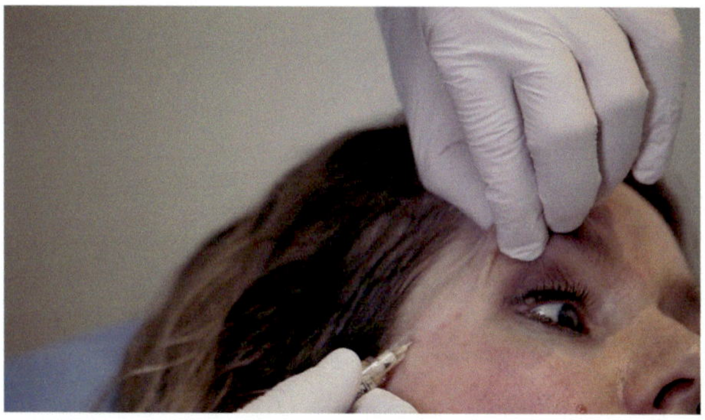

Figure 10.13 Create a path of least resistance to the subgaleal space of the frontal area by lifting the frontalis muscle.

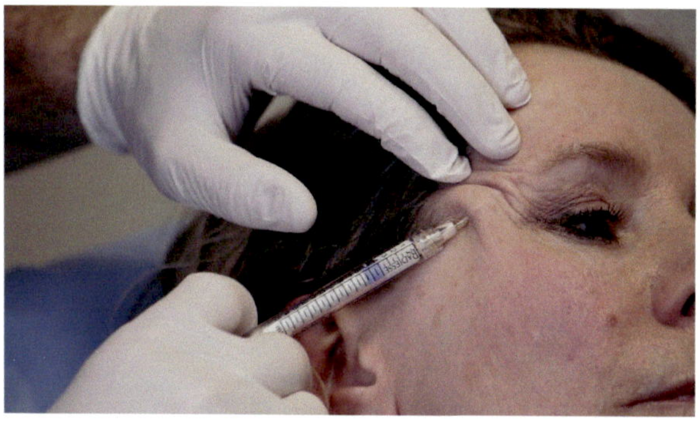

Figure 10.14 Advance the cannula beyond the temporal crest into the frontal area.

10.4 AFTERCARE

If necessary, the area can be manually massaged to even out the product. When doing so, try to massage the product to the immediate lateral temporal crest by purposeful molding ("rocking and rolling") over the skin. After injection, distension of the veins and superficial temporal artery can be observed due to increased pressure in the area. Swelling might be uneven in the temples, so the patient should be advised that any swelling is to be expected and is temporary, usually lasting one day, but can last up to five days. When injecting in the subcutaneous layer, swelling is more severe than injecting in deeper layers. When injecting periosteally with a sharp needle, pain on mastication can be expected, as the product is mostly injected intramuscularly using this technique [3].

10.5 ADDITIONAL TREATMENTS FOR OPTIMAL RESULTS

To further improve the aesthetics of the temporal sharpness and skeletonized appearance, filling the temporal hollows and brow reshaping with botulinum toxin and fillers can be considered. Also, skin improvement with topical creams, peels, and lasers might be advisable depending on the patients and their needs.

See further Figure 10.15 and Videos 10.1–10.3 for before and after results and application techniques, respectively.

Video 10.1 Temporal crest smoothing: needle technique.

Video 10.2 Temporal crest smoothing: cannula technique 1.

Video 10.3 Temporal crest smoothing: cannula technique 2.

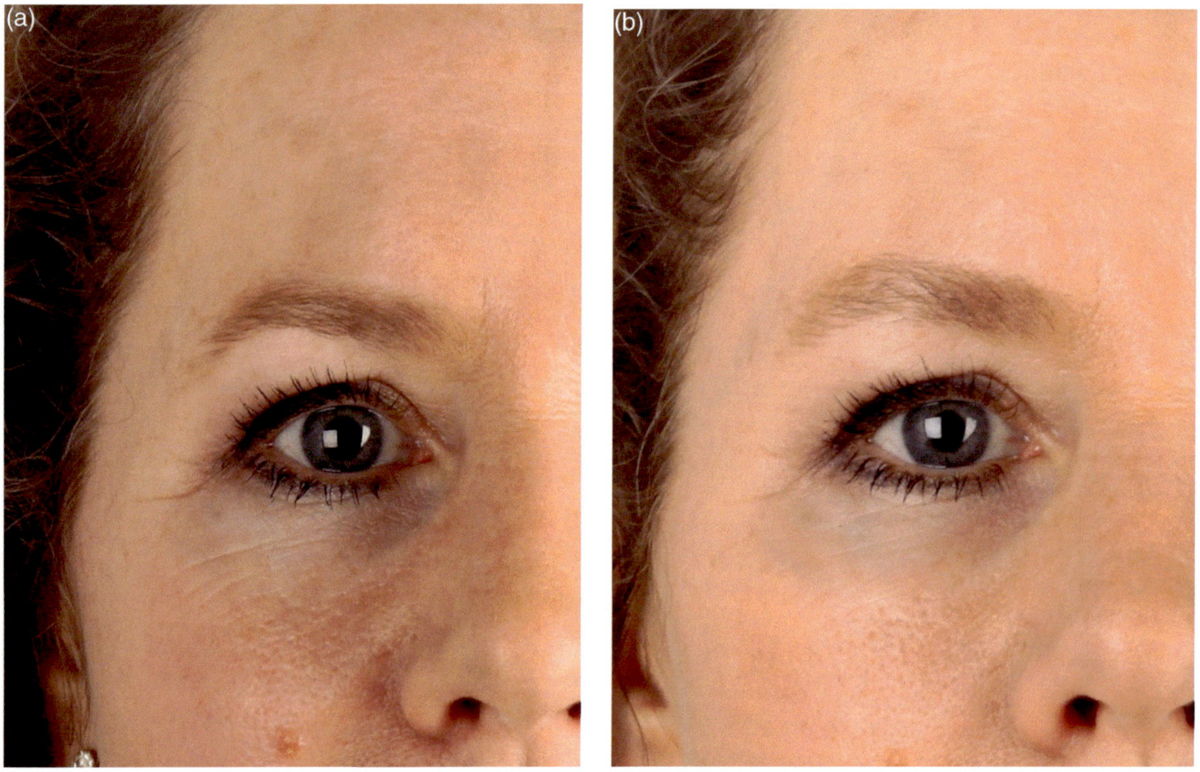

Figure 10.15 Example of a patient before (a) and after (b) treatment with 1.5 mL of CaHA at both the temporal crest and the interfascial space of the temporal hollows.

REFERENCES

[1] J. A. J. van Loghem et al., "Calcium hydroxylapatite: Over a decade of clinical experience," *J Clin Aesthet Dermatol*, vol. 8, no. 1, pp. 38–49, Jan. 2015.

[2] J. A. J. van Loghem et al., "Sensitivity of aspiration as a safety test before injection of soft tissue fillers," *J Cosmet Dermatol*, vol. 17, no. 1, pp. 39–46, Feb. 2018.

[3] J. A. J. van Loghem, "Use of calcium hydroxylapatite in the upper third of the face: Retrospective analysis of techniques, dilutions and adverse events," *J Cosmet Dermatol*, vol. 17, no. 6, pp. 1025–1030, Dec. 2018.

The Middle Third of the Face

11

Cheek Ligament Lift

POLINA HOLOVINA, AINA CERVERA-BAREA, AND JANI VAN LOGHEM

11.1 INTRODUCTION

Ligamentous attachments have been considered important facial structures by plastic surgeons and cosmetic physicians. Their relevance lies in their consistent positioning across individuals and their role in facial aging and rejuvenation due to their retaining and stabilizing functions [1]. The retaining ligaments of the face originate as relatively thick collagenous structures on the periosteum or deep facial fascia, and as they progress more superficially, they sprout into thinner structures penetrating the SMAS, which serve as points supporting the skin and the subcutaneous tissue [2].

These ligaments divide the mobile section of the face from the masticatory structures. From top to bottom, the retaining ligaments are the temporal (adhesion and septa), lateral orbital thickening, zygomatic, masseteric, and mandibular retaining ligaments [3], but only the zygomatic will be discussed in this chapter (Figure 11.1).

For cheek lifting, two relevant ligamentous structures should be considered—the *zygomatic retaining ligament* and the *zygomatic-cutaneous ligament* (ZRL and ZCL, respectively). The ZRL/ZCL ligament is considered a true ligament (originating on periosteum and inserting into skin), with a cylindrical arrangement, originating at the inferior border of the zygomatic arch (ZA) and inserting into the skin [4,5].

Nowadays, cosmetic procedures with minimal downtime are preferred over surgical facial liftings. To reposition the ZRL, Cong *et al.* suggest injecting along the ZA based on the subject's needs, preferably in the posterior portion due to safety reasons [6]. The ZCL is targeted to lift the middle and lower thirds of the face, so it is recommended to inject in the intersection of the mid-cheek groove and the vertical line passing through the lateral canthus [6].

11.2 ANATOMICAL DANGER ZONES

The cheek area is a highly innervated and vascularized region. To tackle ligament liftings in this area, special attention must be paid to the transverse facial artery, the infraorbital artery, the zygomaticofacial artery, the origin of zygomatic major muscles, and the parotid gland (Figure 11.2) [3,6].

11.3 ZYGOMATIC RETAINING LIGAMENT LIFT

For injection placement, see Figure 11.3.

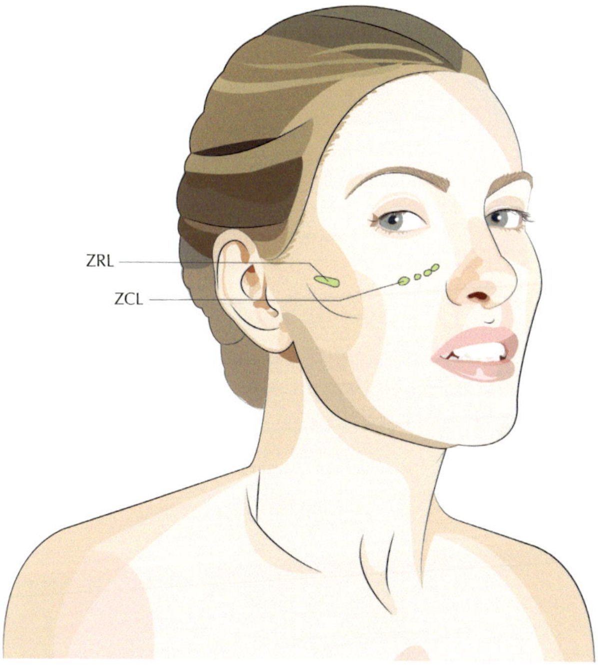

Figure 11.1 The zygomatic retaining and zygomatic-cutaneous ligaments from the upper and middle thirds of the face. The zygomatic retaining ligament (ZRL) is found at the inferior border of the zygomatic arch, whereas the zygomatic-cutaneous ligament (ZCL) is present in the middle of the face.

11.3.1 Step-by-Step Technique

1. Create the markings in the upper and lower borders of the ZA (Figure 11.4).
2. Choose the entry point from the upper border of the ZA.
3. Disinfect and anesthetize the area with adrenalized lidocaine 2% (Figure 11.5).
   NOTE: Consider a zygomaticofacial nerve block (see Chapter 3 for reference).
4. Using a 23G needle, create the entry point into the skin (Figure 11.6).
5. Advance a 25G, 38 mm cannula through the skin towards the lower border of the zygomatic arch while propping up the cheek with the non-dominant hand.
6. Penetrate through the first resistance (SMAS) and the second resistance (ZRL).

DOI: 10.1201/9781003617129-11

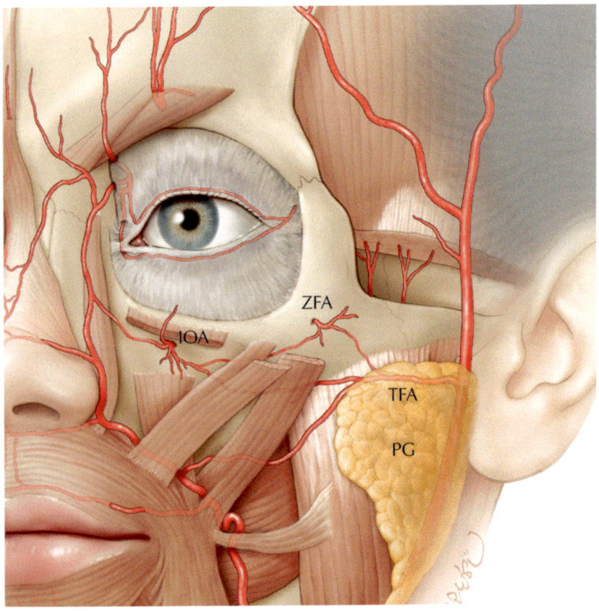

Figure 11.2 Arterial danger zones during a cheek ligament lifting are: transverse facial artery (TFA), the zygomaticofacial artery (ZFA), the infraorbital artery (IOA), and the parotid gland (PG).

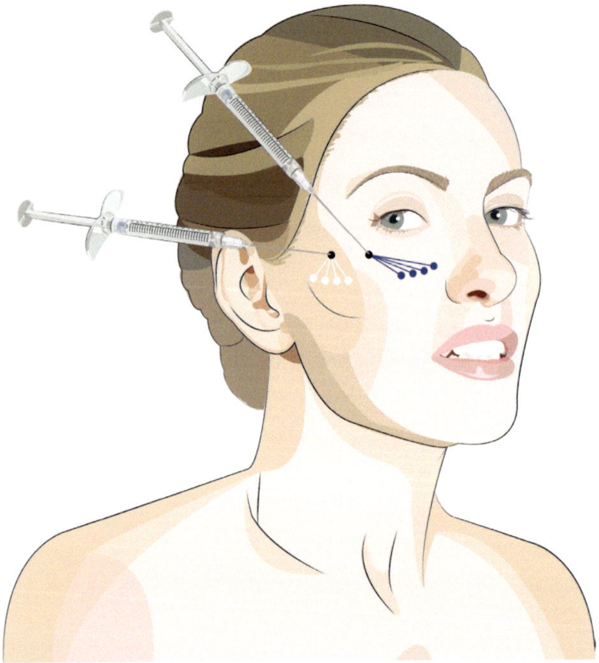

Figure 11.3 Injection techniques to lift the zygomatic retaining and zygomatic cutaneous ligaments. To lift the ZRL, an entry hole (black dot) is created above the origin of the ligament; the needle is advanced to deposit a bolus (white dot); and following a fanning technique, a linear thread (white lines) of CaHA is deposited retrogradely. To lift the ZCL, an entry hole (black dot) is created at the apex of the cheek, and boluses of CaHA (blue dots) are deposited along the cutaneous insertion of the ligament, serving as anchor points, while injecting more product retrogradely (blue lines).

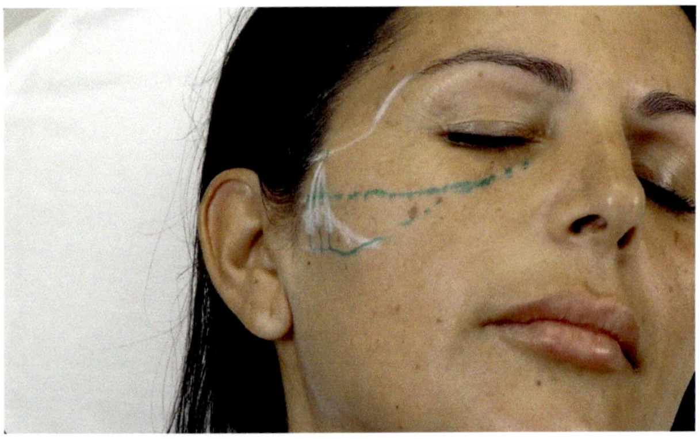

Figure 11.4 Marking of the zygomatic retaining ligament origin (vertical green lines).

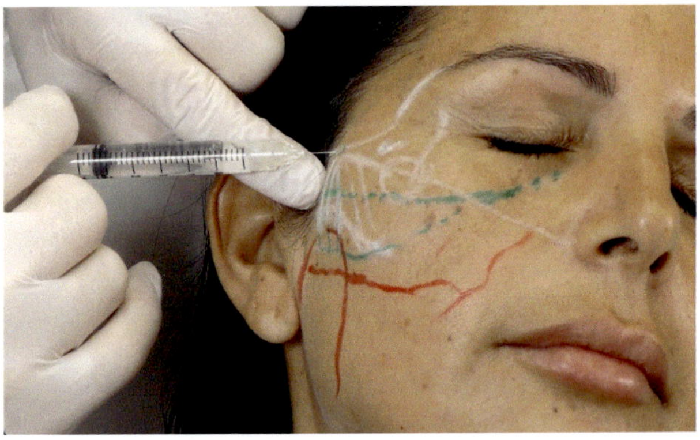

Figure 11.5 Anesthesia administration prior the ligament lift.

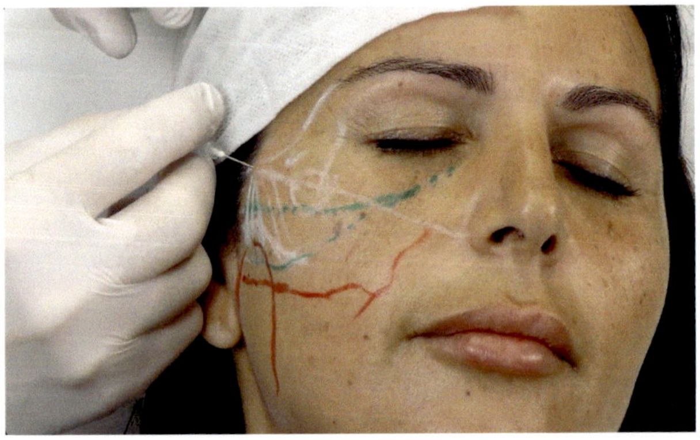

Figure 11.6 Creation of the entry point with a needle.

7. Keep a non-dominant finger on the lower border of the ZA, preventing the cannula from moving too low and injecting into the danger zones (Figure 11.7).
8. Inject a 0.05 mL bolus and then 0.05 mL more in a retrograde fashion.
9. Retract and reorient the cannula towards a medial direction. Penetrate through the ZRL again and

deposit CaHA in the same manner as described in the previous step.

10. Inject a total of 0.3 mL in boluses and retrograde.
11. Mold the boluses by pressing and rolling upwards to reposition the ZRL (Figure 11.8).

11.4 ZYGOMATIC-CUTANEOUS LIGAMENT LIFT

For injection placement, see Figure 11.3.

11.4.1 Step-by-Step Technique

1. Make the markings to select the entry hole. Extend a parallel line starting at the hairline and lining the superior border of the zygomatic arch until the nose, and then draw a vertical line starting at the lateral of the orbital rim and intersecting with the previous marking. The entry hole should roughly coincide with the apex of the cheek (Figure 11.9).
2. Disinfect and anesthetize the area with adrenalized lidocaine 2%.
3. Advance a 25G, 38 mm cannula through the skin towards the zygomatic bone and at the insertion point of the ZCL (Figure 11.10).
4. Lateral to the infraorbital foramen, inject a 0.05 mL bolus and then 0.05 mL in a retrograde fashion (Figure 11.11).
5. Retract and reorient the cannula towards a lateral direction. Penetrate through the ZCL again and inject the product in the same manner as described in the previous step.
6. Move laterally and repeat the step above.
7. Mold the product by pressing and rolling upwards to reposition the ZCL (Figure 11.12).

See further Figure 11.13 and Videos 11.1–11.2 for before and after results and application techniques, respectively.

11.5 AFTERCARE

The area can be manually massaged to even out the product. To improve the placement of the filler material in hope of supporting the retaining ligaments in a more horizontal fashion, a purposeful molding technique is advised, commonly referred to as the "rock 'n' roll technique". When doing do, use an upward molding technique to press the product on the periosteum to the origin of the retaining ligament, and then roll

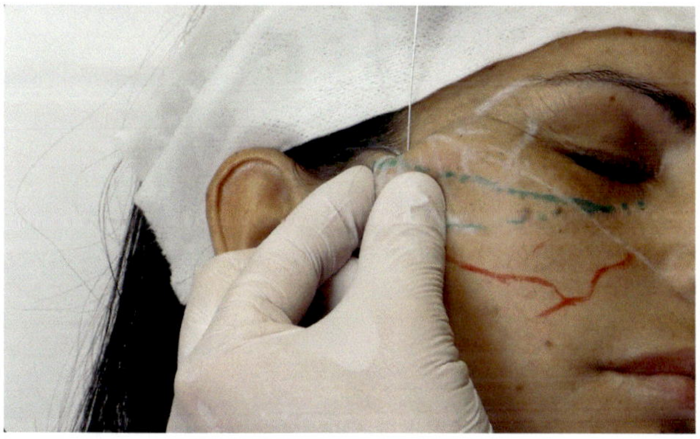

Figure 11.7 Insertion of the cannula to proceed with the injection of CaHA.

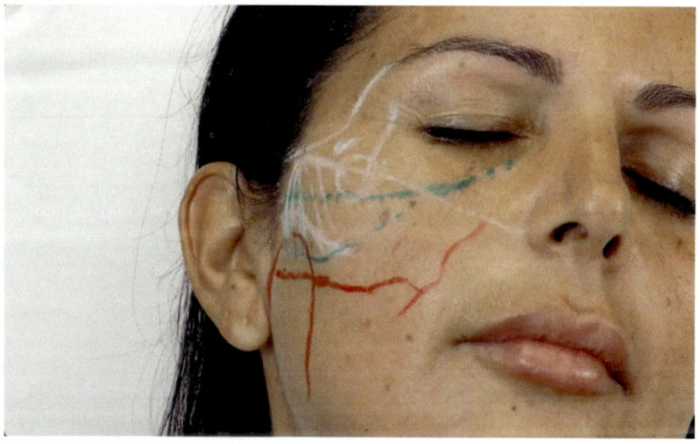

Figure 11.9 Marking of the cheek's apex prior zygomatic cutaneous ligament lifting.

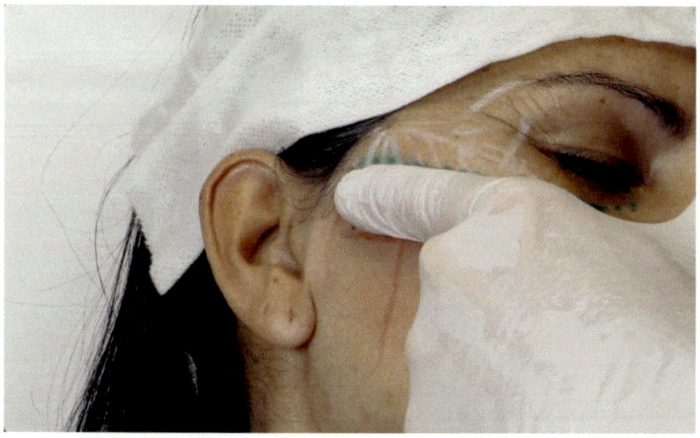

Figure 11.8 Molding of the product to help lift the ligament.

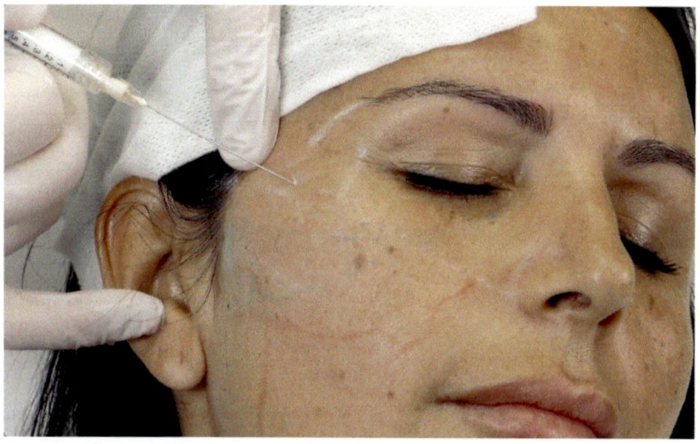

Figure 11.10 Insertion of the cannula at the entry point.

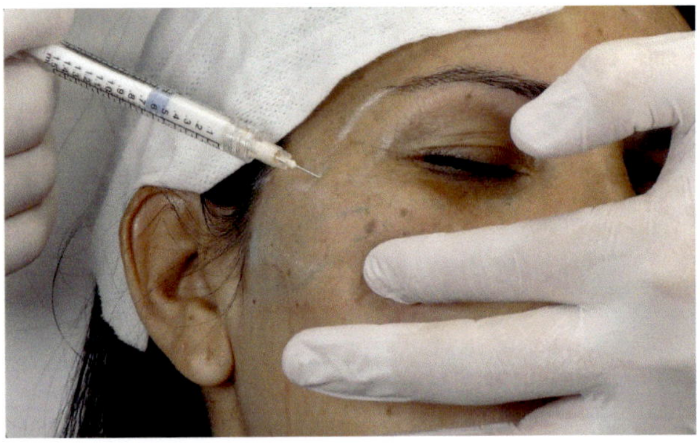

Figure 11.11 Advancement of the cannula towards the zygomatic cutaneous ligament.

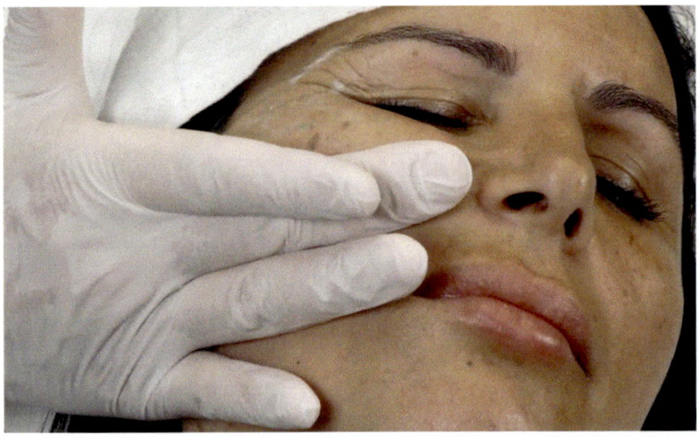

Figure 11.12 Molding of the product to help elevate the ligament.

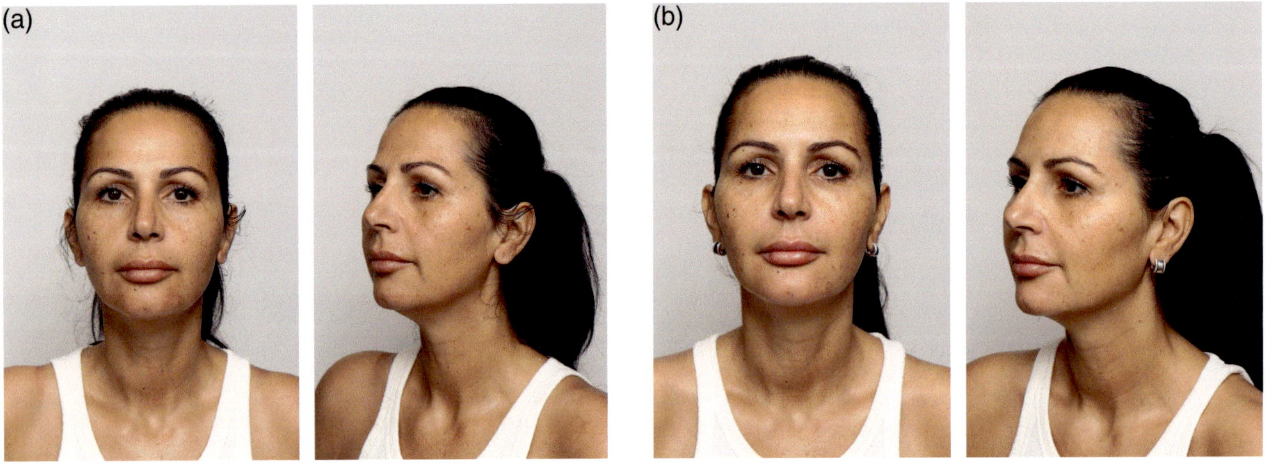

Figure 11.13 Before (a) and 1-month after (b) CaHA treatment to elevate the zygomatic retaining and cutaneous ligaments.

the finger upward to reinforce placement against the ligament origin. Swelling may be uneven and should subside in a day or two.

11.6 ADDITIONAL TREATMENTS FOR OPTIMAL RESULTS

To further improve the aesthetics of the cheeks, skin quality improvement with topical creams, peels, and lasers might be advisable depending on the patients and their needs. Combination with jawline recontouring may also improve clinical jowls.

Video 11.1 ZRL lift.

Video 11.2 ZCL lift.

REFERENCES

[1] M. Alghoul, M. A. Codner, "Retaining ligaments of the face: Review of anatomy and clinical applications," *Aesthet Surg J*, vol. 33, no. 6, pp. 769–782, 2013.

[2] A. Braz et al., "Revisiting the ligament line of the face: A new understanding for filling the fixed and mobile face," *Dermatol Clin*, vol. 42, no. 1, pp. 97–102, 2024.

[3] B. Mendelson, "Facelift anatomy, SMAS, retaining ligaments and facial spaces," in: Aston, J. et al., eds., *Aesthetic Plastic Surgery*. London: Saunders Elsevier, 2009, ch. 6, pp. 53–72.

[4] D. W. Furnas, "The retaining ligaments of the cheek," *Plast Reconstr Surg*, vol. 83, no. 1, pp. 11–16, 1989.

[5] C. J. Moss et al., "Surgical anatomy of the ligamentous attachments in the temple and periorbital regions," *Plast Reconstr Surg*, vol. 105, no. 4, pp. 1491–1498, 2000.

[6] L. Y. Cong et al., "Injectable filler technique for face lifting based on dissection of true facial ligaments," *Aesthet Surg J*, vol. 41, no. 11, pp. NP1571–NP1583, 2021.

The Middle Third of the Face

Cheek Augmentation

12

SHINO BAY AGUILERA, LUIS SORO, AND JANI VAN LOGHEM

12.1 INTRODUCTION

Aging may be inevitable, but an understanding of the aging process grants us the ability to enhance our youth and restore what was lost. Facial aging, previously thought to be the consequence of gravity on the skin and subcutaneous fat, is a multidimensional, multilevel, and multitissue process [1–4]. The progression of an aging face occurs due to intrinsic and extrinsic changes in the skin, absorption of deep fat, and skeletal alterations [5]. The result is a change in the topography, shape, and proportions of the face, all of which are responsible for the characteristics of the aging face [6]. The midface in particular tends to flatten and sag over time [7]. It is the belief of the authors that the cheekbones are a particularly important sign of youth, beauty, and fertility. Some studies have shown that a larger bizygomatic width to facial height ratio is associated with an increased perception of attractiveness. Therefore, the cheekbones must be preserved, restored, or imitated but never deformed, altered, or buried when performing injectable fillers on the midface. The ideal cheekbone is ovoid, not round; has an angle; and has a high point at the lower limbus of the eye, known as the apex. HD-Sculpt is a technique using CaHA that reverses these midface changes by contouring and elevating the midface to create a more chiseled, defined look. The goal is cheekbone enhancement through re-volumization of the midface and augmentation of the zygomatic arch. As a result of lifting this area, the jowls can be notably improved as well. Directly injecting the lower face along the jawline and around the jowl can also be used for further enhancement of jawline definition and rejuvenation of the face.

12.2 SAFETY CONSIDERATIONS

The primary concern with filler injection is the occlusion of arteries, whether by external compression or injection of product into the vessel (Figure 12.1). This is especially true of products that are more difficult to dissolve, such as CaHA. Fortunately, vascular occlusion is rare and easily avoided when injecting in the periosteal region, as in the HD-Sculpt technique. Major midface arteries to be aware of, however, are the infraorbital artery, the transverse facial artery, and the tortuous facial artery with anastomosing angular artery. Although less common, piercing injuries to nerves should be avoided, and the primary nerve to be mindful of with this technique is the infraorbital nerve. Injury to this nerve can cause intractable neuralgia for an extended period.

Prior to injecting CaHA, consider transferring the product to a 1 mL BD syringe, which allows for easier aspiration and assurance the needle tip is not placed intravascularly [8]. Utilizing a retrograde injection technique and avoiding large boluses can also help minimize inadvertent occlusion. Recently, handheld vein finders have become available and can be extremely helpful in lessening risk as well while decreasing ecchymoses.

The ability to differentiate intravascular injection versus ecchymosis is vital. Immediate blanching of the tissue suggests intravascular injection. Icing an area mistaken for a bruise can further compromise blood flow, quickening necrosis. Pain is variable given anesthetic components of some products. Several hours after injecting, a purple-maroon reticulated patch usually appears in the distribution of the injected

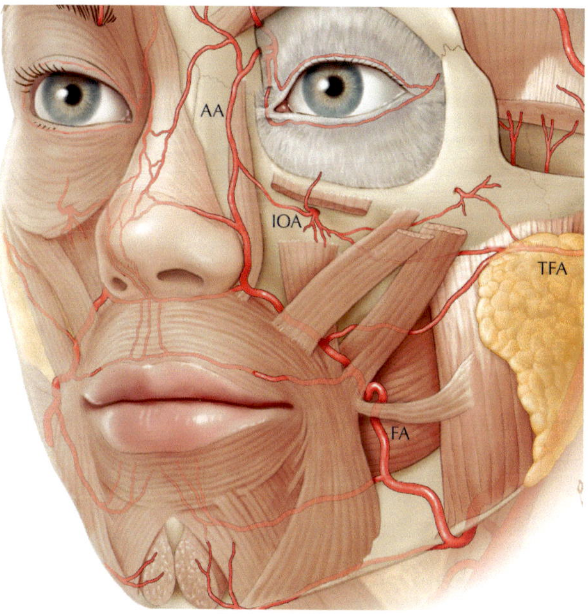

Figure 12.1 Arterial danger zones to consider during cheek augmentation are: infraorbital artery (IOA), transverse facial artery (TFA), facial artery (FA), and angular artery (AA).

DOI: 10.1201/9781003617129-12

vessel. Pustule formation followed by progressive darkening of tissue suggests impending necrosis. Upon suspicion of vascular occlusion, immediate steps should be taken, including injecting the affected area with at least 150 units of hyaluronidase to minimize external compression, applying nitric oxide ointment, using frequent warm compresses, massaging the area vigorously, and recommending aspirin daily until symptoms resolve.

12.3 CHEEK AUGMENTATION—HD-SCULPT TECHNIQUE 1 (MALE)

See Figure 12.2 for injection placement.

12.3.1 Step-by-Step Technique

1. Identify the cheek apex. If unable to locate, use Hinderer's Lines. In males, use a vertical line between the lateral iris and the oral commissure and find the crossing with the alar-tragal line. Numb the area with lidocaine (Figure 12.3) and create a point of entry with a 21G needle (Figure 12.4).
2. Introduce the cannula at a 30° angle (Figure 12.5).
3. Once in the supraperiosteal plane, decrease the angle to 10° and keep the syringe parallel to the zygoma. The tip of the cannula should be 1–2 mm behind the female apex or zygomatic eminence in males.
4. Inject while moving retrograde and laterally toward the hairline, placing 0.1 mL of product continuously, with a final total of 0.5 mL having been placed across the zygoma (Figure 12.6). This accentuates and defines the malar cheek while using the zygoma as a platform to directly lift the mid-face. Parts of the lower face are indirectly lifted as well.

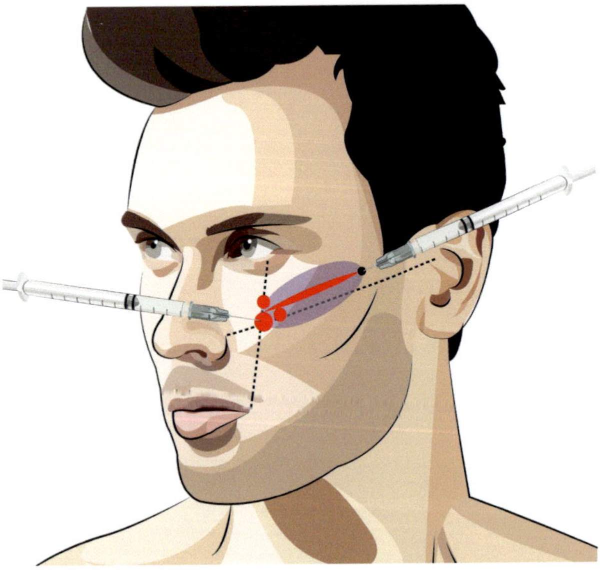

Figure 12.2 Product injection at the midface. The red line represents a single retrograde line consisting of multiple periosteal boluses injected with a nontraumatic cannula. The red dots represent supraperiosteal boluses injected with a 27G sharp needle. The same should be done on the other side.

5. Place 0.2 mL of product perpendicular to the zygoma at the apex with provided needle (Figure 12.7).
6. Continue injecting additional aliquots of 0.05 mL laterally to the hairline until the desired definition and lift are achieved, keeping in mind the zygoma should thin laterally.

See further Video 12.1 to visualize the application technique.

12.4 CHEEK AUGMENTATION—HD-SCULPT TECHNIQUE 2 (FEMALE)

See Figure 12.8 for injection placement.

12.4.1 Step-by-Step Technique

1. Locate the apex of the cheek. If unable to find, use Hinderer's lines (Figure 12.9).
2. Move 1 cm posteriorly to the apex and inject 0.1 mL perpendicular to the periosteum (supraperiosteal; Figure 12.10).
3. Return to the cheek apex located earlier and inject 0.2 mL supraperiosteal (Figure 12.11).
4. Continue following the zygoma with small aliquots of 0.05 mL until reaching the hairline, spacing injections approximately 0.5 cm apart (Figure 12.12).
5. For females, recreate an Ogee curve at the anteromedial cheek by injecting product in the deep medial cheek fat compartment (Figure 12.13).

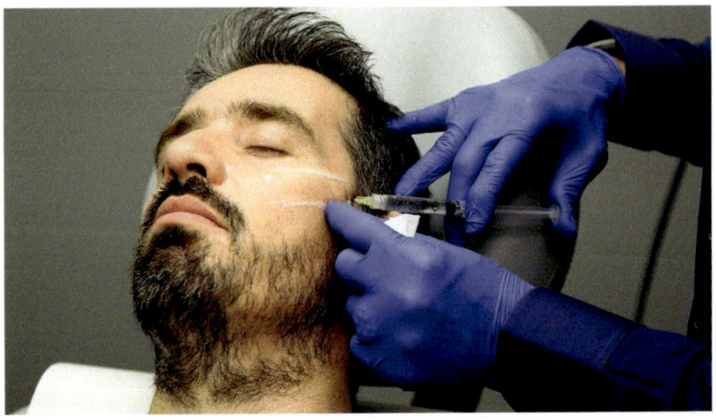

Figure 12.3 Numbing the area with 1% lidocaine.

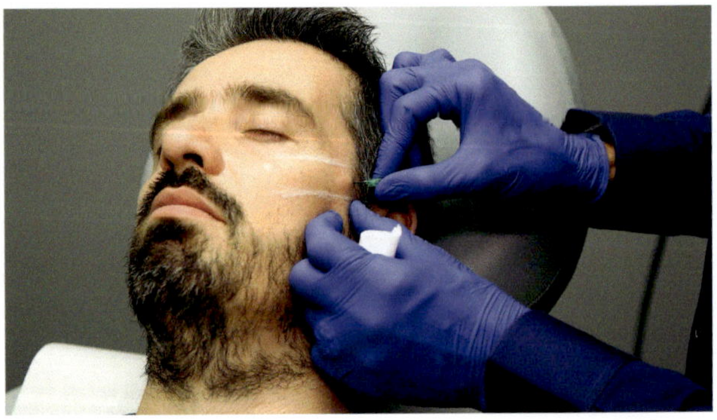

Figure 12.4 Create a point of entrance with a 21G needle.

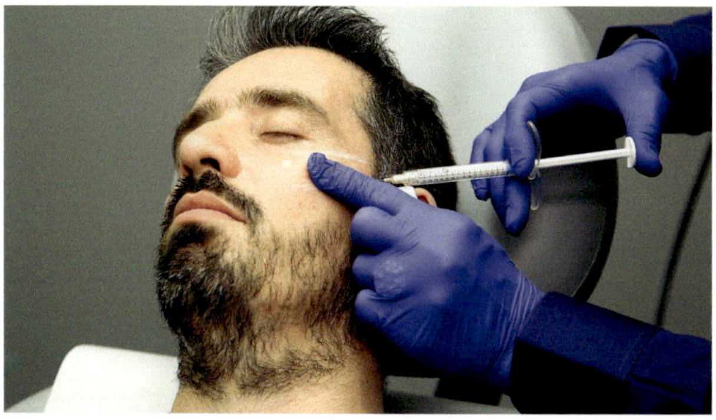

Figure 12.5 Introduce the cannula at a 30° angle. Once in the supraperiosteal plane, decrease the angle to 10° and keep the syringe parallel to the zygoma. The tip of the cannula should be 1–2 mm behind the zygomatic eminence.

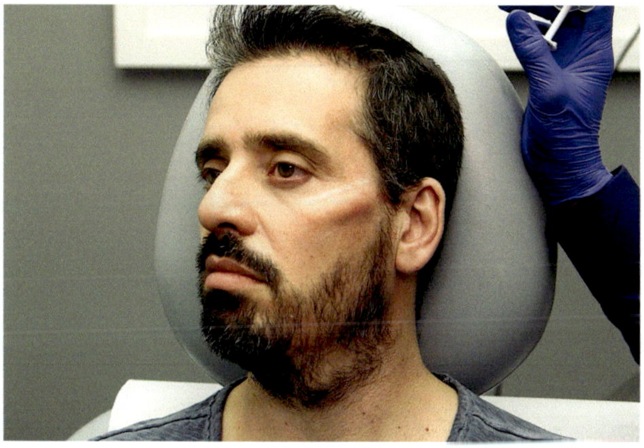

Figure 12.6 Inject while moving retrograde and laterally toward the hairline, placing 0.1 mL of product continuously, with a final total of 0.5 mL having been placed across the zygoma.

6. For males, do not create an Ogee curve. Maximize product placement on the lateral cheeks to create a more angular appearance.
7. The submalar area may be injected using different techniques such as serial puncture or fanning retrograde injections.

See also Video 12.2 to visualize the application technique.

12.5 CHEEK AUGMENTATION: SPERMATOZOA MULTILEVEL CANNULA TECHNIQUE

Descent of the cheeks is caused by many anatomical-based changes. To lift and improve the aesthetic appearance of the cheeks, many of those changes can be corrected with CaHA. Additionally, beauty ideals can be used to enhance certain features of the shape of the cheeks. Bone and fat resorption, as well as skin laxity, allow gravity to pull down the soft tissue of the midface, only to be limited by the retaining ligaments that limit this descent. The spermatozoa technique was

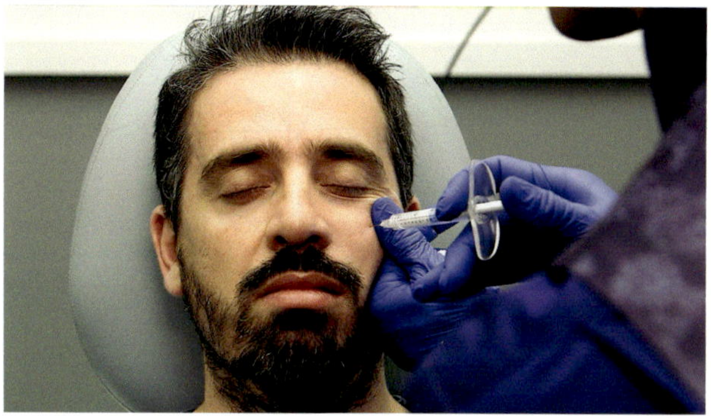

Figure 12.7 Place 0.2 mL of product perpendicular to the zygoma at the apex with provided needle.

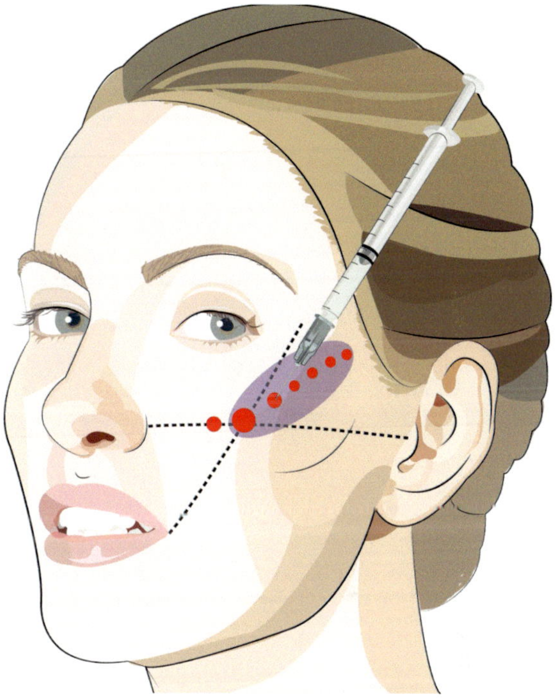

Figure 12.8 Product injection at the midface. The dotted lines are used to find the apex of this Latin/Asian/Indian cheek. A 30–45° angle is used to introduce the syringe from slightly top-down (not perpendicular/horizontal). The red dots indicate supraperiosteal CaHA boluses.

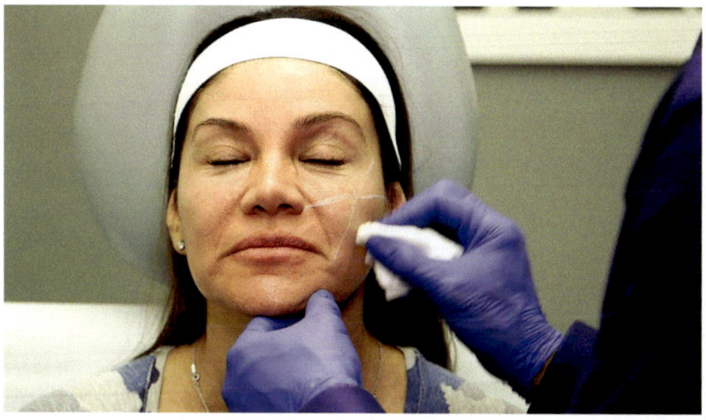

Figure 12.9 Using Hinderer's line to locate the apex of the cheek.

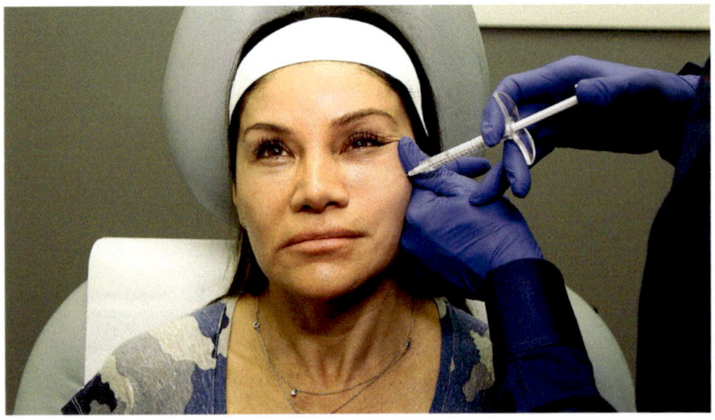

Figure 12.10 Needle is coming from cranial direction in order to give a vertical lift, 1 cm lateral to the apex while pulling up the cheek.

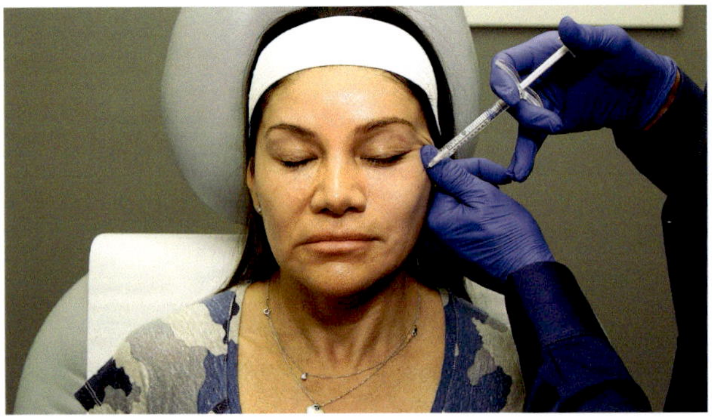

Figure 12.11 Injection of 0.2 mL at the apex while pulling the cheek backward.

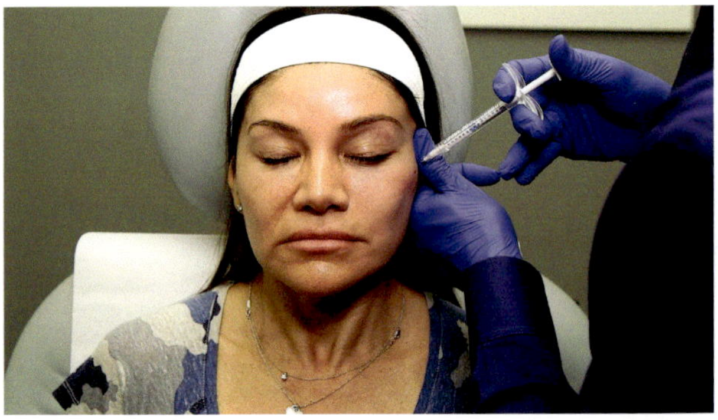

Figure 12.12 Injection of additional 0.05 mL aliquots on the top of the zygomatic arch toward the hairline.

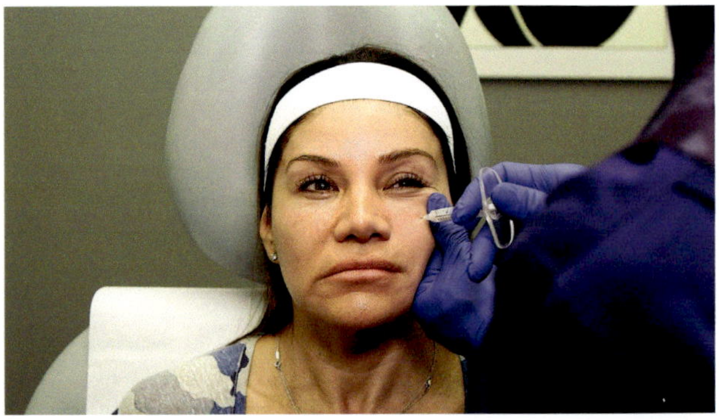

Figure 12.13 Injection of additional 0.1 mL aliquot in the deep medial cheek fat compartment.

named after a comment from a colleague who came to a workshop while the author described the technique: a bolus (head) followed by a retrograde linear thread (tail) of the white-colored product.

For injection placement, see Figure 12.14.

12.5.1 Step-by-Step Technique

1. Disinfect and mark the zygomatic arch entry point immediately medial to the hairline.
2. Mark the alar–tragal line, the zygomatic arch, the infraorbital rim, the insertion of the zygomatic cutaneous ligament, and the vector line (which is anatomically correlated to the position of the facial vein).
3. Mark the medial cheek entry point at the alar–tragal line lateral to the insertion of the zygomatic cutaneous ligament, at the crossing of the vector line and the alar–tragal line.
4. Mark the danger zones: infraorbital rim (to avoid advancing the cannula into the orbit) and the infraorbital foramen.
5. Use full viscosity (undiluted) CaHA or standard dilution for periosteal injection with a 25G, 38 mm cannula and hyperdiluted (1–1.5 mL per syringe of 1.5 mL) CaHA for superficial subcutaneous injection with a 25G, 50 mm cannula.
6. Anesthetize the entry points with adrenalized lidocaine.
7. Use a 23G needle for the pre-hole.
8. At the zygomatic arch entry point, maneuver the cannula through the skin to the subcutaneous fat.
9. Rotate the cannula and press through the resistance of the SMAS to the periosteum (Figure 12.15).
10. Advance the cannula parallel to the alar–tragal line to approximately 1–2 cm inferior to the inferolateral orbital rim.
11. Inject a bolus of 0.1–0.2 mL high-viscosity product. From there, inject a retrograde linear thread of approximately 0.1–0.2 mL over the periosteum back toward the entry point (Figure 12.16).
12. Reorient the cannula at the entry point and repeat these steps twice in a more inferior direction.
13. At the medial entry point, advance the cannula to the periosteum, in between the infraorbital rim and the infraorbital foramen (Figure 12.17).
14. Inject a small bolus of approximately 0.05–0.1 mL; inject an additional retrograde linear thread from the bolus toward the entry point of 0.1–0.2 mL (Figure 12.18).
15. Repeat this step in a more inferior direction with the cannula just lateral to the infraorbital foramen.

16. Change to the hyperdiluted CaHA with the longer cannula.
17. From the lateral entry point, advance the cannula along the vector line at the dermal–subdermal junction. Make sure the product does not get injected cranial to the cutaneous insertion of the zygomatic cutaneous ligament to avoid malar edema.
18. Inject a retrograde linear thread of approximately 0.05–0.1 mL.
19. Repeat retrogrades more inferiorly in a fanning technique (Figure 12.19).
20. From the medial entry point, advance the cannula along the alar–tragal line to the ala.
21. Inject a retrograde linear thread of approximately 0.05–0.1 mL.
22. Repeat retrogrades more inferiorly in a fanning technique (Figure 12.20). Avoid injecting high volumes in the jowls.
23. Even out with manual massage as needed.

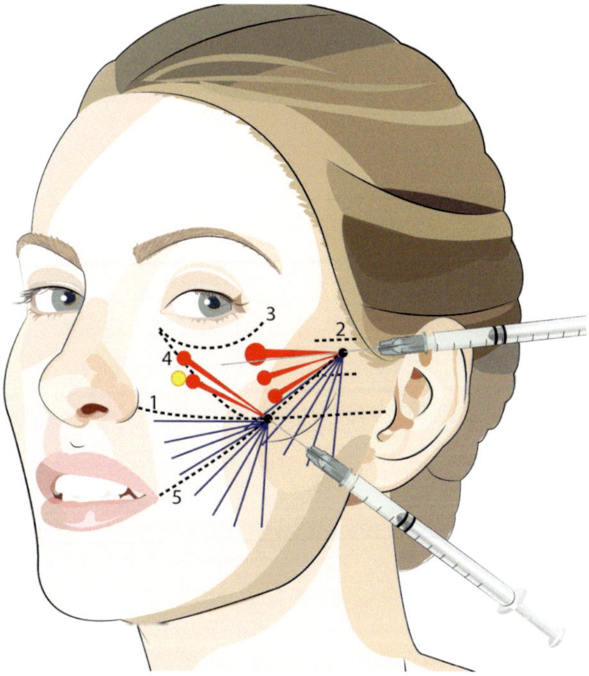

Figure 12.14 The multilevel cannula technique. Red represents periosteal placement; blue represents superficial placement. The black dotted lines indicate the alar-tragal line (1), the zygomatic arch (2), the infraorbital rim (3), the mid face fold (4), and the vector line for the direction of lifting. The yellow dot indicates the infraorbital foramen.

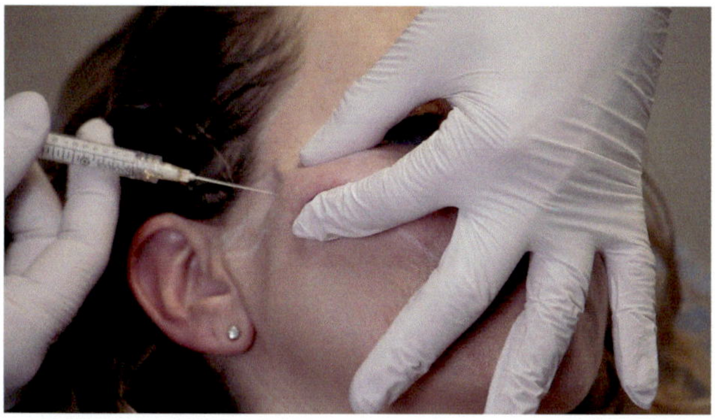

Figure 12.15 Lift the tissue in front of the cannula tip to create a path of least resistance to the deep layer. Rotate to pass the resistance of SMAS and retaining ligaments.

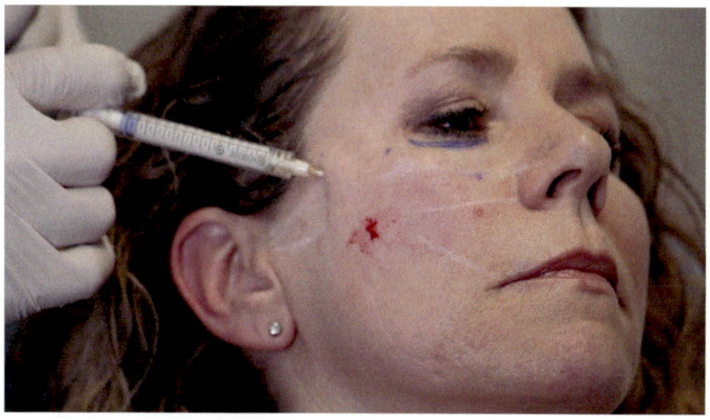

Figure 12.16 Inject a bolus and a retrograde, each approximately 0.1–0.2 mL.

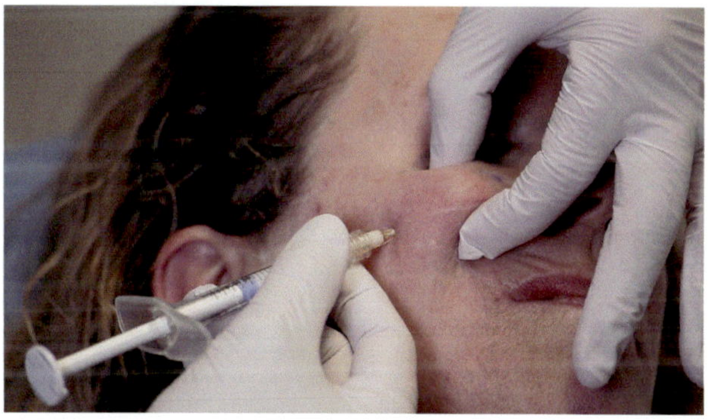

Figure 12.17 Lift the tissue in front of the cannula tip to create a path of least resistance to the deep layer. Rotate to pass the resistance of SMAS and retaining ligaments.

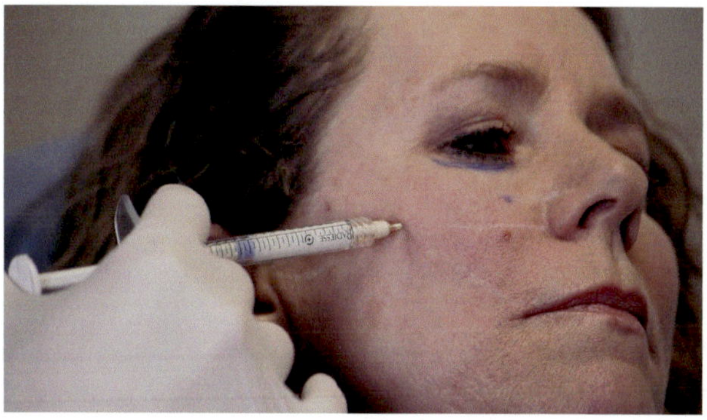

Figure 12.18 Inject a bolus of approximately 0.05–0.1 mL and a retrograde of approximately 0.1–0.2 mL.

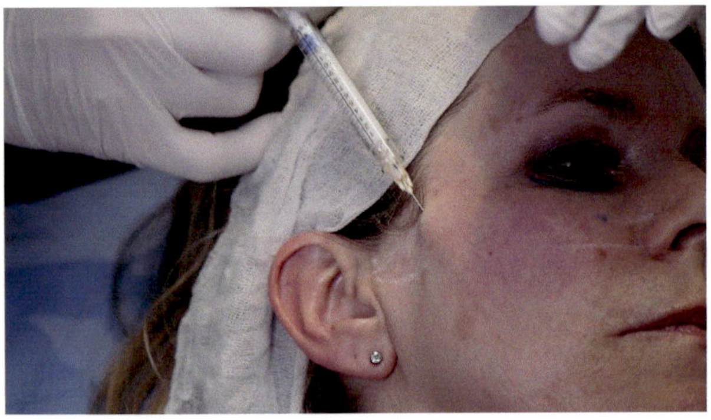

Figure 12.19 With diluted CaHA, inject multiple linear threads in a fanning technique from the lateral entry point.

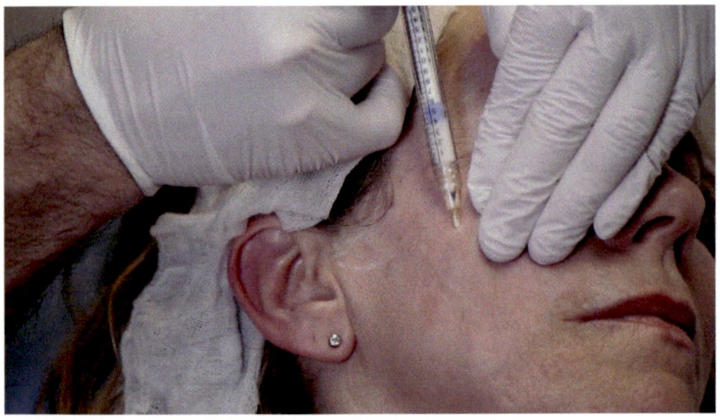

Figure 12.20 With diluted CaHA, inject multiple linear threads in a fanning technique from the medial entry point.

See also Video 12.3 to visualize the product placement using the spermatozoa multilevel cannula technique.

12.6 CHEEK AUGMENTATION: SHARP NEEDLE TECHNIQUE

For injection placement, see Figure 12.21, and for procedure, see Video 12.4.

12.6.1 Step-by-Step Technique

1. Mark the lines and danger zones as indicated in the schematics.
2. Use full viscosity (undiluted) CaHA or standard dilution for periosteal injection with a 27G, 19 mm sharp needle.
3. Lift the cheek on advancement of the needle to reposition the retaining ligaments (Figure 12.22).
4. Use a single skin puncture to place approximately 3–4 boluses on the periosteum to minimize discomfort (Figure 12.23).
5. Work from lateral to medial and inject approximately 0.05–0.1 mL per bolus. At the apex of the cheek, inject more, but do not inject more than 0.1 mL per bolus to prevent vascular complications (Figure 12.24).
6. Lift the zygomatic cutaneous ligament while injecting on the periosteum to push it up with the boluses. Even out the result (Figure 12.25).
7. At the medial cheek, recheck the location of the infraorbital foramen (Figure 12.26).
8. Place boluses superior, lateral, and inferior to the foramen.
9. Even out with manual massage as needed.

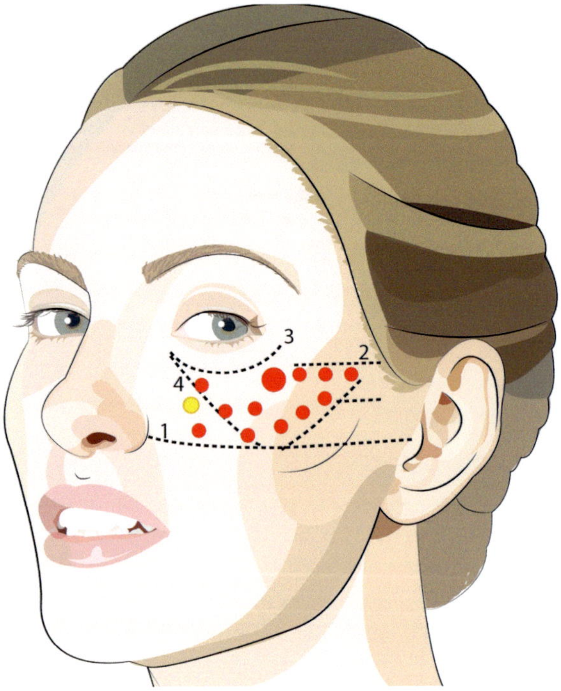

Figure 12.21 The periosteal bolus technique for sharp needle periosteal cheek augmentation. The dotted black lines indicate (1) the alar–tragal line, (2) the zygomatic arch, (3) the infraorbital rim, (4) insertion of the zygomatic cutaneous ligament. The yellow circle represents the infraorbital foramen, and the red dots represent periosteally placed CaHA boluses.

12.7 CHEEK AUGMENTATION: SKIN QUALITY IMPROVEMENT

For injection placement, see Figure 12.27.

12.7.1 Step-by-Step Technique

1. Mark the lines and entry points as indicated in the schematics.
2. Disinfect the skin, the ears, and the hair in front of and above the ear. Place a sterile gauze on the hair.
3. Consider using local anesthesia at the entry points (lidocaine with adrenaline for vasoconstriction).
4. Use hyperdiluted CaHA (0.5–1.5 mL (diluted) lidocaine per 1.5 mL CaHA product) and a 25G, 50 mm cannula.
5. To remain superficial, stretch the skin in the direction of the length of the cannula with one finger in front and one finger behind the entry point (Figure 12.28).

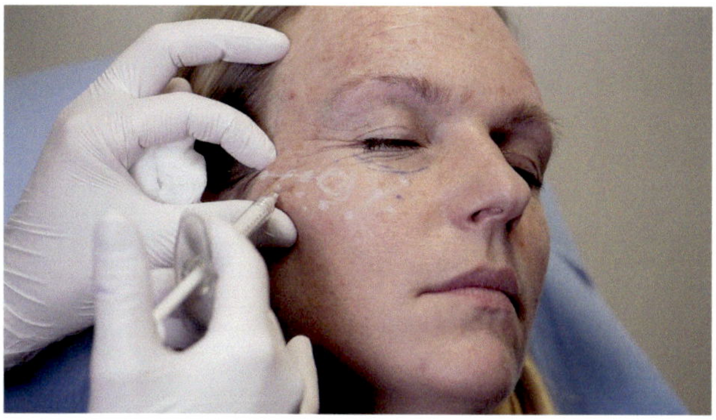

Figure 12.22 Lift the tissue and target the cranial side of the zygomatic arch.

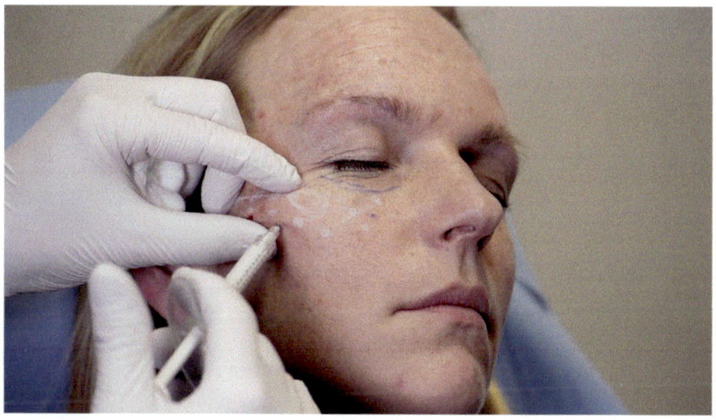

Figure 12.23 Use one entry point for multiple periosteal boluses.

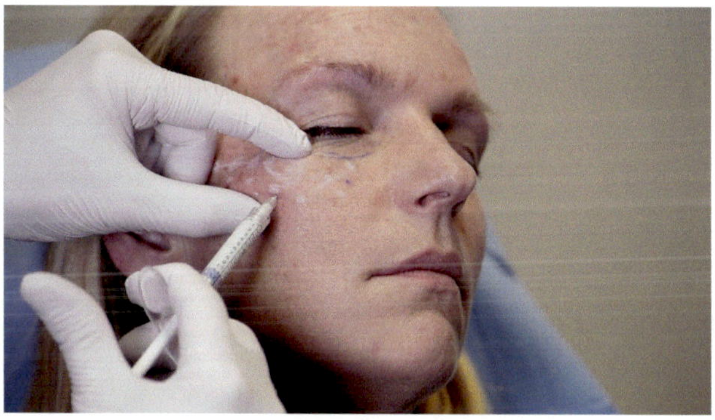

Figure 12.24 At the apex, inject more.

6. Make a fan of retrogrades of approximately 0.05–0.1 mL per line in a fanning technique according to the schematics.
7. From the medial cheek entry point, advance over the alar–tragal line to the nasolabial fold (Figure 12.29). As diluted CaHA is being used, the nasolabial fold can also be injected. Be aware of the facial artery in that area.
8. Place multiple retrogrades of approximately 0.05–0.1 mL per line in a fanning technique according to the schematics.

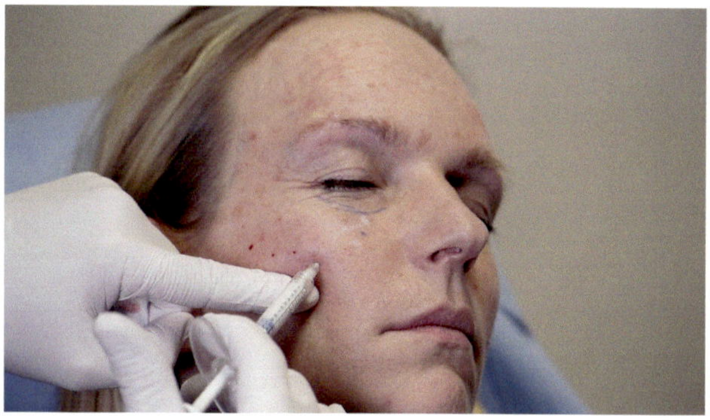

Figure 12.25 Check light reflection and even out the result.

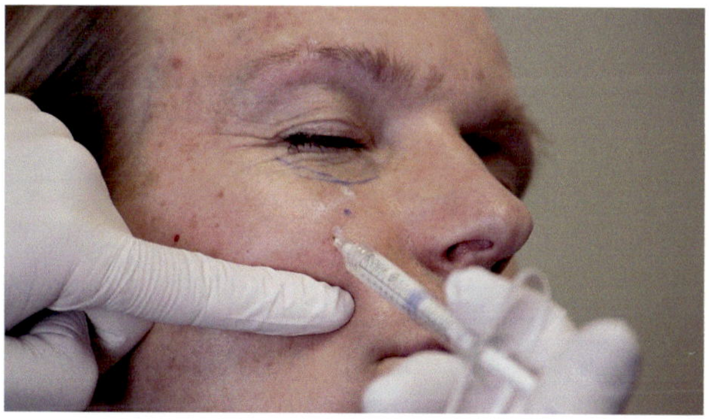

Figure 12.26 Medially, avoid the infraorbital foramen.

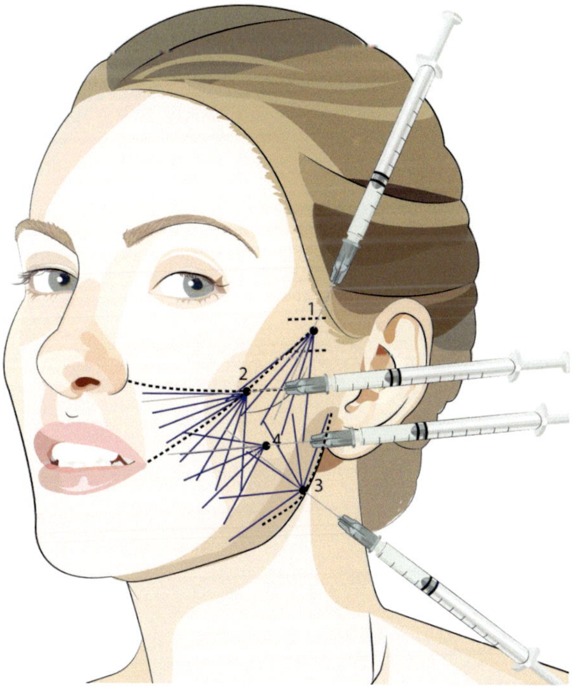

Figure 12.27 The cannula technique for cheek skin quality improvement. The dotted black lines indicate the alar–tragal line, the zygomatic arch, and the mandibular angle. The numbers indicate the four entry points. The blue lines represent hyperdiluted CaHA injected at the dermal–subdermal level.

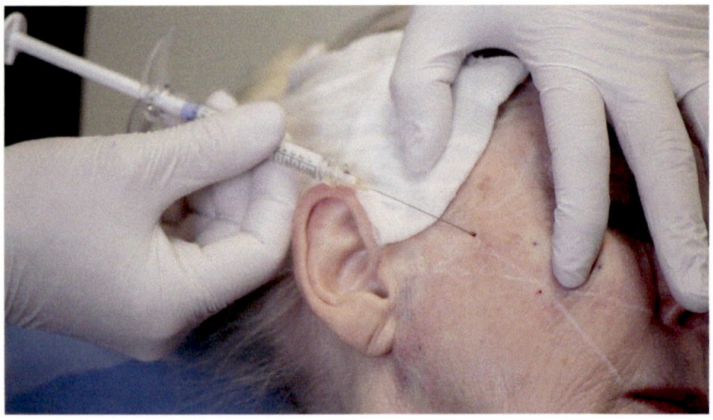

Figure 12.28 First entry point at the zygomatic arch, just in front of the hair line, approximately midway between the tragus and the lateral canthus.

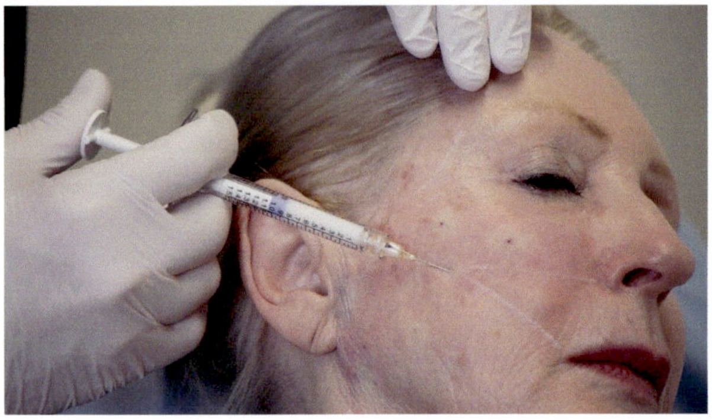

Figure 12.29 Second entry point is on the alar–tragal line and approximately on a vertical line coming from the lateral orbital rim.

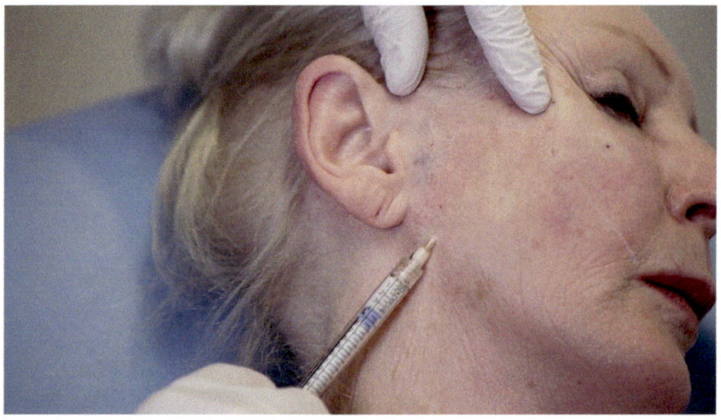

Figure 12.30 The third entry point is on the mandibular angle.

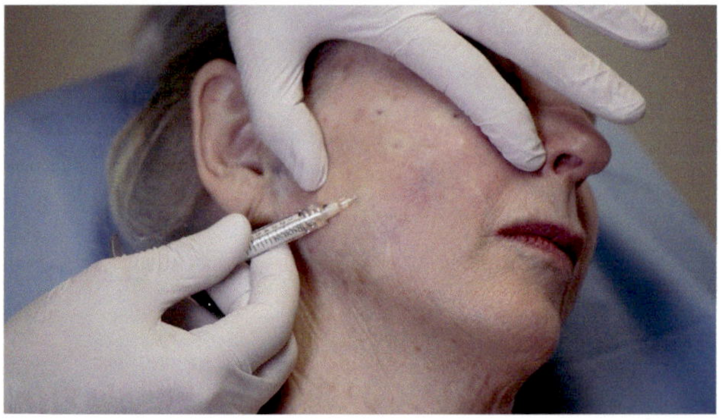

Figure 12.31 The fourth entry point is midway between the second and third entry points.

9. From the mandibular angle entry point (Figure 12.30), pull up the cheek with the nondominant hand to facilitate superficial injection.
10. Make another fan of thin retrogrades.
11. From the middle cheek entry point (Figure 12.31), place multiple retrogrades in a fanning technique according to the schematics.
12. Mold as needed.

See also Video 12.5 to visualize the product placement.

12.8 AFTERCARE

If necessary, the area can be manually massaged to even out the product. When doing so, use an upward molding technique to improve the shape of the injected product and to reposition the retaining ligaments to a more horizontal direction. Swelling may be uneven and should subside in a day or two.

12.9 ADDITIONAL TREATMENTS FOR OPTIMAL RESULTS

Sometimes, due to lateral cheek augmentation, the palpebromalar groove (PMG) becomes more pronounced. Critical assessment after treatment is necessary, and additional injection at the PMG may be indicated (Figure 12.32).

Video 12.1 Cheek augmentation HD sculpture technique (male).

Video 12.2 Cheek augmentation technique (female).

Video 12.3 Cheek augmentation multilevel spermatozoa technique.

Video 12.4 Cheek augmentation sharp needle technique.

Video 12.5 Cheek skin quality improvement.

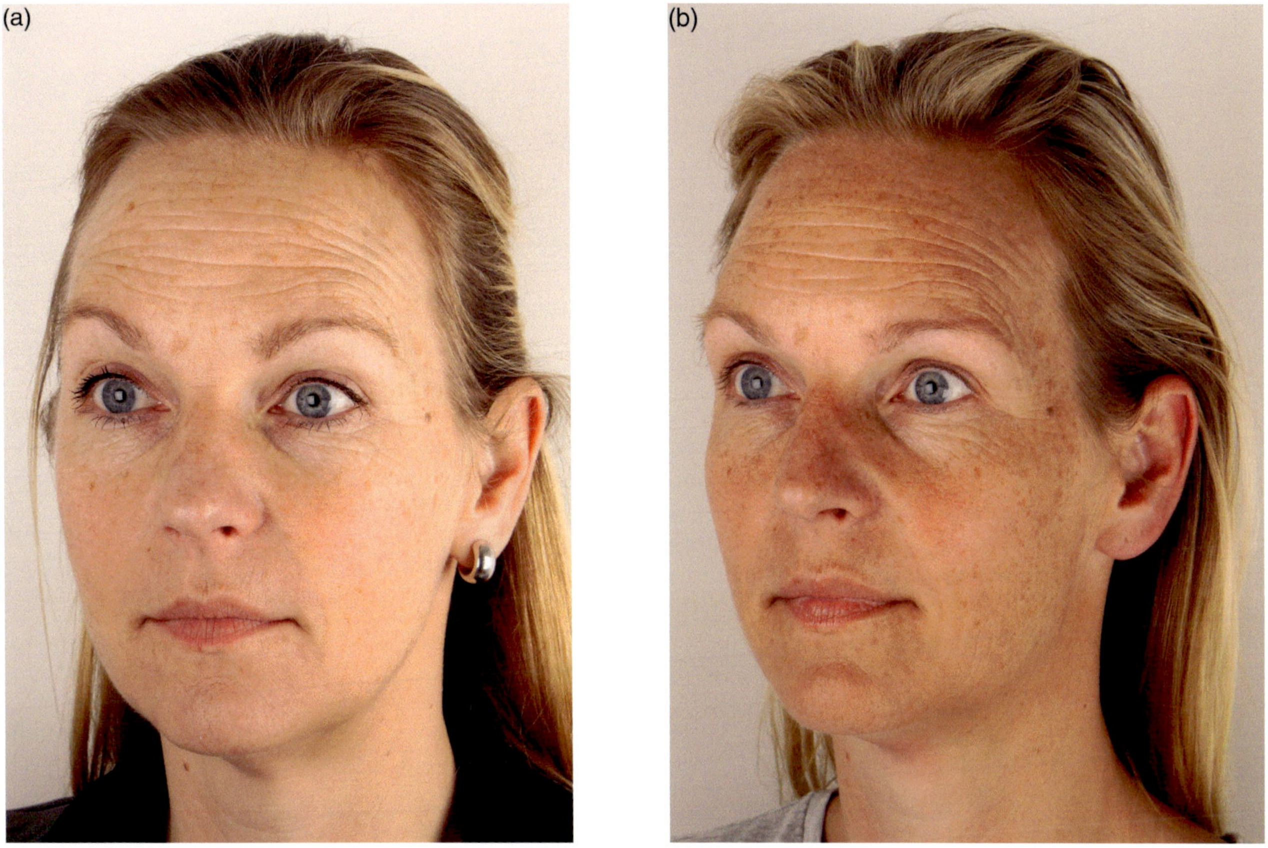

Figure 12.32 Patient treated with CaHA (a) before and (b) after 2 months.

REFERENCES

[1] D. W. Furnas, "The retaining ligaments of the cheek," *Plast Reconstr Surg*, vol. 83, no. 1, pp. 11–16, 1989.

[2] F. E. Barton, "The SMAS and the nasolabial fold," *Plast Reconstr Surg*, vol. 89, no. 6, pp. 1054–1057, 1992.

[3] I. Pitanguy et al., "Numerical modeling of facial aging," *Plast Reconstr Surg*, vol. 102, no. 1, pp. 200–204, Jul. 1998.

[4] D. W. Furnas, "Festoons, mounds, and bags of the eyelids and cheek," *Clin Plast Surg*, vol. 20, no. 2, pp. 367–385, Apr. 1993.

[5] M. Gonzalez-Ulloam, E. S. Flores, "Senility of the face—basic study to understand its causes and effects," *Plast Reconstr Surg*, vol. 36, no. 2, pp. 239–246, Aug. 1965.

[6] R. Fitzgerald et al., "Update on facial aging," *Aesthet Surg J*, vol. 30, no. Suppl 1, 2010.

[7] K. A. Valentine et al., "Judging a man by the width of his face: The role of facial ratios and dominance in mate choice at speed-dating events," *Psychol Sci*, vol. 25, no. 3, pp. 806–811, 2014.

[8] S. Bay Aguilera et al., "How to make calcium hydroxylapatite injections safer," *J Drugs Dermatol*, vol. 13, no. 9, p. 1015, 2014.

The Middle Third of the Face

13

Treatment of Acne Scars

FADI HAMADANI

13.1 PATHOPHYSIOLOGY AND CLASSIFICATION OF ACNE SCARS

Acne is a complex and chronic inflammatory disease of the pilosebaceous unit that involves multiple factors, including genetic predisposition, the immune system, certain skin flora, and environmental factors [1]. One of the main sequelae of acne can be disfiguring scars, which have an impact on both self-confidence as well as cosmesis [2]. Atrophic acne scars exist on a spectrum that ranges from ice-pick scars to deep, tethered scars that atrophy into the subcutaneous tissue [3]. Acne scar revision requires a bespoke approach with a combination of tools suited to the scar type, patient and skin factors, and available physician skills. Nevertheless, it is possible to have a global/regional approach whereby any area with acne scars, regardless of type or depth, can be improved by combining some simple steps. Volume enhancement is a crucial component of such a regional approach, and CaHA has proven to be an effective and reliable tool to this effect [4]. The purpose of this chapter is to highlight the important and effective role that CaHA can play in the management of deep atrophic acne scars by focusing on several combinations in different acne scar types.

13.1.1 The Pathophysiology of Acne Scars

The pathophysiology of acne scars is a complex interplay of inflammatory processes, tissue remodeling, and the body's attempt to heal following acne lesions [3,5]. Acne scars result from the disruption of the pilosebaceous unit, involving intricate cellular and molecular mechanisms [5].

13.1.1.1 Inflammatory Cascade

The journey toward acne scarring begins with the inflammatory cascade triggered by acne lesions. Comedones, inflammatory papules, pustules, and nodules induce an immune response, activating pro-inflammatory cytokines and chemokines. This heightened immune activity contributes to tissue damage, particularly in the dermis [6].

13.1.1.2 Dermal Remodeling

Following the inflammatory phase, the dermal remodeling process takes center stage. Collagen, the structural protein providing skin firmness and support, undergoes alterations. In the context of acne scars, this often leads to an imbalance in collagen production and degradation. The transition from normal collagen architecture to abnormal scar tissue involves changes in collagen types, with an overproduction of disorganized collagen fibers [7].

13.1.1.3 Atrophy and Hypertrophy

Different types of acne scars manifest as a result of varied tissue responses. Atrophic scars, including ice-pick and rolling scars, arise from the loss of collagen, elastin, and subcutaneous tissue. Conversely, hypertrophic scars form when there's an excess of collagen deposition during the healing process, resulting in raised scars [3,5,7].

13.1.1.4 Fibroblast Activation

Central to the pathophysiology is the activation of fibroblasts, key players in collagen synthesis. Dysregulation of fibroblast activity contributes to the aberrant collagen composition seen in acne scars. Moreover, the intricate crosstalk between fibroblasts, inflammatory cells, and extracellular matrix components influences scar morphology [8].

13.1.1.5 Vascular Alterations

Vascular alterations play a role in the pathogenesis of acne scars. The increased blood flow and angiogenesis during the inflammatory phase contribute to tissue damage. Persistent vascular changes may further impact scar appearance and texture. Understanding the pathophysiology of acne scars is crucial for developing targeted interventions. By unraveling the intricacies of these molecular and cellular processes, therapeutic approaches can be tailored to modulate inflammation, promote balanced tissue remodeling, and ultimately mitigate the long-term impact of acne on skin integrity [9].

13.1.2 Classification of Acne Scars

Acne scars manifest in a variety of forms, each characterized by distinct features and presenting unique challenges in terms of treatment. These scars are broadly categorized into several types, providing a comprehensive framework for understanding their varied characteristics.

DOI: 10.1201/9781003617129-13

13.1.2.1 Atrophic Scars

- Description: Depressed scars resulting from the loss of tissue.
- Pathophysiology: Involves the depletion of collagen, elastin, and subcutaneous fat.
- Appearance: Includes ice-pick, boxcar, and rolling scars, collectively characterized by tissue loss.

Understanding the types and classifications of acne scars is instrumental in tailoring effective treatment strategies. A nuanced approach, considering the specific characteristics of each scar type, ensures optimal outcomes in the complex landscape of acne scar revision.

13.1.2.2 Ice-Pick Scars

- Description: Narrow, deep scars resembling small puncture wounds.
- Pathophysiology: Result from the loss of tissue and collagen in a localized manner.
- Appearance: Often gives the skin an appearance similar to that of being punctured by an ice-pick.

13.1.2.3 Boxcar Scars

- Description: Broad, box-like depressions with well-defined edges.
- Pathophysiology: Arise from the destruction of collagen, creating a depressed area with distinct borders.
- Appearance: Resembles a box or rectangular shape, impacting skin texture.

13.1.2.4 Rolling Scars

- Description: Broad, undulating depressions with sloping edges.
- Pathophysiology: Result from tethering of the epidermis to the underlying subcutaneous tissue.
- Appearance: Creates a rolling or wave-like contour on the skin [10].

13.1.2.5 Hypertrophic Scars

- Description: Raised, thickened scars that extend beyond the original wound site.
- Pathophysiology: Excessive collagen production during the healing process.
- Appearance: Elevated and often red or hyperpigmented, in contrast to the surrounding skin [11].

13.1.2.6 Keloid Scars

- Description: Elevated, irregularly shaped scars extending beyond the original wound.
- Pathophysiology: Aberrant collagen synthesis, exceeding the boundaries of the initial injury.
- Appearance: Extends beyond the original wound site, often with a firm and rubbery texture [11].

13.2 TREATMENT STRATEGIES FOR ACNE SCARS BASED ON SCAR TYPE

Acne scars manifest in diverse forms, necessitating targeted treatment approaches. The following outlines strategic interventions tailored to specific scar types:

13.2.1 Atrophic Scars

Atrophic scars, including ice-pick, boxcar, and rolling scars, demand precision in treatment.

Laser Therapy: Fractional laser treatments, such as fractional CO_2 or erbium lasers, target damaged skin areas, promoting collagen remodeling and skin rejuvenation [12].

13.2.1.1 Microneedling

This minimally invasive procedure induces micro-injuries, triggering the body's natural healing response and stimulating collagen production [13].

13.2.1.2 Dermal Fillers

Injectable fillers, like hyaluronic acid or collagen, can temporarily improve the appearance of atrophic scars by plumping up the depressed areas [14].

13.2.2 Hypertrophic and Keloid Scars

Elevated scars require specialized interventions to reduce excess tissue formation.

13.2.2.1 Corticosteroid Injections

Intralesional corticosteroids help flatten hypertrophic or keloid scars by reducing inflammation and inhibiting collagen synthesis [15].

13.2.2.2 Surgical Removal

Excision of hypertrophic or keloid scars may be considered for cases resistant to other treatments, followed by meticulous wound closure and a series of laser sessions to remodel the scar. Silicone sheets or gel may prevent scar recurrence [16].

13.2.2.3 Hyperpigmentation

Post-inflammatory hyperpigmentation necessitates targeted depigmenting strategies.

13.2.2.4 Topical Retinoids

Retinoids, such as tretinoin, promote skin cell turnover, aiding in the fading of hyperpigmented areas [15–17].

13.2.2.5 Chemical Peels

Chemical exfoliants, like glycolic or salicylic acid peels, can help remove superficial pigmentation and improve overall skin tone [17].

13.2.3 Individualized Plans

Combination therapies and individualization treatments render optimal outcomes and often result from tailored, multifaceted approaches. Specialists should tailor treatment plans based on scar type, skin type, and patient preferences.

13.2.4 Patient Education

Emphasize the importance of consistent treatment and realistic expectations, as improvements may be gradual.

In conclusion, a comprehensive strategy for acne scar treatment involves a nuanced understanding of scar types and a personalized, multidimensional approach to address the unique needs of each patient.

13.3 GLOBAL ENHANCEMENT PROTOCOL UTILIZING SUBCISION AND DILUTED CAHA

See Video 13.1 on enhancement protocol of the skin and before-and-after procedures in three different individuals (Figures 13.1–13.3).

Video 13.1 Subcision of acne scars with CaHA.

13.3.1 Step-by-Step Technique

NOTE: Maintain sterility at all times.

1. Anesthesia is accomplished with a series of round blocks using 1% lidocaine and adrenaline (1:100000) with optional addition of conscious sedation.
2. The scars are demarcated clearly by drawing regional circles around areas involved with scarring.
3. An introductory hole is made with a 22G needle. It is best to plan a triangular approach to the scars.
4. A 22G blunt cannula is introduced through the hole and is used to subcise and break down any tethering of scars. The depth of submission depends on the depth of the fibrosis. Multiple back-and-forth passes are made to ensure a good release of the bands. This also serves the purpose of tunneling for the CaHA. It is best to triangulate the scars, i.e., to subcise from three different directions. This ensures a more comprehensive release.
5. A 2:1 dilution of CaHA is accomplished by diluting the CaHA with 1.5 mL of 1% lidocaine without adrenaline. A series of 30 back-and-forth motions is accomplished to ensure a uniform suspension of CaHA.
6. The material is injected in small aliquots of 0.025 mL each as the cannula is withdrawn slowly.
7. This is done until a 40 cm^2 area receives 1.5 mL of the diluted CaHA [18,19].

13.4 COMBINATION PROTOCOL UTILIZING SUBCISION, ENERGY-BASED DEVICES, AND DILUTED CAHA

13.4.1 Step-by-Step Technique

NOTE: Maintain sterility at all times.

1. Anesthesia is accomplished with a series of round blocks using 1% lidocaine and adrenaline (1:100000) with the optional addition of conscious sedation.
2. The scars are demarcated clearly by drawing regional circles around areas involved with scarring.
3. An introductory hole is made with a 22G needle. It is best to plan a triangular approach to the scars.

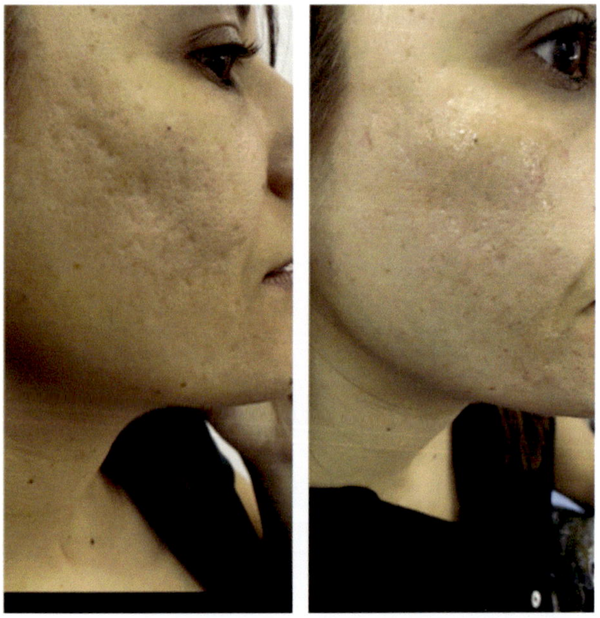

Figure 13.1 A 36-year-old woman underwent two sessions of global subcision with one syringe of CaHA diluted 1:1 spaced two months apart. The results are three months after the last session.

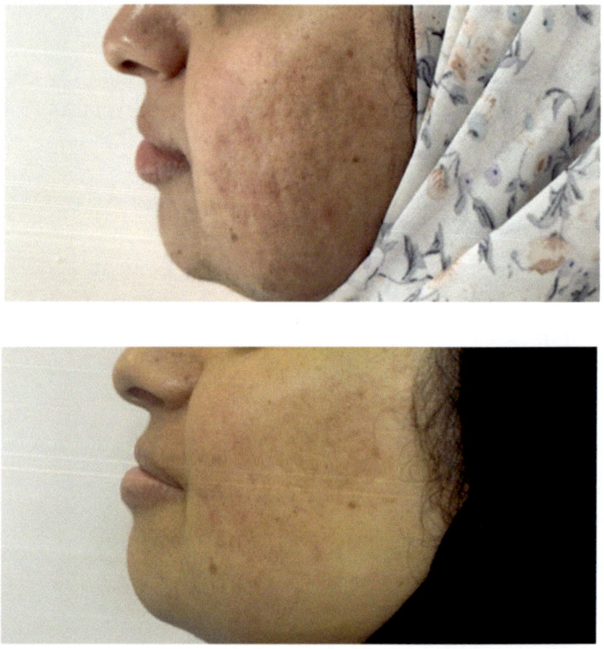

Figure 13.2 A 27-year-old woman six months after one session of global subcision with one syringe of diluted CaHA diluted 1:1.

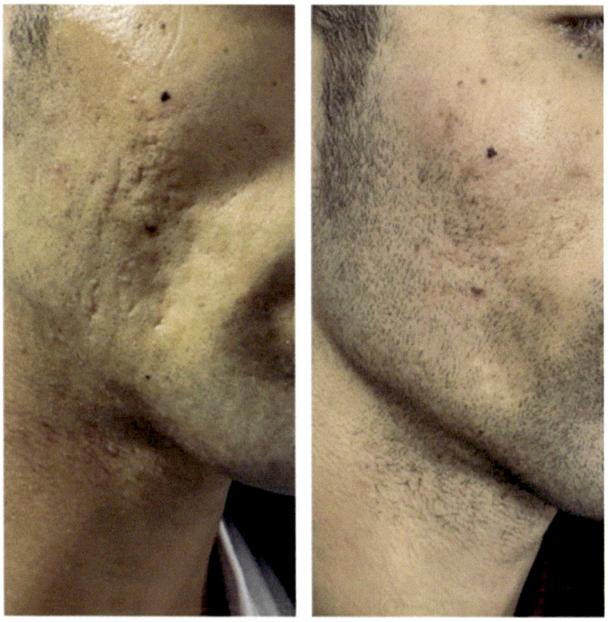

Figure 13.3 A 29-year-old male after three sessions of global subcision, the last two including one syringe of diluted CaHA diluted 1:1.

4. A 22G blunt cannula is introduced through the hole and is used to subcise and break down any tethering of scars. The depth of submission depends on the depth of the fibrosis. Multiple back-and-forth passes are made to ensure a good release of the bands. This also serves the purpose of tunneling for the CaHA. It is best to triangulate the scars, i.e., to subcise from three different directions. This ensures a more comprehensive release.
5. At this point the energy-based device is utilized. If the modality is a laser or radiofrequency microneedling it is best to be performed prior to the injection of CaHA.
6. A 2:1 dilution of CaHA is accomplished by diluting the CaHA with 1.5 mL of 1% lidocaine without adrenaline. A series of 30 back-and-forth motions is accomplished to ensure a uniform suspension of CaHA.
7. The material is injected in small aliquots of 0.025 mL each as the cannula is withdrawn slowly.
8. This is done until a 40 cm^2 area receives 1.5 mL of the diluted CaHA.

13.5 COMBINATION PROTOCOL UTILIZING TCA CROSS/PHENOL CROSS, SUBCISION, EBD, AND CAHA (FIGURES 13.4–13.5)

13.5.1 Step-by-Step Technique

NOTE: Maintain sterility at all times.

1. Ice-pick scars are marked, and an 80% TCA formula is inserted into each scar using a small paintbrush or toothpick.
2. An 80% formula of TCA can be obtained by mixing 0.8 mL of a 100% TCA solution with 0.2 mL of sterile distilled water.
3. When applying the TCA solution, make sure excess TCA is discarded from the paintbrush by gently running it on the wall of the solution container.
4. The TCA formula should be placed well within the borders of the scar with minimal spill-over.
5. The clinical endpoint to look for is a sharp white/gray color within the confines of the scar.
6. Following completion of the targeted TCA CROSS treatment of the scars, anesthesia and subcision of the scars is performed, as described above [20,21].
7. This is followed by the injection of diluted CaHA, as described above.

13.6 TIPS TO OPTIMIZE SUBCISION

Subcision is a vital procedure in acne scar revision, involving the insertion of a blunt, semi-blunt, or sharp device to break down scar formations between the dermis and underlying muscular fascia.

The extent of scar tissue varies among patients, often occurring after acne scars, with nearly all cases exhibiting some degree of tethering. Precise demarcation of the area and determining access points for the subcision tool are crucial. Caution must be taken to avoid ligamentous origins to prevent potential ptosis [22]. Depth assessment of scar tissue is essential, and tumescent is crucial for nerve protection, reducing ecchymosis, bruising, and hematomas [23].

When using a blunt device like a cannula (ranging from 16–22G), multiple passes at various levels are necessary for proper scar tissue release. Cross-hatching and triangulating the scar with the subcision tool are

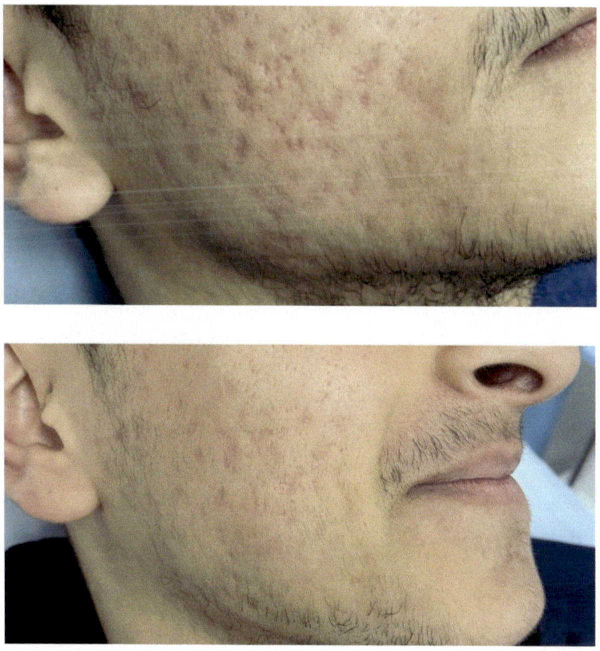

Figure 13.4 A 22-year-old male six months after two sessions of subcision, TCA CROSS (80%), and one syringe of diluted CaHA with 1:1 dilution. Two months between first and second session.

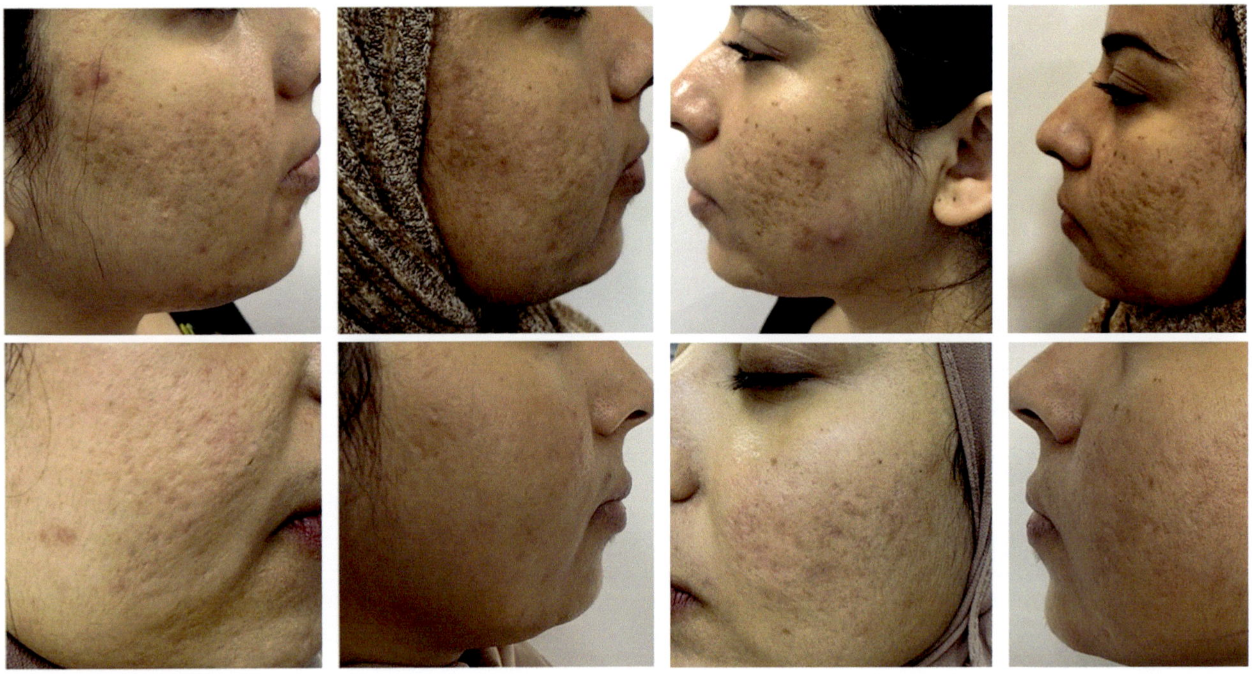

Figure 13.5 Evolution of 18 months of treatment. Upper left pictures are prior to commencing treatment. The upper right pictures are after active acne control and prior to commencing scar revision (low dose isotretinoin and erbium:glass laser). Lower left photos are three months after two sessions of TCA CROSS (80%), subcision, fully ablative CO_2, and two syringes of diluted CaHA (1:1). Lower right photos are six months after an additional two sessions, but fractional RF was used instead of CO_2. The patient still had post-inflammatory hyperpigmentation in the final photo, which resolved three months later with topical whitening agents.

important. For semi-blunt tools like a Taylor liberator or liposuction V-dissector, gentle strokes are necessary to prevent deep injuries. Sharp subcision, involving an 18G hypodermic needle or corneal knives, is reserved for specific areas with significant tethering [23,24].

Post-subcision, buffering the tissue is crucial to prevent scar tissue reforming. CaHA is a preferred choice, though some use fillers or normal saline injections [25]. Recovery typically spans seven to ten days, with edema and chemosis possible. Patients are advised to apply cold compresses for the first 24 hours, followed by warm compresses. Standard pain medications may be used. Depending on acne scar severity, one to six sessions of subcision, spaced six to eight weeks apart, may be necessary, with gradual but consistent results expected.

Performing an effective subcision prior to injecting diluted CaHA is crucial to prevent non-scar tissue from elevating more than scar tissue, avoiding an uneven appearance at the scars or deeper levels. Proper release ensures a smoother result.

13.7 COMMENTARY ON CAHA DILUTION

Diluted CaHA can stimulate collagen in scarred areas and skin depressions. Dilution ranges of 1:1, 1:2, and 1:3 are possible. Typically, a 1:2 or 1:3 dilution is suitable for thinner skin, while a 1:1 dilution is used for thicker skin. When injected retrogradely in small micro boluses rather than linear threads, it is less likely to produce nodules.

13.8 COMMENTARY ON CAHA AS DRUG DELIVERY

CaHA is effective as a drug delivery modality. Following the application of a CO_2 laser, it becomes feasible to topically administer diluted CaHA. Wang *et al.* demonstrated that after CO_2 treatment, micro-channels stay open for approximately 24 hours, enabling the effective delivery of diluted CaHA into these channels [26]. This presents an alternative approach for treating acne scars.

REFERENCES

[1] P. Ghasemiyeh et al., "The role of different factors in pathophysiology of acne and potential therapeutic options: A brief review," *Trends Pharmacol Sci*, vol. 8, no. 2, pp. 107–118, 2022.

[2] K. Chilicka et al., "Methods for the improvement of acne scars used in dermatology and cosmetology: A review," *J Clin Med*, vol. 11, no. 10, 2022.

[3] D. A. Agrawal, N. Khunger, "A morphological study of acne scarring and its relationship between severity and treatment of active acne," *J Cutan Aesthet Surg*, vol. 13, no. 3, pp. 210–216, 2020.

[4] A. Antonino, A. Francesco, "Prospective and randomized comparative study of calcium hydroxylapatite vs calcium hydroxylapatite

plus HIFU in treatment of moderate-to-severe acne scars," *J Cosmet Dermatol*, vol. 20, no. 1, pp. 53–61, 2021.

[5] T. Jennings et al., "Acne scarring-pathophysiology, diagnosis, prevention and education: Part I," *J Am Acad Dermatol*, vol. 90, no. 6, pp. 1123–1134, 2024.

[6] Y. ElAttar et al., "Study of interleukin-1 beta expression in acne vulgaris and acne scars," *J Cosmet Dermatol*, vol. 21, no. 10, pp. 4864–4870, 2022.

[7] M. R. Roh, K. Y. Chung, "Acne scars: How they form and how to undo them," in: Ogawa, R., ed., *Total Scar Management: From Lasers to Surgery for Scars, Keloids, and Scar Contractures*. Springer, 2019, pp. 97–103.

[8] B. Chancheewa et al., "Myofibroblasts, B cells, and mast cells in different types of long-standing acne scars," *Skin Appendage Disord*, vol. 8, no. 6, pp. 469–475, 2022.

[9] D. M. K. El-Sayed et al., "Brief overview about updated management lines of post acne erythema: Review article," *Egypt J Hosp Med*, vol. 91, no. 1, pp. 4294–4297, 2023.

[10] M. Boen, C. Jacob, "A review and update of treatment options using the acne scar classification system," *Dermatol Surg*, vol. 45, no. 3, pp. 411–422, 2019.

[11] G. Fabbrocini et al., "Acne scars: Pathogenesis, classification and treatment," *Dermatol Res Pract*, vol. 2010, no. 1, 2010.

[12] B. E. Cohen et al., "Acne scarring: A review of available therapeutic lasers," *Lasers Surg Med*, vol. 48, no. 2, pp. 95–115, 2016.

[13] N. Mujahid et al., "Microneedling as a treatment for acne scarring: A systematic review," *Dermatol Surg*, vol. 46, no. 1, pp. 86–92, 2020.

[14] E. Forbat et al., "The role of fillers in the management of acne scars," *Clin Exp Dermatol*, vol. 42, no. 4, pp. 374–380, 2017.

[15] M. Jalali, A. Bayat, "Current use of steroids in management of abnormal raised skin scars," *Surgeon*, vol. 5, no. 3, pp. 175–180, 2007.

[16] P. Durani, A. Bayat, "Levels of evidence for the treatment of keloid disease," *J Plast Reconstr Aesthet Surg*, vol. 61, no. 1, pp. 4–17, 2008.

[17] A. Jackson, "Chemical peels," *Facial Plast Surg*, vol. 30, no. 1, pp. 26–34, 2014.

[18] J. A. J. van Loghem et al., "Calcium hydroxylapatite: Over a decade of clinical experience," *J Clin Aesthet Dermatol*, vol. 8, no. 1, pp. 38–49, 2015.

[19] A. T. De Almeida et al., "Consensus recommendations for the use of hyperdiluted calcium hydroxyapatite (Radiesse) as a face and body biostimulatory agent," *Plast Reconstr Surg Glob Open*, vol. 7, no. 3, 2019.

[20] J. B. Lee et al., "Focal treatment of acne scars with trichloroacetic acid: Chemical reconstruction of skin scars method," *Dermatol Surg*, vol. 28, no. 11, pp. 1017–1021, 2002.

[21] M. Dalpizzol et al., "Comparative study of the use of trichloroacetic acid and phenolic acid in the treatment of atrophic-type acne scars," *Dermatol Surg*, vol. 42, no. 3, pp. 377–383, 2016.

[22] F. Araghi et al., "The importance of facial retaining ligaments' preservation during the subcision," *Aesthet Surg J*, vol. 42, no. 1, pp. NP87–NP88, 2022.

[23] S. Dadkhahfar et al., "Subcision: Indications, adverse reactions, and pearls," *J Cosmet Dermatol*, vol. 19, no. 5, pp. 1029–1038, 2020.

[24] M. B. Taylor et al., "Single session treatment of rolling acne scars using tumescent anesthesia, 20% trichloracetic acid extensive subcision, and fractional CO2 laser," *Dermatol Surg*, vol. 43, no. Suppl 1, pp. S70–S74, 2017.

[25] K. Balighi et al., "Subcision in acne scar with and without subdermal implant: A clinical trial," *J Eur Acad Dermatol Venereol*, vol. 22, no. 6, pp. 707–711, 2008.

[26] J. V. Wang et al., "Evaluation of device-based cutaneous channels using optical coherence tomography: Impact for topical drug delivery," *Dermatol Surg*, vol. 48, no. 1, pp. 120–125, 2022.

The Middle Third of the Face 14

Tear Trough

NIAMH CORDUFF AND JANI VAN LOGHEM

14.1 INTRODUCTION

The tear trough (TT) is one of the most requested filler treatments, but due to the anatomy of the area, it is considered an advanced indication, as improper (superficial) placement of CaHA can result in malar edema that is resistant to treatment [1]. TT deformity (TTD) is essentially the result of the anatomy of the orbicularis retaining ligament (ORL), the zygomatic cutaneous ligament (ZCL), and the anatomical layers in between them. The ORL runs from the periosteum of the orbital rim and inserts into the orbicularis oculi muscle at the junction of the palpebral and orbital parts of the muscle. The ORL is, therefore, a false retaining ligament, as it does not extend from the periosteum to the skin. The ZCL runs from the periosteum of the maxilla to its skin insertion, making it a true retaining ligament. Medially, the ZCL origin runs just below and parallel to the ORL. From the medial canthus, they run to just cranial to the infraorbital foramen. There, the origin of the ZCL takes a turn and travels away from the ORL, laterally and horizontally over the bone of the maxilla and zygoma toward McGregor's patch.

In between these ligaments from the medial canthus to the foramen, we find the TTD. Below the skin, an almost nonexistent subcutaneous fat compartment is located just over the orbicularis oculi muscle. Below the muscle, the sub-orbicularis oculi fat (SOOF) compartment is found, then, deep to the SOOF, a glide space made of two sliding membranes, also known as the malar septum or premaxillary space, is found, and below the malar septum, we find the preperiosteal fat (also sometimes called the deep SOOF), the periosteum, and the bone. Placement of CaHA superficial to the malar septum (so even deep to the muscle) can result in malar edema [2]. With proper injection techniques, however, malar edema can be avoided. This means injecting CaHA deep on the periosteum underneath the malar septum in the preperiosteal fat. Using a deep plane, CaHA is an excellent choice for TT injection, as the product does not attract water, and therefore the risk of edema is much lower than with HA fillers. This was documented very well in a case series published in 2009 by Oscar Hevia, who injected 301 patients and saw transient edema in only 2% of the cases [3].

Often accompanying TTD are dark under-eye circles, which arise from contour deficits and changes in skin quality. Contour deficits include maxillary hypoplasia, recessed inferomedial orbital rims, and herniation of orbital fat which lead to shadowing. Concurrently, skin quality changes, including hyperpigmentation and thin, translucent lower eyelid skin, exacerbate the appearance of dark circles. In this context, patients with deep TT pigmentation may continue to experience persistent or increasingly noticeable discoloration, even after undergoing successful contour correction. Of note, due to its distinct rheological and biostimulatory effects, careful placement of CaHA in small amounts beneath a prolapsed TT ORL was shown to effectively lift and support the area without adding excess volume. Furthermore, subcutaneous wash with diluted CaHA (1:5) led to improved skin thickness and pliability in patients with hyperpigmentation [4].

14.2 SAFETY CONSIDERATIONS

When injecting the TT with a needle, care should be taken not to inject too much product in a single bolus, as backflow through the tunnel created with the needle can be expected [5]. When the product flows back to more superficial layers, malar edema is more likely to occur. Funt described a good technique for using sharp needles while avoiding malar edema [1].

The arterial dangers are represented by the infraorbital artery, the angular artery, and their branches, plus the inferior marginal arterial arcade (Figure 14.1).

14.3 TEAR TROUGH CANNULA TECHNIQUE

For injection placement, see Figure 14.2.

1. Identify and mark the skin insertion of the ZCL and the ORL. Realize that the superficial insertions of these ligaments are lower than the bony origins.
2. Mark the entry point in between the two ligaments, so that the cannula can reach the medial side of the TT.
3. Disinfect. Consider giving an infraorbital nerve block and local anesthesia at the entry point.
4. Make a pre-hole with a 23G needle.
5. Use nondiluted CaHA or standard dilution of CaHA (0.3 mL 1% lidocaine with adrenaline 1:200000 per 1.5 mL CaHA) and a 25G, 38 mm cannula.
6. Point the cannula in the direction of the medial TT (Figure 14.3).

DOI: 10.1201/9781003617129-14

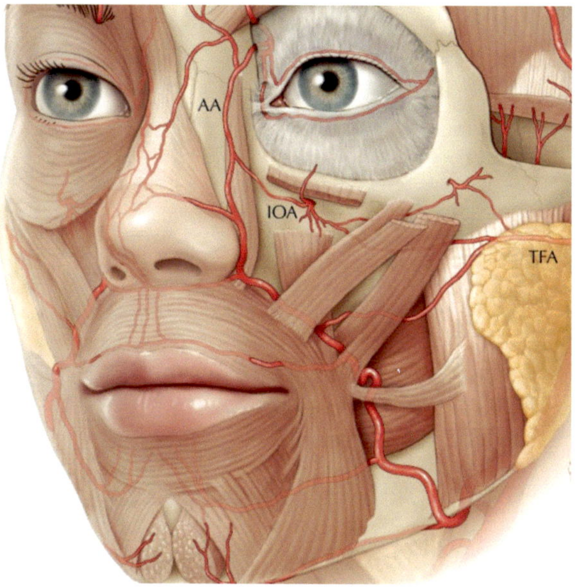

Figure 14.1 Arterial danger zones of the tear trough are: infraorbital artery (IOA), transverse facial artery (TFA), and angular artery (AA).

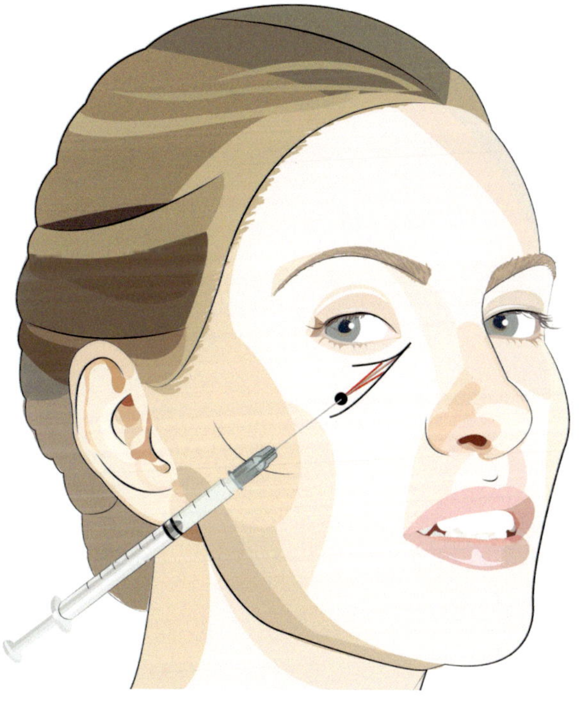

Figure 14.2 Product injection at the TT. The two black lines represent the ORL and the ZCL. Red lines indicate CaHA product placement at the periosteal level in between the two ligaments.

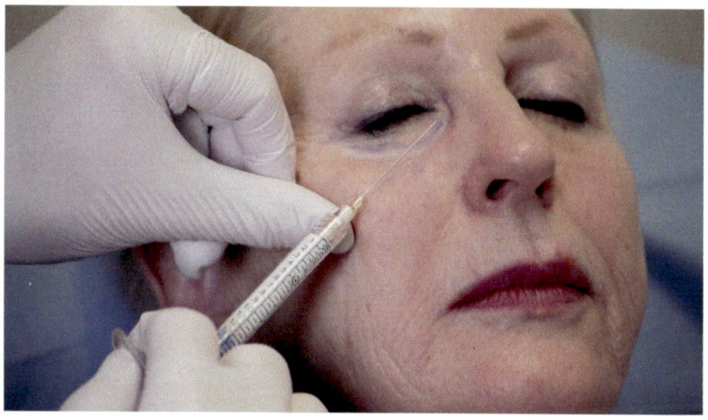

Figure 14.3 The entry point can be approximately at the vertical line going down from the lateral orbital rim. Check cannula length to see if medial TT can be reached.

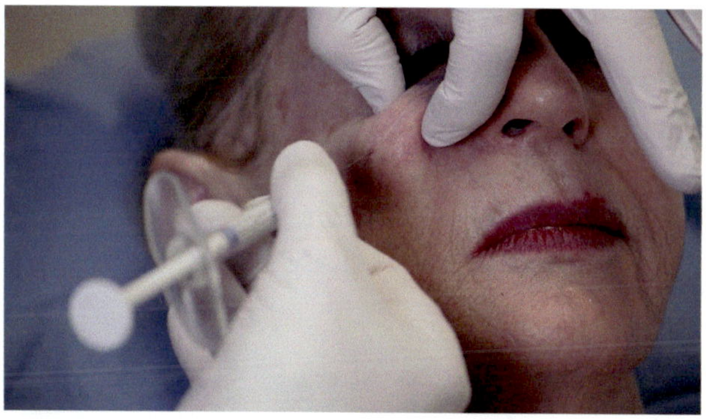

Figure 14.4 Make sure the cannula direction is toward the target (medial TT) while lifting the skin in front of the cannula.

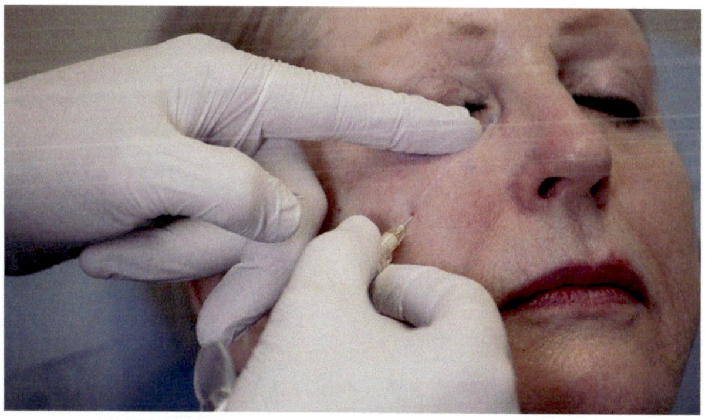

Figure 14.5 While advancing the cannula over the periosteum, keep a finger of the nondominant hand on the infraorbital rim to avoid placing the cannula in the intraorbital space.

7. With the nondominant hand, lift the tissue up in front of the cannula tip, and maneuver the cannula through resistances to the periosteum (Figure 14.4).
8. On the periosteum, slide the cannula medially into the funnel created by the two ligaments (Figure 14.5).
9. Inject small amounts while retracting.
10. Mold and check.
11. Readvance and place additional deposits as needed. Do not overcorrect (Figure 14.6).
12. Even out with manual massage as needed.

14.4 TEAR TROUGH NEEDLE TECHNIQUE

For injection placement, see Figure 14.7.

1. Identify and mark the skin insertion of the ZCL, the ORL and the infraorbital foramen. Realize that the superficial insertions of these ligaments are lower than the bony origins.
2. Disinfect. Consider giving an infraorbital nerve block.
3. Use nondiluted CaHA or standard dilution of CaHA (0.3 mL 1% lidocaine with adrenaline 1:200000 per 1.5 mL CaHA) and a 27G needle supplied with the product.
4. Lift the cheek and keep a finger of the nondominant hand on the infraorbital rim to avoid inadvertent intraorbital injection.
5. Use a skin entry point inferior to the ZCL skin insertion (Figure 14.8).
6. With the bevel down and a 45° direction to the bone surface, advance the needle slowly to the periosteum.
7. With a soft touch to the periosteum, inject a series of three small aliquots of approximately 0.025 mL each. Small amounts will reduce the risk of malar edema and vascular complications (Figure 14.9).
8. Remove the needle, reinsert the needle more medially, and repeat.
9. Do not overcorrect.
10. Even out with manual massage as needed.

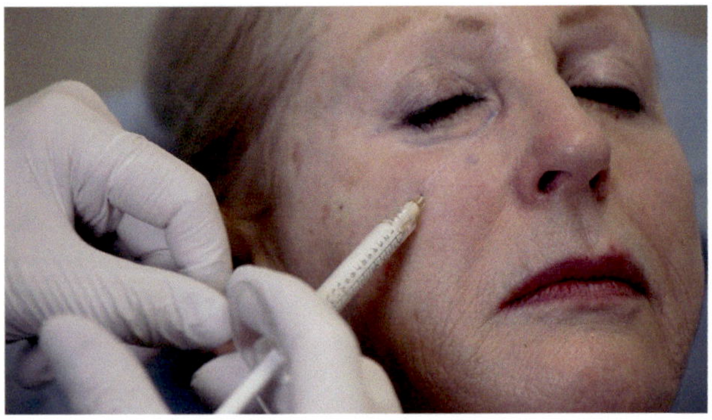

Figure 14.6 Place small aliquots. Do not overcorrect.

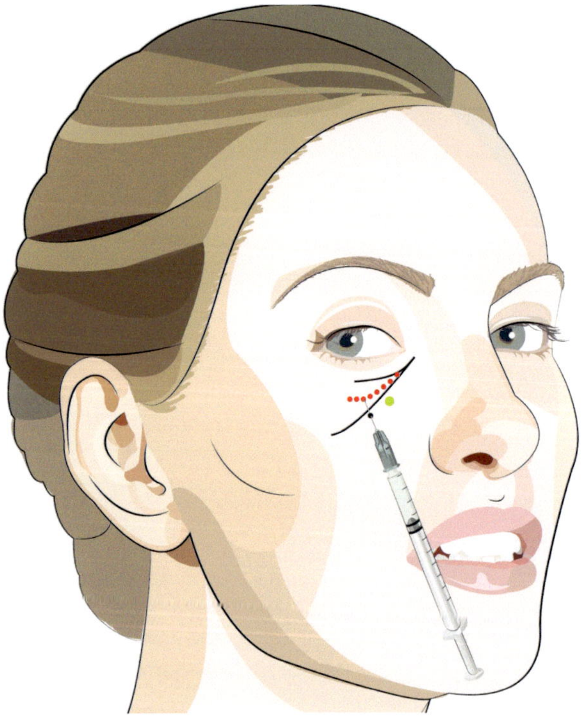

Figure 14.7 CaHA injection at the TT using sharp needle. The two black lines represent the ORL and the ZCL. Red dots indicate CaHA product placement at the periosteal level in between the two ligaments. The black dot indicates entry of the needle inferior to the skin insertion of the ZCL. Green dot indicates approximate location of the infraorbital foramen.

14.5 SUBDERMAL DILUTED CAHA TECHNIQUE

1. 0.1 mL CaHA is thoroughly mixed with 0.5 mL of 1% lidocaine.
2. A 27G cannula should be passed subcutaneously from a lateral point below the lateral canthus to access the lower eyelid, and this hyperdiluted wash should be flushed across the lower eyelid and lid-cheek junction

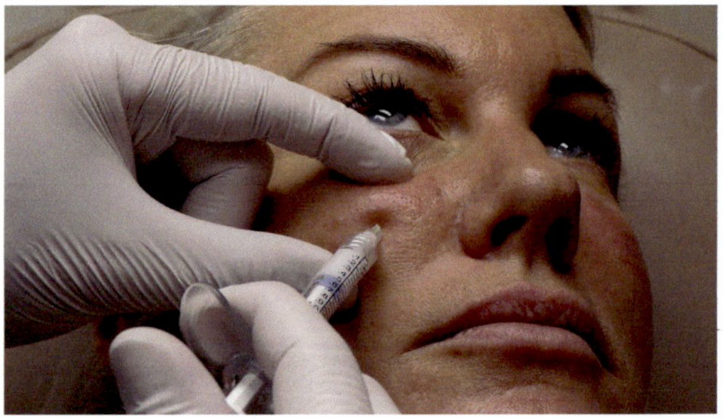

Figure 14.8 The needle should be inserted inferior to the ZCL to prevent a needle trajectory perpendicular to the skin surface (that can give more edema). Placing a finger on the infraorbital rim with the nondominant hand will make the injection safer.

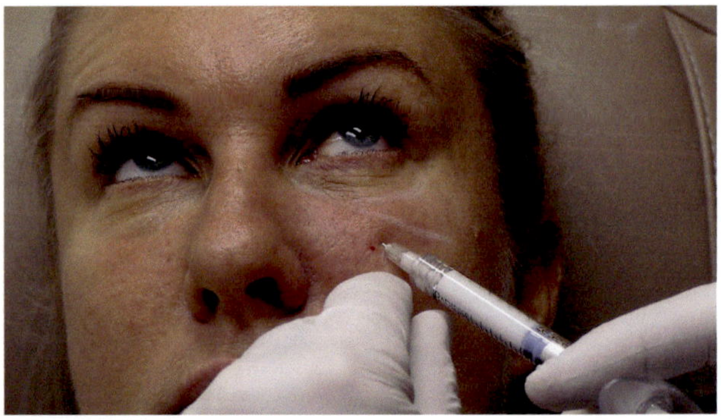

Figure 14.9 Place small aliquots on the periosteum.

periorbital area in the subcutaneous plane. 0.3 mL of the mix is the maximum used per side.
3. The cannula should be visible throughout the procedure, as the skin is very thin in this area.
4. The position of the cannula should be maintained superficial to the orbicularis muscle, just under the dermis, to avoid clumping of CaHA in the mobile muscle, which might lead to nodule formation.
5. To distribute the CaHA wash evenly, the area should be gently massaged with the fingertips or a Q-tip.

Note: The improvement in skin quality is a biological process that will gradually take place over the ensuing six months and is unlikely to be as successful in immunosuppressed patients, smokers, and those with poor diets or chronic health conditions. This treatment is suitable for patients of Fitzpatrick skin type 4 and above with melanotic pigmentation of the skin associated with the TTD and in whom the skin is not excessively thin. It is not suitable for patients with dark circles that are due to the visibility of underlying muscle and vessels through transparent skin. This area is prone to bruising, and patients need to have ceased all medications and supplements that can affect blood coagulation.

All patients (who are likely wearing concealer already to camouflage the hyperpigmentation) need to be advised of this risk and prepared to continue wearing concealer in case of visibility issues until they resolve. Based on the author's experience, all cases of visibility complications have eventually resolved without the need for additional interventions, though the resolution can sometimes take up to 12 months. No visibility issues have been encountered by the author in patients with Fitzpatrick 4 and above skin types.

14.6 VISIBILITY RISKS

There is a risk of prolonged erythema and or visibility of the CaHA crystals through thin skin that has the appearance of cream patches.

See also Figures 14.10–14.11 and Videos 14.1–14.4 to visualize before and after results and application techniques, respectively.

14.7 AFTERCARE

If necessary, the area can be manually massaged to even out the product. With an upward molding technique, the product may be advanced more medially. For 24 hours, keep area clean and proceed with a gentle washing with water. Swelling may be uneven and should subside in a day or two. Oral antihistamines can help keep the swelling to a minimum.

14.8 ADDITIONAL TREATMENTS FOR OPTIMAL RESULTS

Before addressing the TT, cheek augmentation may be considered, as deep injection of CaHA or other volumizers to the cheek will usually reduce the TT. For more natural and even correction of the infraorbital area, the palpebromalar groove may be indicated for treatment as well.

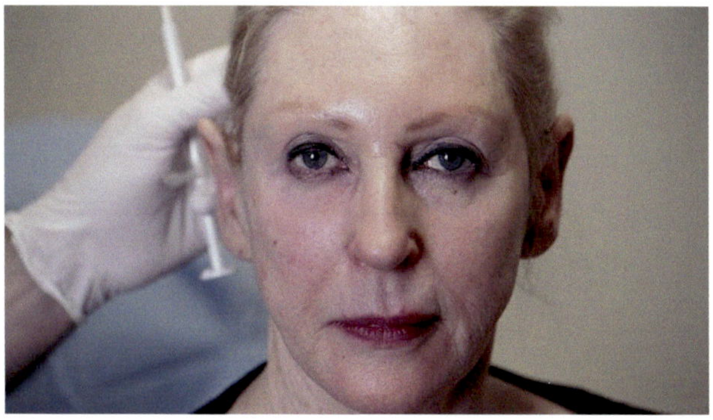

Figure 14.10 TT treatment with CaHA. Right side directly after treatment, left side untreated.

Since the skin at the TT is significantly thinner than the skin inferior to the ZCL, the color of the TT is usually darker than that of the skin below it, due to transparency of the thin skin through which bluish blood vessels can be seen. To improve skin thickness and therefore reduce dark color, chemical peels or other dermal collagen stimulating treatments may be considered. Moreover, topical skin care including growth factors can be applied after a few days of treatment.

Video 14.1 Tear trough: cannula technique.

Video 14.2 Tear trough: sharp needle technique.

Video 14.3 Periorbital Radiesse.

Video 14.4 Periorbital Radiesse wash.

REFERENCES

[1] D. K. Funt, "Avoiding malar edema during midface/cheek augmentation with dermal fillers," *J Clin Aesthet Dermatol*, vol. 4, no. 12, p. 32, Dec. 2011.

[2] D. Funt, T. Pavicic, "Dermal fillers in aesthetics: An overview of adverse events and treatment approaches," *Clin Cosmet Investig Dermatol*, vol. 6, pp. 295–316, Dec. 2013.

[3] J. A. J. van Loghem et al., "Cannula versus sharp needle for placement of soft tissue fillers: An observational cadaver study," *Aesthet Surg J*, vol. 38, no. 1, pp. 73–88, Dec. 2017.

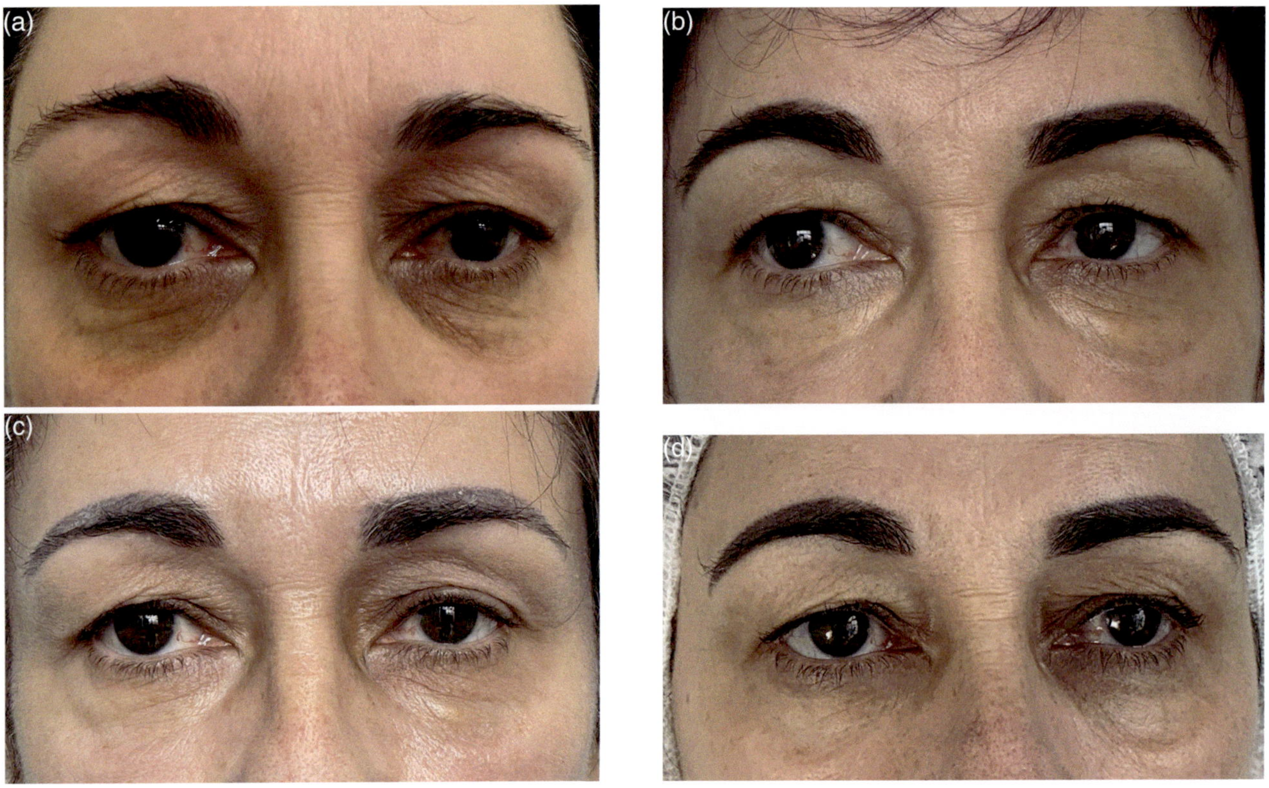

Figure 14.11 Patient (a) prior to treatment showing TTD associated with pigmentation, (b) 3 months post-treatment showing xanthelasma-like appearance of CaHA particles, (c) 12 months, and (d) 4 years post-treatment demonstrating maintenance of the outcome (correction of hyperpigmentation and improvement of rhytids and skin quality).

[4] N. Corduff, "An alternative periorbital treatment option using calcium hydroxyapatite for hyperpigmentation associated with the tear trough deformity," *Plast Reconstr Surg Glob Open*, vol. 8, no. 2, 2020.

[5] O. Hevia, "A retrospective review of calcium hydroxylapatite for correction of volume loss in the infraorbital region," *Dermatol Surg*, vol. 35, no. 10, pp. 1487–1494, Oct. 2009.

The Middle Third of the Face

Nasolabial Folds

15

JANI VAN LOGHEM

15.1 INTRODUCTION

The nasolabial folds are probably the most requested filler indication, and it is often the indication that is treated as a first choice by novel filler injectors. The nasolabial fold is located at the medial border of the nasolabial fat compartment and extends from the lateral ala, where we find the deepest point, to lateral to the oral commissures. At the nasolabial fold, different facial muscles insert into the skin, making it not only a static fold but also one with a dynamic component. The aging process results in descent of soft tissue of the cheeks, and the nasolabial fold is where the superficial nasolabial fat compartment gets stopped in this descent, causing it to fall over the muscle insertions in the skin. Bone resorption at the maxilla adds to a deepened aspect of the superior part of the nasolabial fold, dermal loss of collagen adds to sharpness of the fold, and subcutaneous volume loss adds to deepening of the fold itself [1].

15.2 SAFETY CONSIDERATIONS

When injecting the nasolabial folds with a needle, care should be taken not to inject too laterally, as the facial artery usually runs just lateral to the fold in the subcutaneous plane. At the top of the fold, close to the ala, deep injection is recommended, as superficially, the lateral nasal artery is a danger zone (Figure 15.1).

15.3 NASOLABIAL FOLD CANNULA TECHNIQUE

For injection placement, see Figure 15.2.

15.3.1 Step-by-Step Technique

1. Identify and mark the nasolabial fold.
2. Mark the entry point at the low end of the fold, so that the cannula can reach the top of the fold.
3. Disinfect. Consider giving local anesthesia at the entry point.
4. Make a pre-hole with a 23G needle (Figure 15.3).
5. Use non-diluted CaHA or standard dilution of CaHA (0.3 mL lidocaine 1% with adrenaline 1:200000 per 1.5 mL CaHA) and a 25G, 38 mm, or 50 mm cannula.
6. Point the cannula in the direction of the ala. Make sure it will stay medial to the nasolabial fat compartment.
7. Make sure that the cannula is placed below the skin, medial to the fold or in the fold, but never lateral to the fold in the nasolabial fat compartment.
8. Slowly and delicately advance the cannula to the top of the fold. If resistance is encountered, do not force the canula through, but rather rotate the syringe so that the cannula tip will find the path of least resistance past the danger zones (Figure 15.4).
9. Inject multiple retrograde linear threads of max 0.1 mL per retrograde, just medial to the fold itself.
10. Without exiting, retract the cannula to the entry point.
11. With the non-dominant hand, lift the skin in front of the cannula and maneuver the cannula through the SMAS to the periosteum of the maxilla at the lateral border of the pyriform fossa (Figure 15.5).
12. On the periosteum, the cannula tip will meet resistance of the adhesions to the pyriform fossa.
13. Do not force the cannula through these adhesions, but rather use the resistance as a marking that the ideal place for injection has been reached.

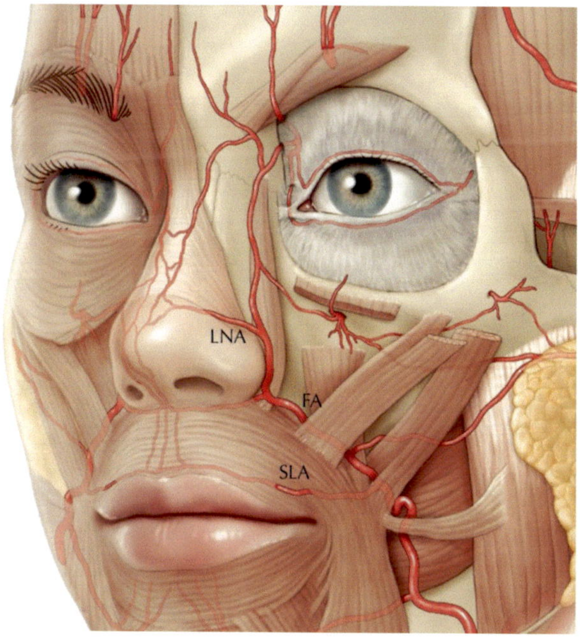

Figure 15.1 Arterial danger zones of the nasolabial fold: lateral nasal artery (LNA), facial artery (FA), and superior labial artery (SLA).

DOI: 10.1201/9781003617129-15

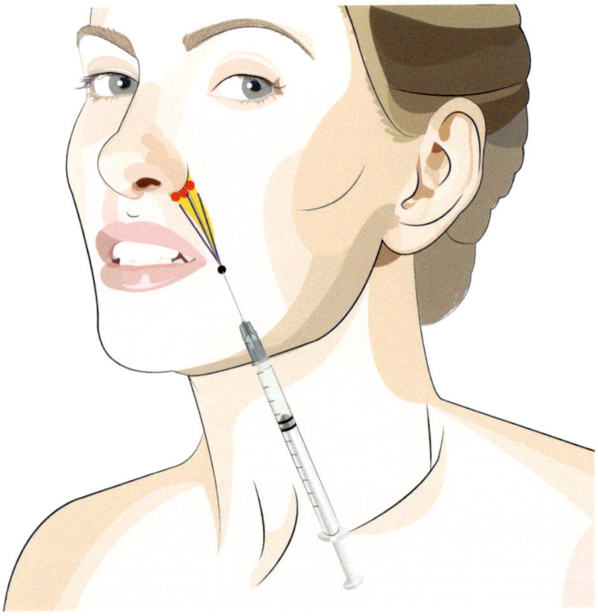

Figure 15.2 CaHA injection at the nasolabial folds using cannula. Yellow indicates the nasolabial fold. Red dots indicate deep periosteal placement at the pyriform fossa. Blue lines indicate retrograde linear threads of CaHA, medial to the nasolabial fat compartment.

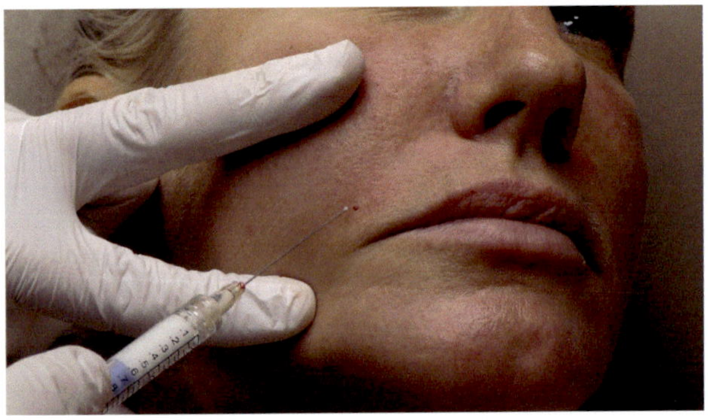

Figure 15.3 Stretch the skin to open the pre-hole.

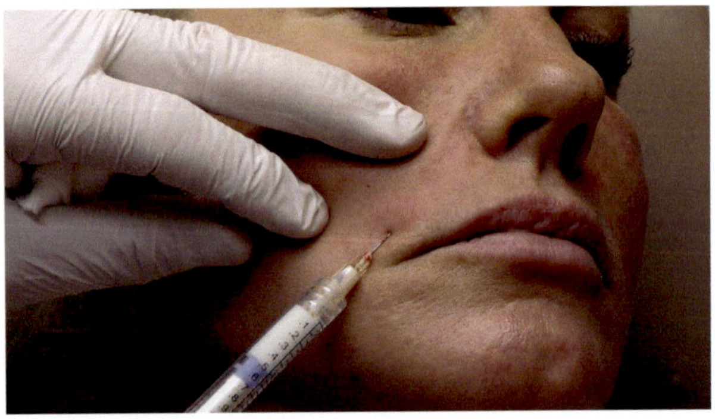

Figure 15.4 Subcutaneous injection.

14. Inject a slow bolus of approximately 0.1 mL (Figure 15.6).
15. Retract the cannula, evaluate, and readvance if needed. Inject additional boluses of CaHA.

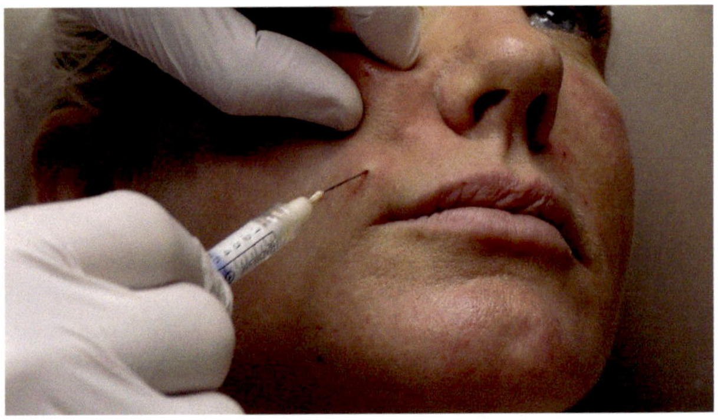

Figure 15.5 Lift the tissue to go deep.

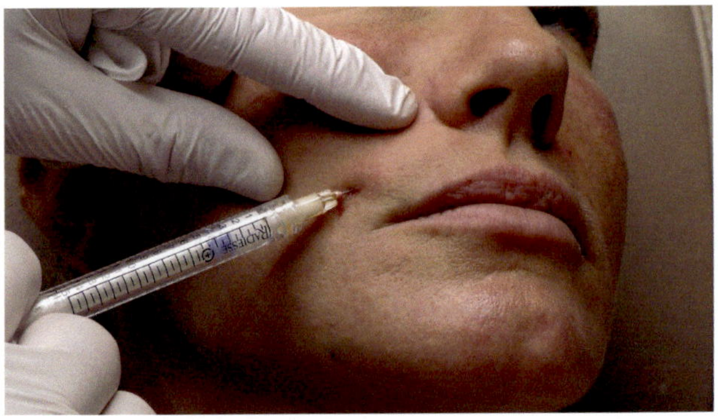

Figure 15.6 Deep periosteal injection.

16. Do not overcorrect.
17. Even out with manual massage as needed.

15.4 NASOLABIAL FOLD NEEDLE TECHNIQUE

For injection placement, see Figure 15.7.

15.4.1 Step-by-Step Technique

1. Use non-diluted CaHA or standard dilution of CaHA (0.3 mL lidocaine 1% with adrenaline 1:200000 per 1.5 mL CaHA) and a 27 or 28G needle (e.g. as supplied with the package).
2. Identify the fold by pinching the skin.
3. Start at the lower end of the nasolabial fold close to the oral commissure.
4. Introduce the needle in an angle of approximately 45° until the tip has reached the dermal–subdermal junction.
5. Reorient the needle to parallel to the skin.
6. Advance the needle cranially along the fold.
7. Make sure that during the retrograde injections, the product is never injected lateral to the fold (Figure 15.8).
8. Inject two or three retrograde linear threads of 0.05 mL each (Figure 15.9).
9. Remove the needle from the skin.
10. Repeat these fans, moving cranially, always moving the needle while injecting small quantities.

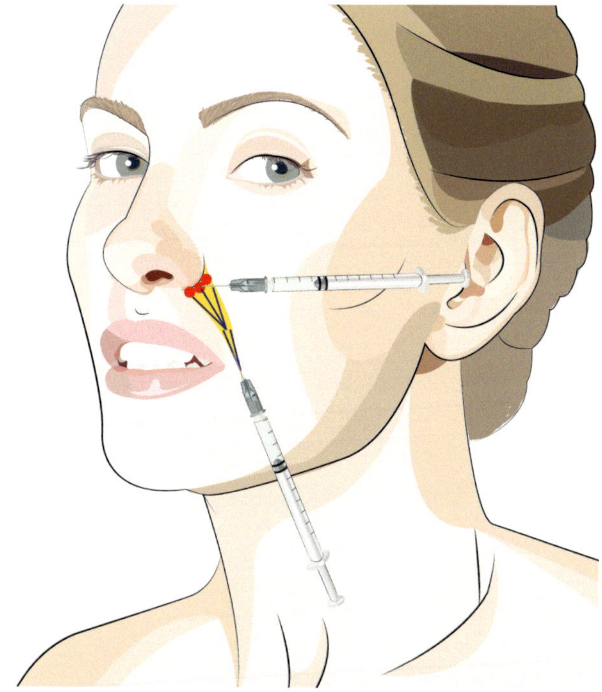

Figure 15.7 CaHA injection at the nasolabial folds using sharp needle. Depending on the length of the needle, two or three fans can be injected.

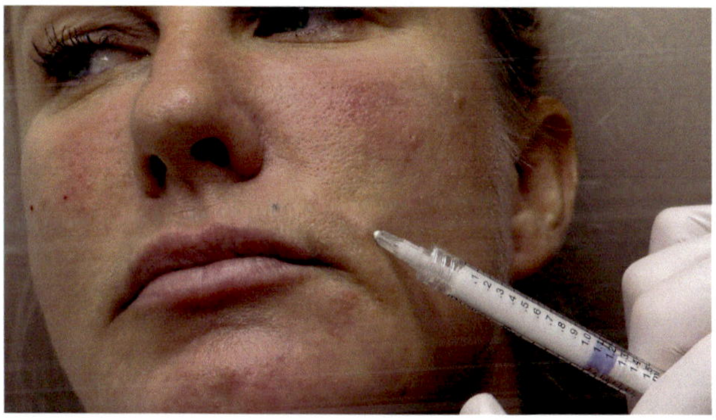

Figure 15.8 Injection depth is at the deep dermal–subdermal level. The gray of the needle should not be visible through the skin to avoid visible product.

11. Remove the needle and readvance it from the top of the fold, perpendicular to the skin toward the periosteum of the maxilla.
12. Inject a small bolus of 0.05–0.1 mL with the needle tip in contact with the maxilla.
13. If the needle is felt passing the maxilla, it may be inside the pyriform aperture. Retract it and readvance to the periosteum (Figure 15.10).
14. Always inject slowly with the bolus technique.

See also Videos 15.1–15.2 for application techniques.

15.5 AFTERCARE

If necessary, the area can be manually massaged to even out the product. With one finger inside the mouth

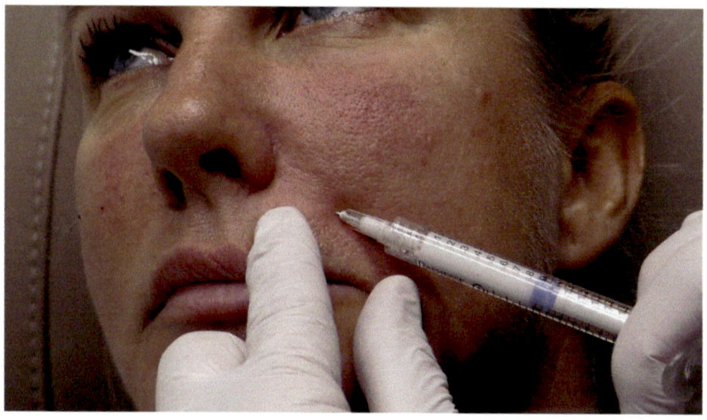

Figure 15.9 Close to the ala, more retrograde linear threads may be injected medially, as the fold is wider here.

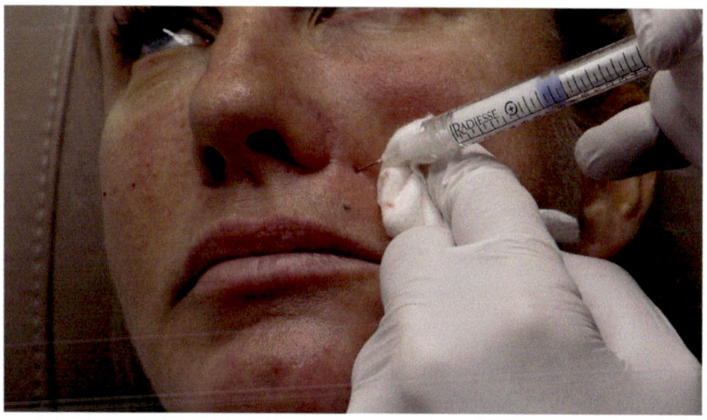

Figure 15.10 A soft touch to the periosteum will reduce discomfort.

and the thumb on the skin, the product can easily be evened out. Swelling may be uneven and should subside in a day or two.

15.6 ADDITIONAL TREATMENTS FOR OPTIMAL RESULTS

Before addressing the nasolabial folds, cheek augmentation may be considered, as deep injection of CaHA or other volumizers to the cheek will usually reduce the nasolabial folds.

Video 15.1 Nasolabial folds: cannula technique.

Video 15.2 Nasolabial folds: sharp needle technique.

REFERENCE

[1] R. B. Shaw et al., "Aging of the facial skeleton: Aesthetic implications and rejuvenation strategies," *Plast Reconstr Surg*, vol. 127, no. 1, pp. 374–383, 2011.

The Middle Third of the Face

Palpebromalar Groove

16

JANI VAN LOGHEM

16.1 INTRODUCTION

The palpebromalar groove (PMG), also known as the lid–cheek junction, is located laterally in the infraorbital area. It is an indication with a very strong rejuvenating power, as correction of the PMG hides evidence of aging. During the ageing process, the orbits widen most significantly at the inferolateral side due to bone resorption [1]. The orbicularis retaining ligament (ORL), which has its origin at the orbital rim, is therefore pulled inward and in inferolateral direction during ageing. The ligament is oriented downward from its origin and inserts into the orbicularis oculi muscle that is attached to the skin. Placement of filler product just below the ORL can push the ORL into a more horizontal orientation and therefore reduce the groove created by the ORL insertion. Treating the PMG can reduce evidence of bone resorption and can therefore trick the observer into estimating a lower age. An additional advantage of treating this area is the effect on the canthal tilt; by injecting CaHA on the periosteum of the inferolateral orbital rim, a non-surgical cantho-modulation can be observed.

16.2 SAFETY CONSIDERATIONS

When injecting the PMG with a needle, care should be taken not to inject too much product in a single bolus, as backflow through the tunnel created with the needle can be expected and could accumulate in the lateral sub-orbicularis oculi fat compartment (SOOF) [2]. When the product flows back to more superficial layers, edema or accumulation of product in a confined space (SOOF) is more likely to occur. Funt described a good technique for using sharp needles while avoiding malar edema [3].

The arterial dangers are represented by the zygomaticofacial artery, the lateral palpebral artery, the transverse facial artery, and their branches, plus the inferior marginal arterial arcade branches (Figure 16.1).

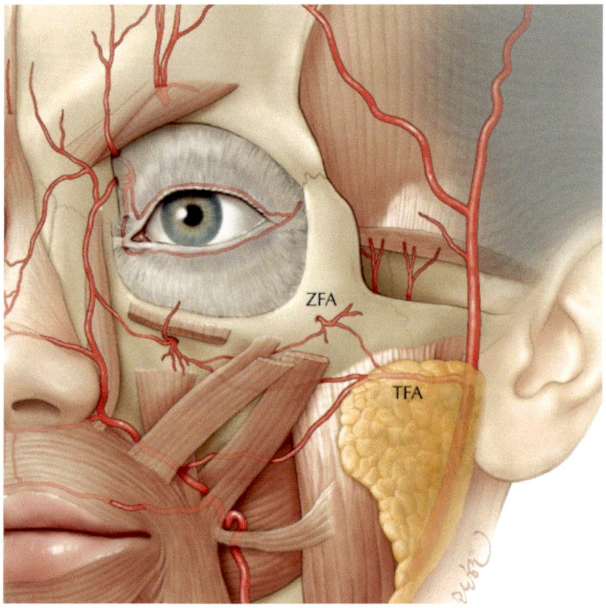

Figure 16.1 Arterial danger zones to consider in the palpebromalar groove are the zygomaticofacial artery (ZFA) and transverse facial artery (TFA).

16.3 PALPEBROMALAR GROOVE CANNULA TECHNIQUE 1

For injection placement, see Figure 16.2.

16.3.1 Step-by-Step technique

1. Identify and mark the skin insertion of the ORL, and mark the inferior orbital rim. It should show that the superficial insertion of this ligament is lower than the bony origin.
2. Mark the entry point lateral from the skin insertion of the orbicularis oculi muscle, so that the cannula can reach the PMG (Figure 16.3).
3. Disinfect. Consider applying a zygomaticofacial nerve block and local anesthesia at the entry points (refer to Chapter 3).
4. Make a pre-hole with a 23G needle.
5. Use non-diluted CaHA or standard dilution of CaHA (0.3 mL 1% lidocaine with adrenaline 1:200000 per 1.5 mL CaHA) and a 25G, 38 mm cannula.
6. Point the cannula in the direction of the PMG (Figure 16.4).
7. With the non-dominant hand, lift the tissue in front of the cannula tip and maneuver the cannula through resistances to the periosteum. Take the convexity of the bone into consideration as well as the danger of puncturing through the ORL and damaging the globus.
8. On the periosteum, guide the cannula with a non-dominant finger on the infraorbital rim and slide the cannula directly to the ORL origin on the periosteum (Figure 16.5).

DOI: 10.1201/9781003617129-16

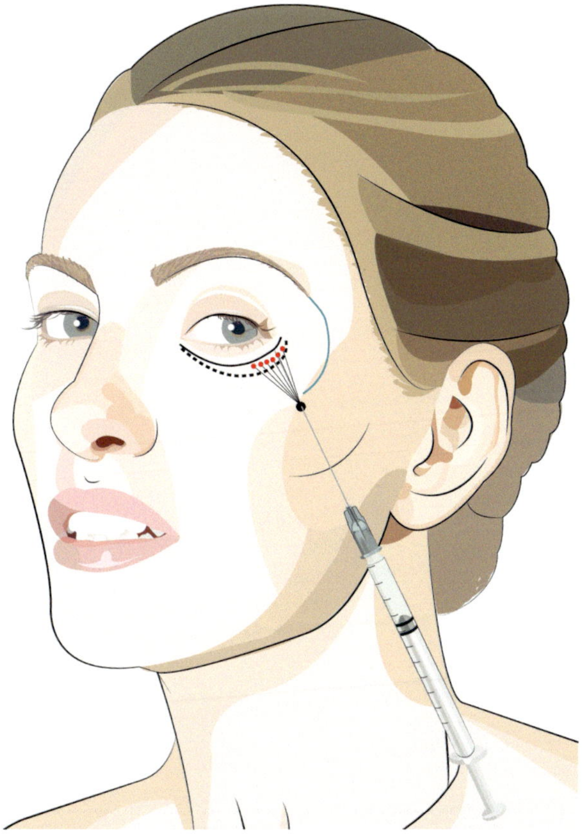

Figure 16.2 Product injection at the PMG. The black line represents the origin of the ORL on the rim, and the dotted black line indicates the superficial insertion. Red lines indicate CaHA product placement at the periosteal level underneath the ORL. Entry point is lateral to orbicularis oculi skin insertion (blue line).

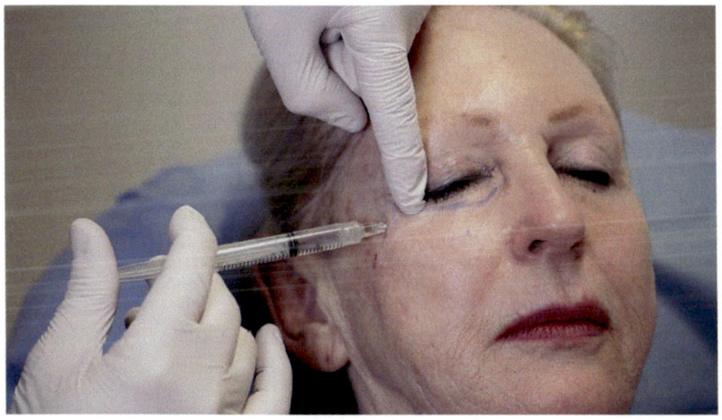

Figure 16.3 Local anesthesia at the periosteal level can be injected to reduce discomfort and to create space in the target area (hydrodissection).

9. Inject a small aliquot (approximately 0.025–0.05 mL per bolus) on the infraorbital rim.
10. Retract the cannula partially, readvance to just beside the previous bolus, and reinject a small bolus.
11. Do not overcorrect (Figure 16.6).
12. Even out with manual massage toward the ORL as needed.

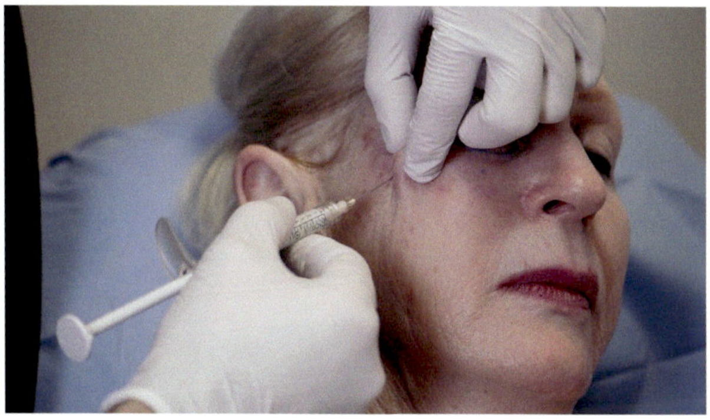

Figure 16.4 Make sure the cannula direction is toward the target (PMG) while lifting the skin in front of the cannula.

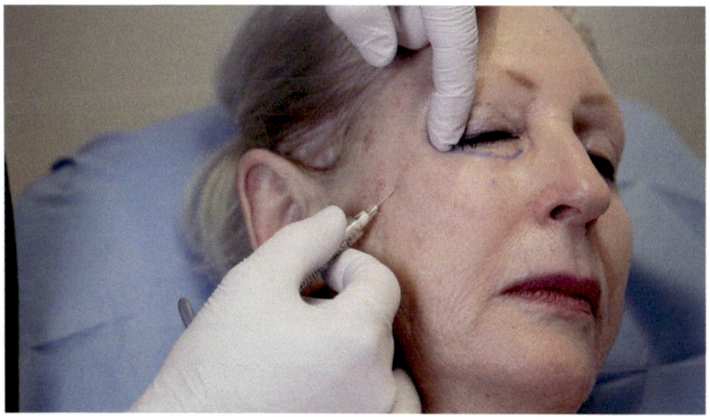

Figure 16.5 Use finger of the non-dominant hand to avoid advancing the cannula too far (into the orbital area).

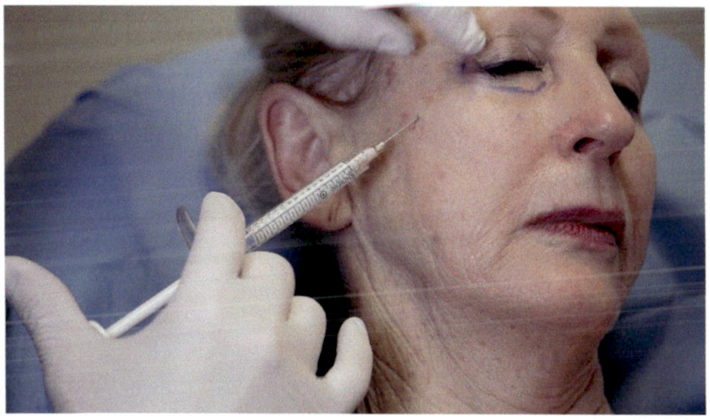

Figure 16.6 Place small aliquots. Do not overcorrect.

16.4 PALPEBROMALAR GROOVE CANNULA TECHNIQUE 2

For injection placement, see Figure 16.7.

16.4.1 Step-by-Step Technique

1. Identify and mark the skin insertion of the ORL, and mark the inferior orbital rim. It should show that the superficial insertion of this ligament is lower than the bony origin.
2. Mark the entry points lateral from the skin insertion of the orbicularis oculi muscle, so that the cannula can reach the PMG without pointing directly to the globus (Figure 16.8).

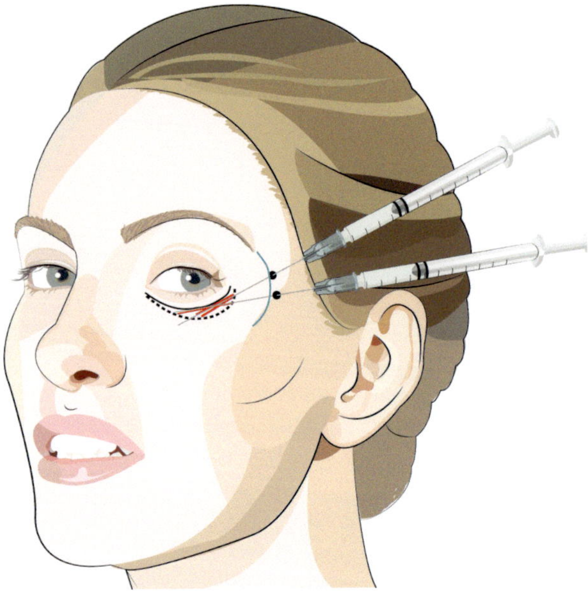

Figure 16.7 Product injection at the PMG. The black line represents the origin of the ORL on the rim and the dotted black line indicates the superficial insertion. Red lines indicate CaHA product placement at the periosteal level underneath the ORL. Entry points are lateral to orbicularis oculi skin insertion (blue line).

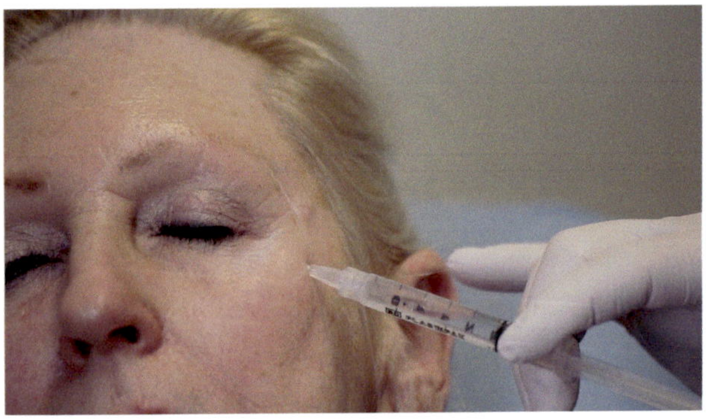

Figure 16.8 Local anesthesia at the periosteum for patient comfort and hydrodissection.

3. Disinfect. Consider giving a zygomaticofacial nerve block and local anesthesia at the entry points.
4. Make a pre-hole with a 23G needle.
5. Use non-diluted CaHA or standard dilution of CaHA (0.3 mL 1% lidocaine with adrenaline 1:200000 per 1.5 mL CaHA) and a 25G, 38 mm cannula.
6. Point the cannula in the direction of the PMG (Figure 16.9).
7. With the non-dominant hand, lift up the tissue in front of the cannula tip and maneuver the cannula through resistances to the periosteum. As the lateral orbital thickening is a strong structure, the high entry point may be more difficult, as some force is needed to pass this ligamentous structure.
8. On the periosteum, guide the cannula with a non-dominant finger on the rim and slide the cannula medially just below the infraorbital rim (Figure 16.10).

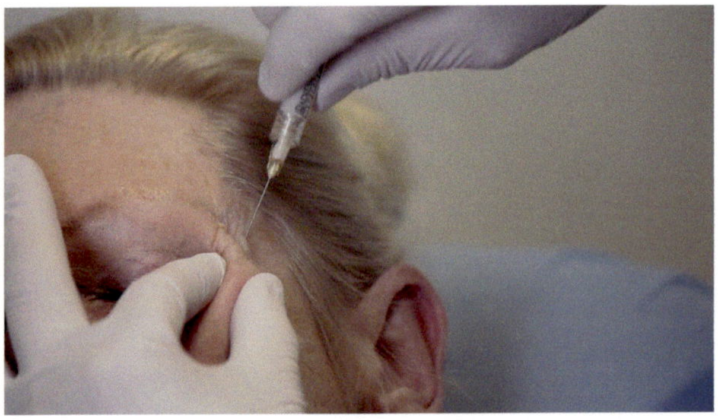

Figure 16.9 Make sure the cannula direction is toward the target (medial tear trough) while lifting the skin in front of the cannula.

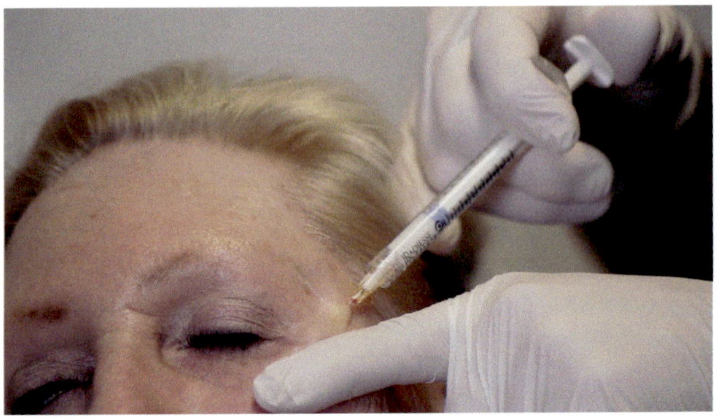

Figure 16.10 Keeping some pressure with the non-dominant finger inferior to the cannula may improve positioning of product adjacent to the ORL.

9. Inject small amounts while retracting (approximately 0.1–0.2 mL should suffice).
10. If necessary, from the second entry point, repeat these steps and place additional deposits as needed.
11. Do not overcorrect.
12. Even out with manual massage as needed.

16.5 PALPEBROMALAR GROOVE NEEDLE TECHNIQUE

For injection placement see Figure 16.11.

16.5.1 Step-by-Step Technique

1. Identify and mark the skin insertion of the ORL, the rim, and the zygomaticofacial foramen. Realize that the superficial insertions of these ligaments are lower than the bony origins.
2. Mark the area (Figure 16.12).
3. Disinfect. Consider giving a zygomaticofacial nerve block.
4. Use non-diluted CaHA or standard dilution of CaHA (0.3 mL 1% lidocaine with adrenaline 1:200000 per 1.5 mL CaHA) and a 27G needle supplied with the product.

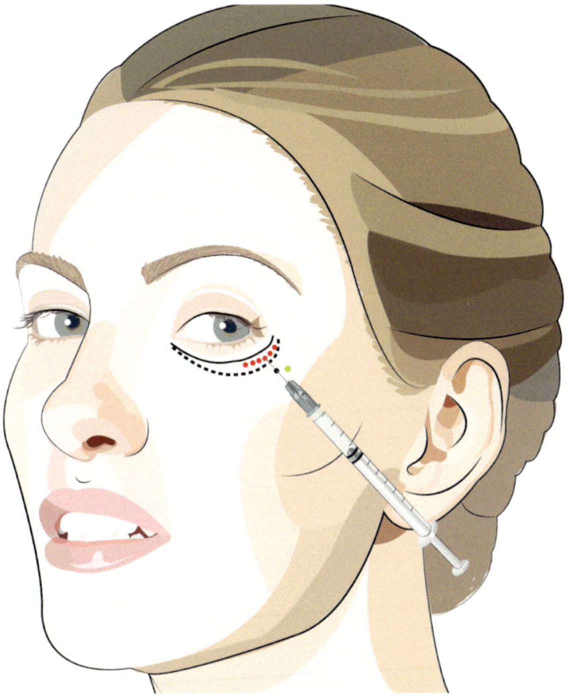

Figure 16.11 CaHA injection at the PMG using sharp needle. The black line represents the origin of the ORL on the rim, and the dotted black line indicates the superficial insertion. Red dots indicate CaHA product placement at the periosteal level underneath the ORL. Entry point is at about 45 degrees to the periosteum. Green dot: approximate location of zygomaticofacial foramen.

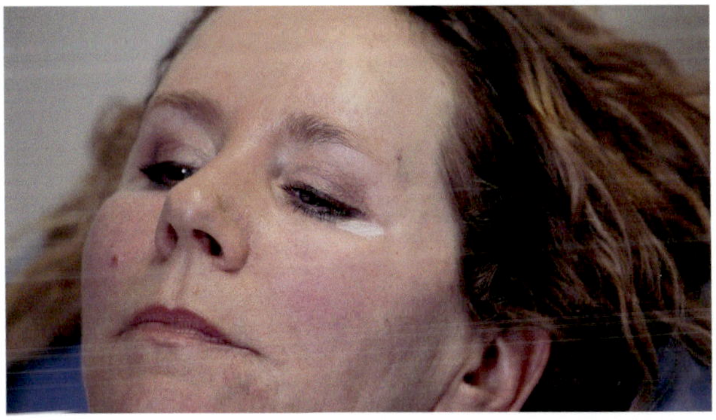

Figure 16.12 Palpate and mark the inferolateral orbital rim and mark the skin depression at the location of the muscular insertion of the ORL.

5. Lift the cheek and keep a finger of the non-dominant hand on the infraorbital rim to avoid inadvertent intraorbital injection (Figure 16.13).
6. Use a skin entry point approximately 1 cm inferior to the PMG.
7. With the bevel down and a 45° direction to the bone surface, advance the needle slowly to the periosteum.

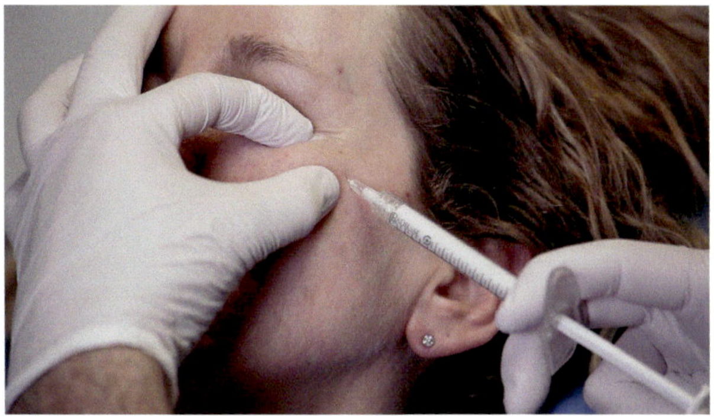

Figure 16.13 Place small aliquots. Do not overcorrect.

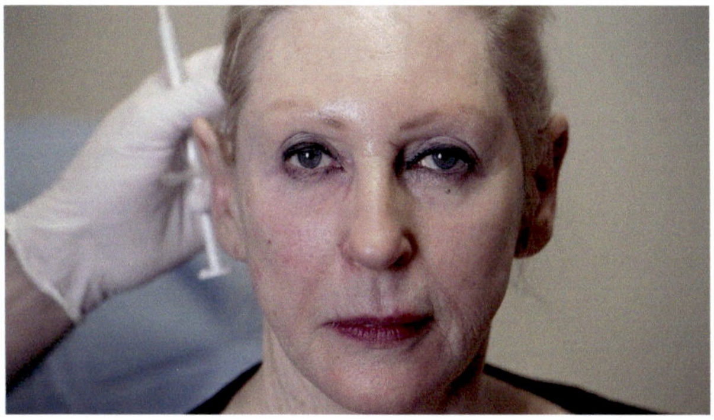

Figure 16.14 Immediate results of one side treated (anatomical right side); note the improvement of canthal tilt. Notice that the tear trough deformity was also treated here.

8. With a soft touch to the periosteum, inject a series of small aliquots of approximately 0.025–0.05 mL each.
9. If necessary, remove the needle, reinsert the needle more medially, and repeat.
10. Do not overcorrect (Figure 16.13).
11. Even out with manual massage as needed.

See also Figure 16.14 and Videos 16.1–16.3 for post-treatment results and application techniques, respectively.

16.6 AFTERCARE

If necessary, the area can be manually massaged to even out the product. With an upward molding technique, the product may be advanced more cranially. Edema may be uneven and should subside in a day or two.

16.7 ADDITIONAL TREATMENTS FOR OPTIMAL RESULTS

Before addressing the PMG, cheek augmentation should be considered, as deep injection of CaHA or other volumizers to the lateral cheek can potentially worsen the PMG. For more natural and even correction of the infraorbital area, the tear trough may be indicated for treatment as well.

Video 16.1 Palpebromalar groove: cannula technique 1.

Video 16.2 Palpebromalar groove: cannula technique 2.

Video 16.3 Palpebromalar groove: sharp needle technique.

REFERENCES

[1] D. K. Funt, "Avoiding malar edema during midface/cheek augmentation with dermal fillers," *J Clin Aesthet Dermatol*, vol. 4, no. 12, p. 32, Dec. 2011.
[2] J. A. J. van Loghem et al., "Cannula versus sharp needle for placement of soft tissue fillers: An observational cadaver study," *Aesthet Surg J*, vol. 38, no. 1, pp. 73–88, Dec. 2017.
[3] R. B. Shaw et al., "Aging of the facial skeleton: Aesthetic implications and rejuvenation strategies," *Plast Reconstr Surg*, vol. 127, no. 1, pp. 374–383, 2011.

The Middle Third of the Face

17

Nose Augmentation

STEVEN DAYAN, THUY-VAN TINA HO AND JANI VAN LOGHEM

17.1 INTRODUCTION

The nose is an important element in the face that contributes to male attractiveness. Although the value of nose augmentation is evident, there are serious adverse events (SAEs) reported after nose augmentation with fillers, such as necrosis and blindness secondary to intravascular injection [1]. CaHA can be used to improve nasal shape by injecting it into the dorsum of the nose in the sub-SMAS plane, below the level of the blood vessels that are typically associated with these SAEs (Figures 17.1 and 17.2) [2]. The nasofrontal and nasolabial angles and supratip region, as well as areas of dorsal irregularity, are routinely addressed with filler injection to improve the nasal appearance (Figure 17.3).

The ideal instrument for injection is a nontraumatic cannula of 22G or thicker to reduce the chance of inadvertent intra-arterial injection of the nasal arteries and branches. Notice that there is still a debate on the safest product deposition techniques for non-surgical rhinoplasty between cannulas and sharp needles [3]. The practitioner should be educated on nasal anatomy and product volumes before conducting this practice [4]. Pre-infiltration and hydrodissection with non-adrenalized 1–2% lidocaine from multiple entry points can reduce the risk of intravascular injection even further. For greater control over precise amounts of CaHA, the contents of the original syringe can be transferred to a disposable 1 mL Luer-lock syringe using a female-to-female Luer-lock connector. Taking into account the contouring capacity of CaHA is an important consideration for nose augmentation; the full viscosity product can be used without premixing with lidocaine. This reduces the risk of the "Avatar nose" deformity, where less viscous products can migrate to the lateral sides of the nose.

17.2 NOSE AUGMENTATION IN MEN, CANNULA TECHNIQUE (FOUR-POINT CANNULA TECHNIQUE)

For injection placement, see Figure 17.4.

17.2.1 Step-by-Step Technique

1. Mark the dorsal hump in the midline and create a port site with a 20G sharp needle (1 in Figure 17.4).
2. Introduce the cannula attached to a 1% lidocaine-filled syringe into the port site and advance it through the SMAS toward the periosteum. Infiltrate approximately 0.3 mL to hydrodissect the plane and create space for the CaHA product (Figure 17.5).
3. Create a second port site with the 20G sharp needle at the nasofrontal angle (2 in Figure 17.4).
4. Advance the cannula perpendicular to the skin toward the periosteum and infiltrate approximately 0.2 mL 1% lidocaine with the cannula tip touching the periosteum. Apply lateral pressure to the nasal root with thumb and index finger of the non-dominant hand to prevent lateral spread of infiltration (Figure 17.6).
5. Create a third port site with the 20G needle at the base of the columella (3 in Figure 17.4).
6. Advance the cannula deeper into the columella base and inject approximately 0.2 mL of 1% lidocaine to create a space in the tissue (Figure 17.7).
7. Create a fourth port site with the 20G needle at the tip of the nose (4 in Figure 17.4).
8. Switch from lidocaine to product-filled syringe with undiluted CaHA for maximum viscosity in a 1 mL disposable syringe for greater control.
9. Introduce the cannula through the nasal tip port site and advance it inferiorly to the base of the columella and inject in retrograde fashion from the base of the columella toward the nose tip (Figure 17.8). This technique should improve the nasolabial angle of the nose.
10. Introduce the cannula through the port site at the nasofrontal angle. With the cannula tip touching the periosteum, inject approximately 0.2–0.3 mL of CaHA until the nasofrontal angle is satisfactorily corrected (Figure 17.9).

17.3 NOSE AUGMENTATION, CANNULA TECHNIQUE (ONE-POINT CANNULA TECHNIQUE)

For injection placement, see Figure 17.10.

17.3.1 Step-by-Step Technique

1. Mark the supraciliary line and determine the area of the nasofrontal angle, the supratip angle, and the nasolabial angle to be augmented. This technique can be used in patients with minimal or no dorsal hump.
2. Consider anesthetizing the nose tip before making a pre-hole with a 23G needle.

DOI: 10.1201/9781003617129-17

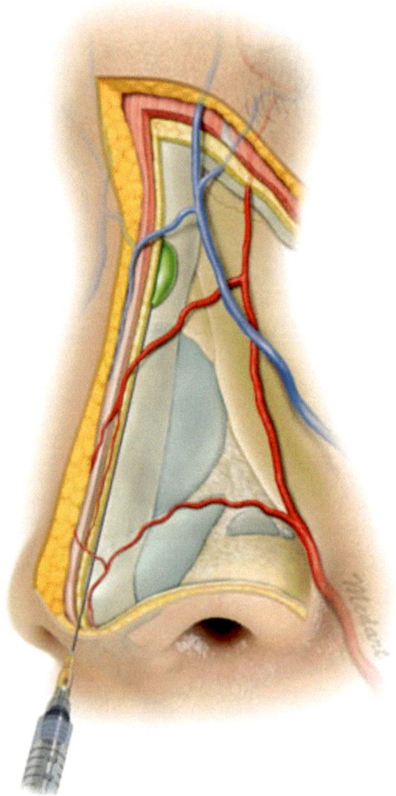

Figure 17.1 Safest plane for filler material (depicted in green) into the nasal dorsum: sub-SMAS in the midline of the nose. (Reproduced from Kim HJ *et al. Clinical Anatomy of the Face for Filler and Botulinum Toxin Injection*, Springer: Singapore, 2016; with permission) [5].

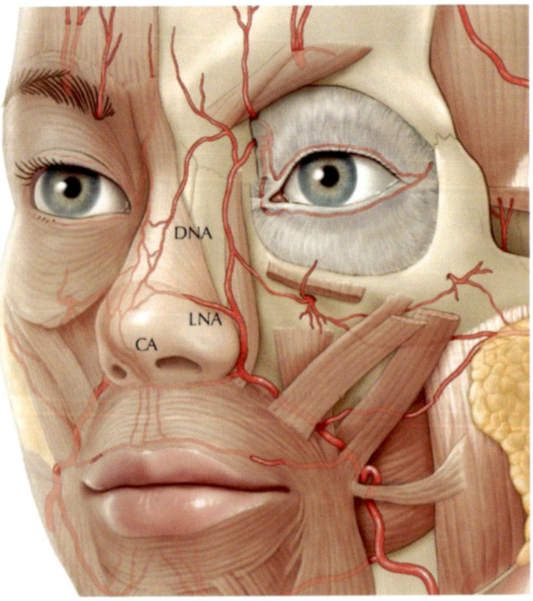

Figure 17.2 Arterial danger zones to consider in nose augmentation are: columellar artery (CA), lateral nasal artery (LNA), and dorsal nasal artery (DNA).

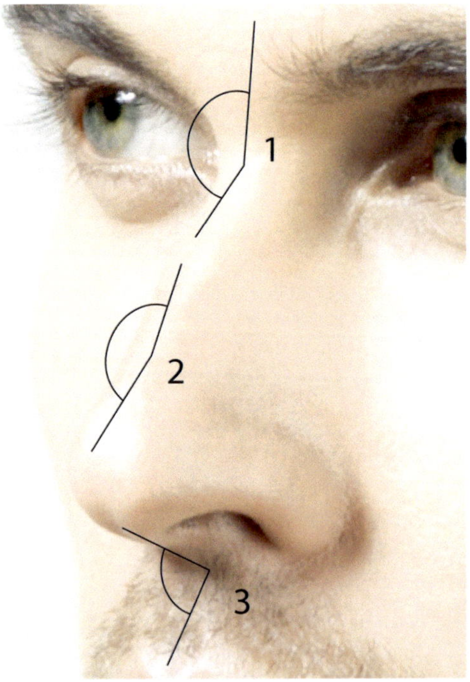

Figure 17.3 Targeted nasal areas for filler injection: (1) nasofrontal angle (ideally 115–135°), (2) supratip break, and (3) nasolabial angle (typically 90–95° in males, 95–110° in females).

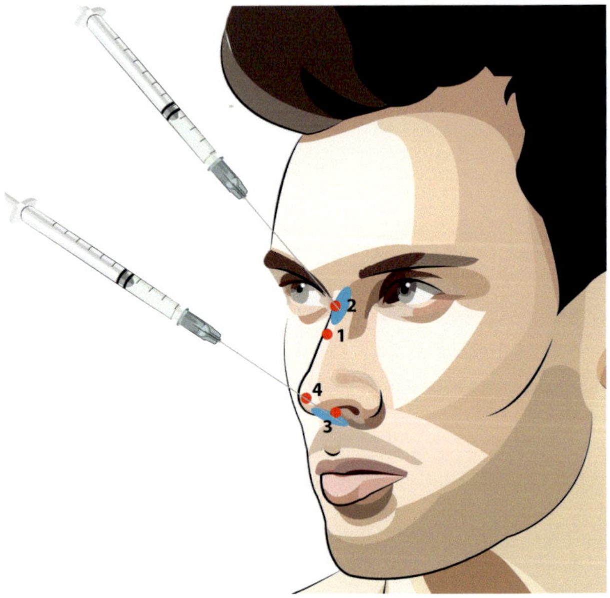

Figure 17.4 Product injection at the nasofrontal and nasolabial angles in males. Red dots indicate the entry points for the nontraumatic cannulas being (1) dorsal hump, (2) nasofrontal angle, (3) base of the columella, and (4) tip of the nose. Blue areas mark designated depositions of CaHA.

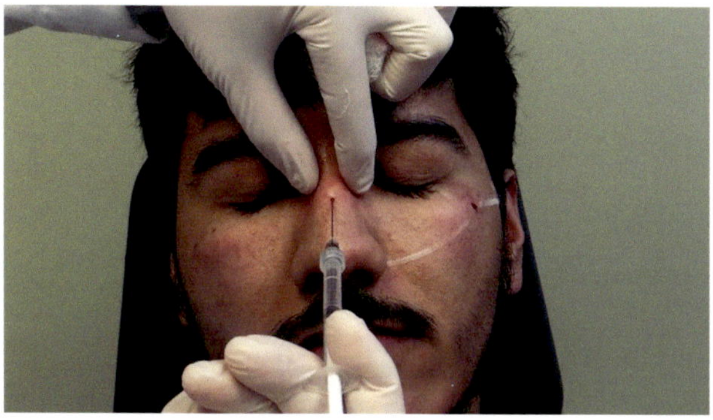

Figure 17.5 Entry of cannula into dorsal hump, followed by lidocaine pre-infiltration in sub-SMAS plane.

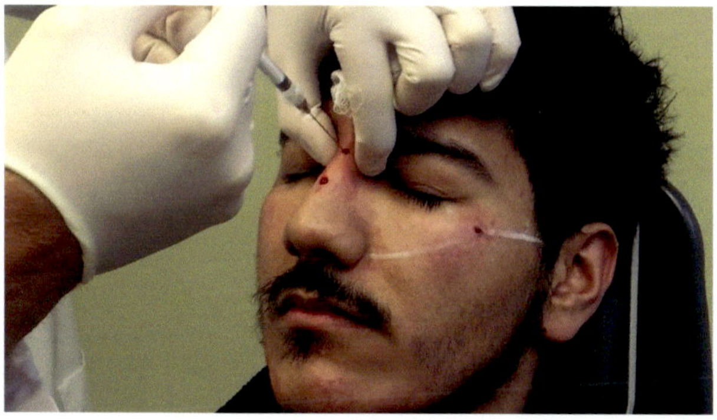

Figure 17.6 Second port site at the nasofrontal angle with lidocaine pre-infiltration.

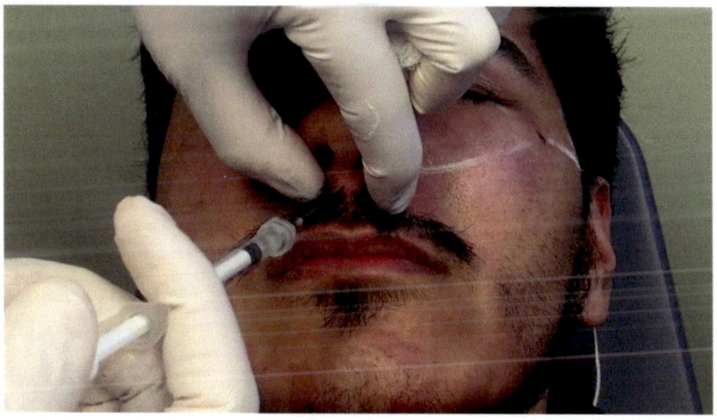

Figure 17.7 Third port site at the base of the columella with lidocaine pre-infiltration.

3. Use non-diluted CaHA and a 25G, 38 mm cannula.
4. Introduce the cannula and advance it through the SMAS to the perichondrium of the nose tip (Figure 17.11).
5. Keep lifting the skin with the nondominant hand in order to smoothly advance the cannula cranially over the perichondrium and periosteum of the nasal bone.
6. Maneuver the cannula through the origin of the procerus muscles and make sure the cannula is placed periosteally at the nasofrontal angle.

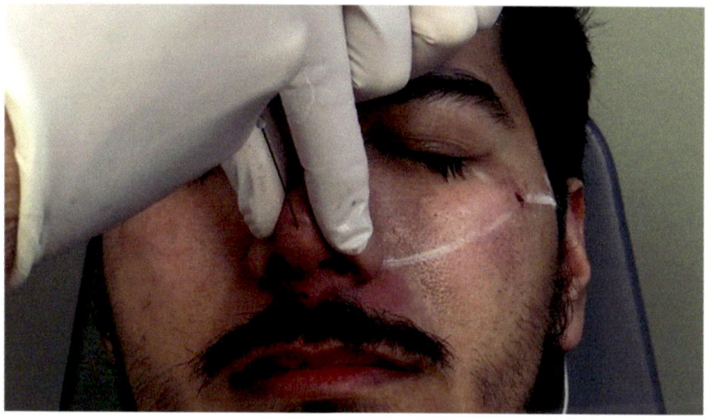

Figure 17.8 Fourth port site at the nasal tip with retrograde injection of CaHA.

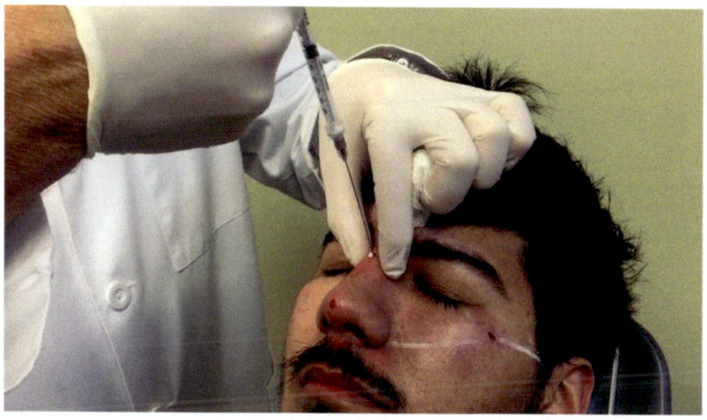

Figure 17.9 Injection of CaHA at the nasofrontal angle with cannula tip in contact with periosteum.

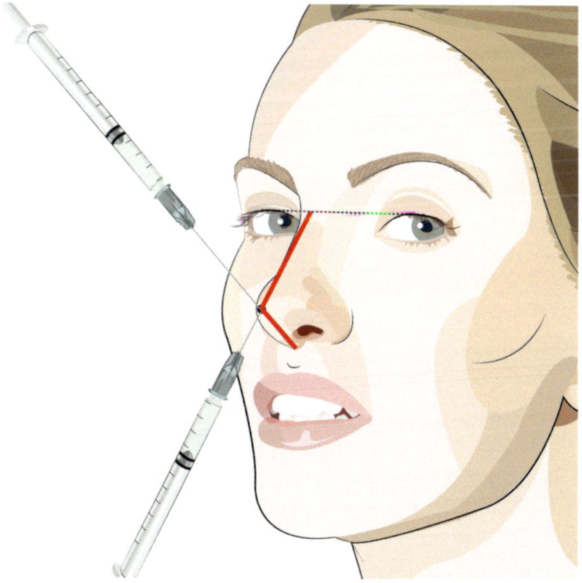

Figure 17.10 Nose augmentation with cannula at the periosteal or perichondral level in females. The red lines indicate placement of CaHA product in the midline. The dotted line indicates the supraciliary line (the ideal horizontal location of the nasofrontal angle).

7. Place the thumb and index fingers of the nondominant hand on the location of the supratrochlear notches and press to the bone in order to temporarily reduce blood flow (Figure 17.12).
8. Inject small amounts of CaHA (the author advises 0.025 mL per deposit or retrograde to minimize risk of blindness).
9. Retract to the supratip angle and place additional deposits at the sub-SMAS level.
10. Check and mold (Figure 17.13). Repeat steps if necessary.
11. Now move the cannula down to the nasolabial angle.
12. Advance below the SMAS to the angle.
13. Inject small amounts of CaHA (the author advises 0.025 mL per deposit or retrograde to minimize risks).

See further Figure 17.14 and Videos 17.1–17.2 for before and after results in male and application techniques, respectively.

17.4 AFTERCARE

After injection, transient swelling or bruising of the nose may be observed. The patient should be counseled that any swelling or bruising may last up to three days and is temporary. Ice packs may be applied the evening after treatment to help reduce swelling and bruising. The patient should not wear any glasses that might rest on the treated area (e.g. nasofrontal angle) for at least two weeks. The patient should be advised not to touch any of the injection port sites with unclean fingers for two hours after the treatment.

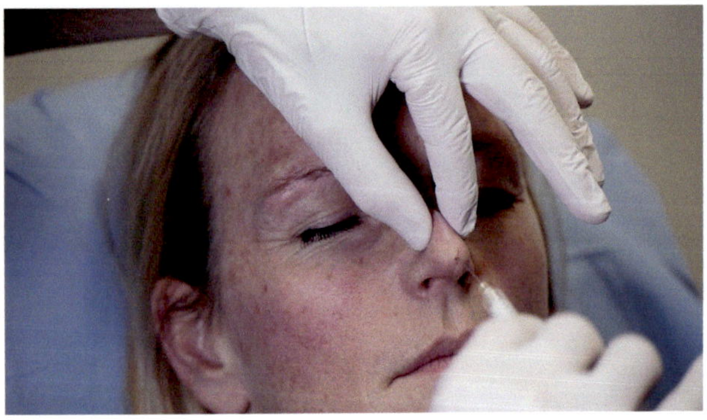

Figure 17.11 Use nondominant hand to advance the cannula to the sub-SMAS level.

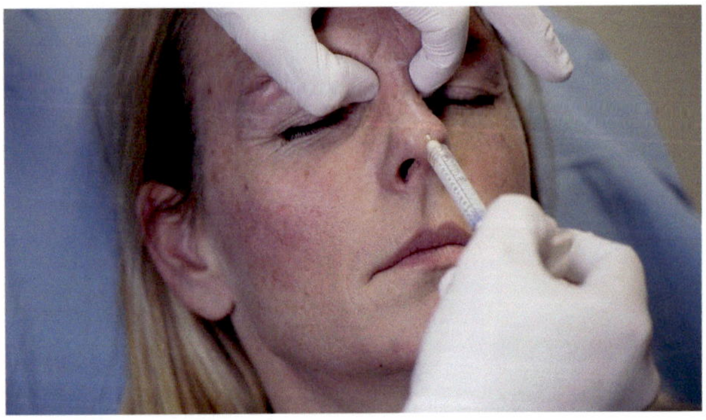

Figure 17.12 Use pressure of thumb and index finger to reduce blood flow of the supratrochlear arteries.

17.5 ADDITIONAL TREATMENTS FOR OPTIMAL RESULTS

Skin problems that occur often in the nasal area such as visible pores, blood vessels, and pigmentation spots can be addressed with other treatment modalities, including chemical peels, laser, and microdermabrasion.

Video 17.1 Nose augmentation, 4 entry points: cannula.

Video 17.2 Nose augmentation, 1 entry point: cannula.

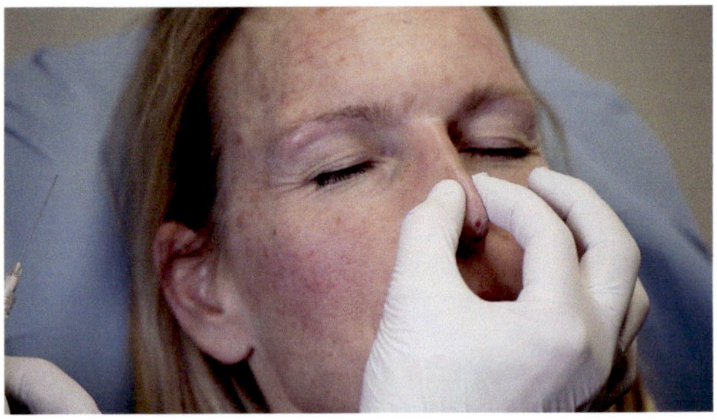

Figure 17.13 After injection, mold the product into the desired shape.

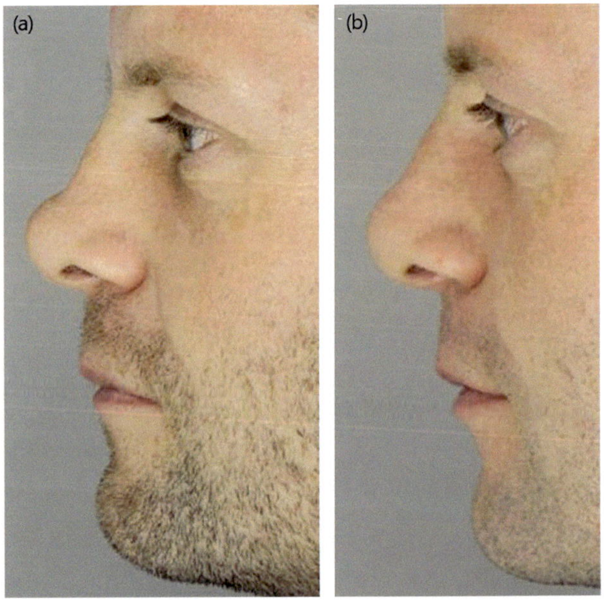

Figure 17.14 Example of a patient before (a) and after (b) treatment with 0.3 mL of CaHA along the dorsum, resulting in a more optimal dorsal contour.

REFERENCES

[1] J. A. J. van Loghem et al., "Cannula versus sharp needle for placement of soft tissue fillers: An observational cadaver study," *Aesthet Surg J*, vol. 38, no. 1, pp. 73–88, Dec. 2017.
[2] C. Delorenzi, "Complications of injectable fillers, part 2: Vascular complications," *Aesthet Surg J*, vol. 34, no. 4, pp. 584–600, 2014.
[3] G. S. Jung et al., "A safer non-surgical filler augmentation rhinoplasty based on the anatomy of the nose," *Aesthetic Plast Surg*, vol. 43, no. 2, pp. 447–452, Apr. 2019.
[4] F. Rosengaus, A. Nikolis, "Cannula versus needle in medical rhinoplasty: The nose knows," *J Cosmet Dermatol*, vol. 19, no. 12, pp. 3222–3228, Dec. 2020.
[5] H.-J. Kim et al., "Clinical anatomy of the face for filler and botulinum toxin injection," in: *Clinical Anatomy of the Face for Filler and Botulinum Toxin Injection*. Springer, 2016.

The Middle Third of the Face

Preauricular Wrinkles

JANI VAN LOGHEM

18

18.1 INTRODUCTION

Preauricular wrinkles occur during the ageing process and are the result of both volume loss, skin laxity, and pull of masseteric cutaneous ligaments from a resorbing mandible moving anteriorly [1]. The ideal correction of preauricular wrinkles focuses on all age-related anatomical changes and therefore should contain volume replacement and skin rejuvenation. The danger zones are the external carotid artery and the parotid gland (both located sub-SMAS) (Figure 18.1). Safe and effective injection planes are therefore the subcutaneous and dermal levels [2]. Theoretically, the bone resorption of the mandible should also be addressed. Practically, this is not always necessary. Injection of CaHA at the mandible (periosteal plane) is discussed in more detail in the chapter on masseter augmentation.

18.2 PREAURICULAR WRINKLES, MULTILEVEL TECHNIQUE

For injection placement, see Figure 18.2.

18.2.1 Step-by-Step Technique

1. Mark and disinfect the area to be treated.
2. Make a pre-hole with a 23G needle at the mandibular angle.
3. Use undiluted or normal dilution CaHA and a 25G, 38 mm, or 50 mm cannula for subcutaneous injection.
4. Advance the cannula through the skin into the subcutaneous fat (lateral temporal cheek fat compartment) (Figure 18.3).
5. Place multiple retrograde linear threads in a fanning technique until sufficient volume correction is achieved.
6. Mold as needed.
7. Determine the necessity of intradermal injection (thin skin with wrinkles remaining visible after subcutaneous injection).
8. Use hyperdiluted CaHA (1.5 mL CaHA with 0.5–1.5 mL of (diluted) lidocaine) and a sharp needle (27–28G, 19 mm cannula) (Figure 18.4).

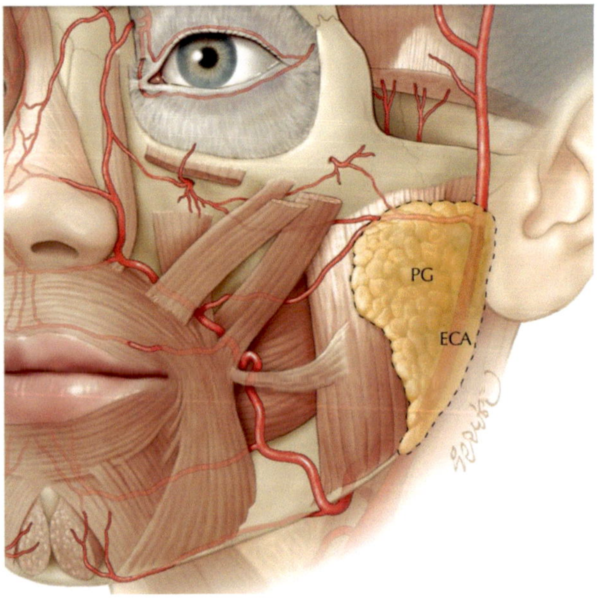

Figure 18.1 Arterial danger zones during the treatment of preauricular wrinkles are: external carotid artery (ECA) and the parotid gland (PG; dashed line).

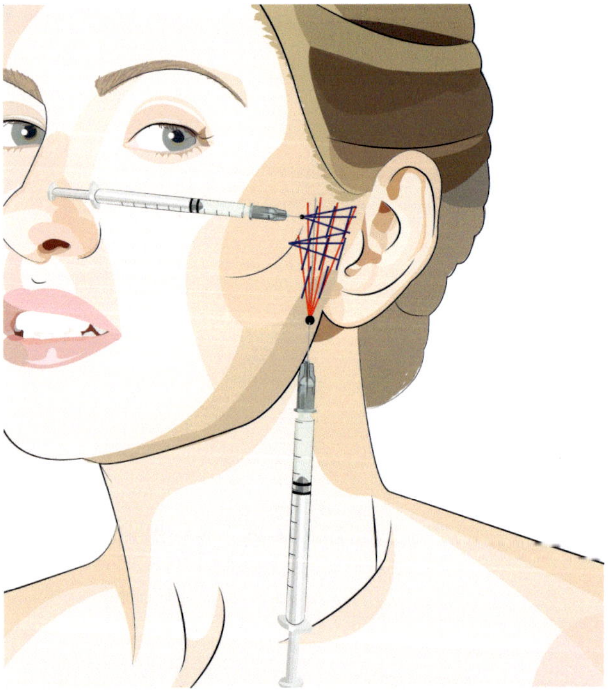

Figure 18.2 Treatment of preauricular wrinkles. Red indicates subcutaneous placement of normally diluted CaHA. Blue indicates intradermal sharp needle retrogrades of hyperdiluted CaHA.

DOI: 10.1201/9781003617129-18

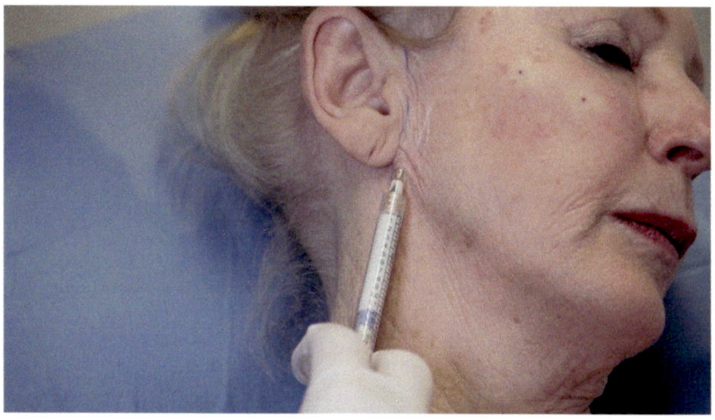

Figure 18.3 Blunt cannula volumizing in the subcutaneous plane.

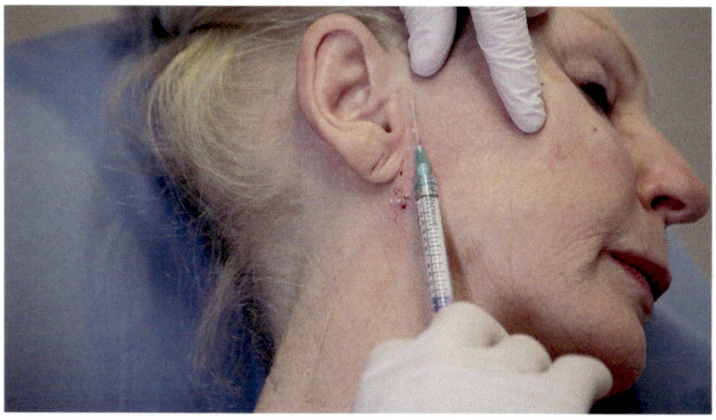

Figure 18.4 Sharp needle wrinkle filling in the deep dermis.

9. Inject directly into the wrinkles (weak spots in the skin) intradermally.
10. Inject fanning in a cross hatching fashion from medial to lateral, intradermally (Figure 18.5).
11. Mold as needed.

See further Video 18.1 to visualize the application technique.

18.3 AFTERCARE

After injection, transient swelling of the treated area can be observed. Swelling might be uneven, so the patient

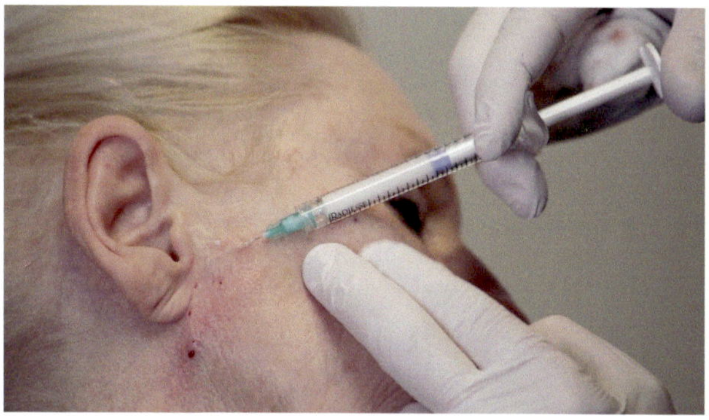

Figure 18.5 Sharp needle cross-hatching intradermally.

should be advised that any swelling is to be expected and is temporary but can last up to three days. Bruising is common in patients with thin skin who get treated with sharp needles for preauricular wrinkles. Sunblock is recommended in these cases.

18.4 ADDITIONAL TREATMENTS FOR OPTIMAL RESULTS

As the skin is a main concern in this indication, many modalities exist for improving the skin such as TCA peels, phenol peels, CO_2 lasers, IPL, and others.

> **Video 18.1** Preauricular wrinkles, multilevel technique.

REFERENCES

[1] R. B. Shaw et al., "Aging of the facial skeleton: Aesthetic implications and rejuvenation strategies," *Plast Reconstr Surg*, vol. 127, no. 1, pp. 374–383, 2011.

[2] J. A. J. van Loghem et al., "Calcium hydroxylapatite: Over a decade of clinical experience," *J Clin Aesthet Dermatol*, vol. 8, no. 1, pp. 38–49, 2015.

The Middle Third of the Face

Accordion Lines

19

JANI VAN LOGHEM

19.1 INTRODUCTION

Accordion lines can be observed in the cheeks, lateral to the nasolabial folds and marionette lines. These lines are the direct result of anterior and inferior descent of the cheeks during the ageing process, combined with skin laxity. The ideal treatment for this indication therefore includes a lifting technique to reposition the cheeks to their original anatomic location. Lifting of the cheeks is discussed in more detail in the chapter on cheek augmentation. In this chapter, we focus exclusively on the wrinkles themselves.

19.2 SAFETY CONSIDERATIONS

When injecting into the accordion wrinkles, care should be taken not to inject too deep, as the facial artery runs close to the skin in the subcutaneous level lateral to the nasolabial folds. Precautions should also be taken to avoid the superior labial artery and the inferior labial artery (Figure 19.1).

19.3 ACCORDION LINE SHARP NEEDLE TECHNIQUE

For injection placement, see Figure 19.2.

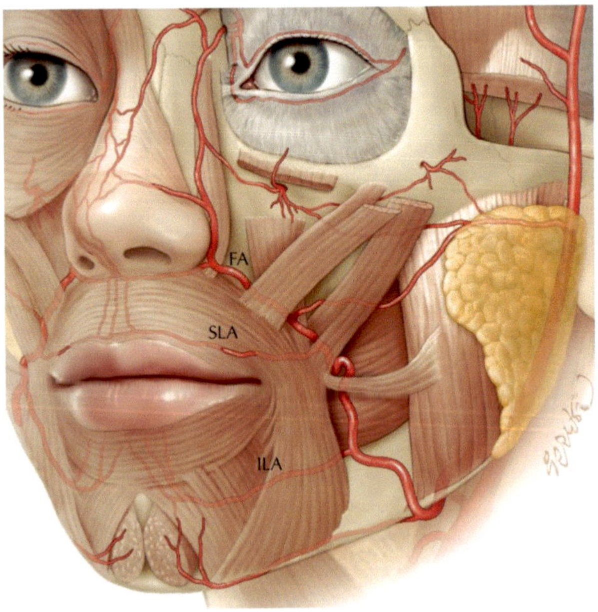

Figure 19.1 Arterial danger zones for the treatment of accordion lines: facial artery (FA), superior labial artery (SLA), and inferior labial artery (ILA).

19.3.1 Step-by-Step Technique

1. Check and mark the location of the vertical wrinkles.
2. Use hyperdiluted CaHA (0.5–1.5 mL lidocaine per 1.5 mL CaHA) and a sharp 28G needle.
3. Carefully place intradermal retrograde linear threads in the most visible wrinkles. Make sure the product is not placed too superficially (the gray of the needle should not be seen through the skin) (Figure 19.3).
4. Direct the needle perpendicular to the wrinkles and place multiple retrograde linear threads in a fanning technique at the dermal–subdermal junction (Figure 19.4).
5. Even out with manual massage as needed.

See also Figure 19.5 and Video 19.1 for before and after results and application techniques, respectively.

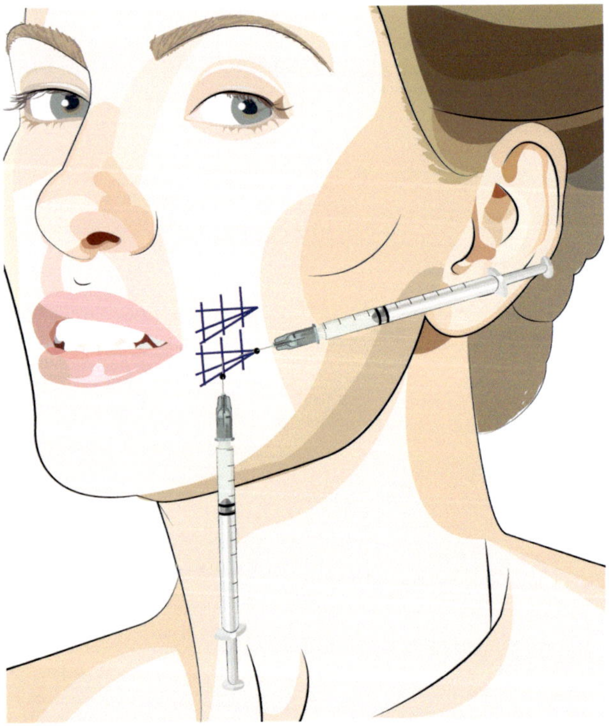

Figure 19.2 Treating accordion lines. Vertical lines indicate direct retrograde intradermal wrinkle correction. Horizontal fans indicate dermal–subdermal junction placement for skin quality improvement.

DOI: 10.1201/9781003617129-19

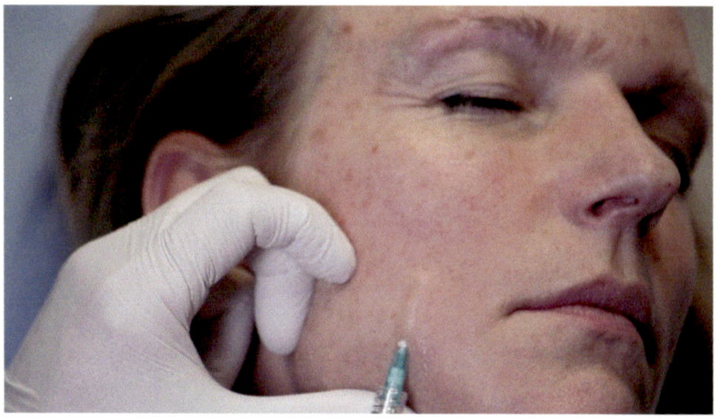

Figure 19.3 Intradermal wrinkle correction.

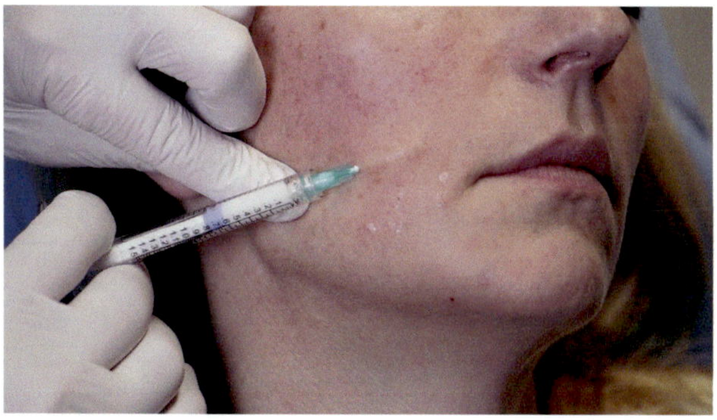

Figure 19.4 Skin rejuvenation.

19.4 AFTERCARE

If necessary, the area can be manually massaged to even out the product, one finger inside the mouth and one outside. Edema may be uneven but should subside in a day or two, and bruises can be observed, especially when using sharp needles.

19.5 ADDITIONAL TREATMENTS FOR OPTIMAL RESULTS

Before addressing accordion lines, a lifting procedure should be considered (see Chapter 12 on cheek augmentation). Also, to aid dermal improvement and tightening, lasers and peels can be considered. Intradermal injection of soft hyaluronic acid may be a good choice to improve results even further.

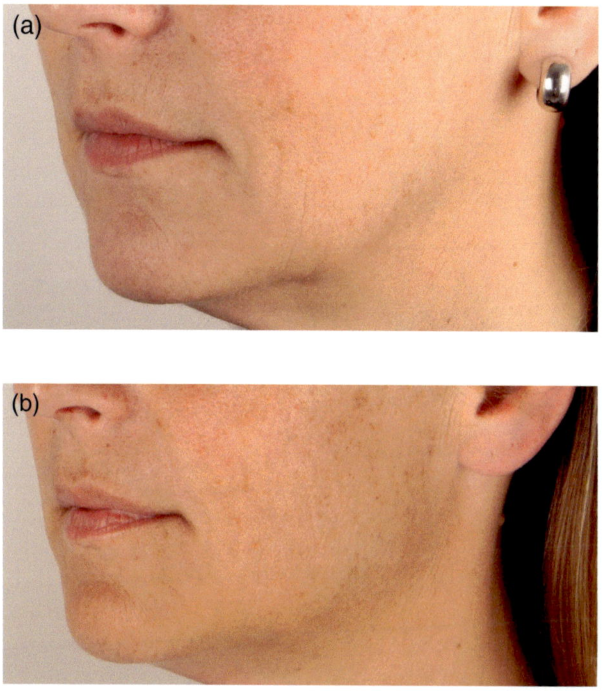

Figure 19.5 Example of a patient (a) before and (b) two months after accordion line rejuvenation.

Video 19.1 Accordion lines: sharp needle technique.

The Lower Third of the Face

Pre-Jowl Sulcus and Marionette Lines

20

NABILA AZIB AND JANI VAN LOGHEM

20.1 INTRODUCTION

The development of the pre-jowl sulcus (PJS) and marionette lines (ML) results from both bone resorption, tissue atrophy, and descent of soft tissue around fixed folds [1,2]. The progressive structural changes in the area just anterior to the jowls were originally called the geniomandibular groove but have been termed the pre-jowl sulcus by Mittleman [3,4].

PJS augmentation allows the camouflage of the jowl by contouring the mandibular border and adding support for the area and for the corners of the mouth.

CaHA appears to be the filler of choice for both lower face contouring and skin stimulation.

20.2 ANATOMY

The depressor *anguli oris* (DAO) muscle, the depressor *labii inferioris* muscle, and the mentalis muscle are all connected superiorly to the orbicularis oris muscle, and inferiorly, the DAO is connected to the platysma muscle (Figure 20.1).

The mandibular ligament remains the fixed point with a deep bony insertion and a skin insertion that limits the jowl anteriorly.

The mandibular septum, along the mandibular bone, is the limit between the superior fat compartment and the inferior fat compartment.

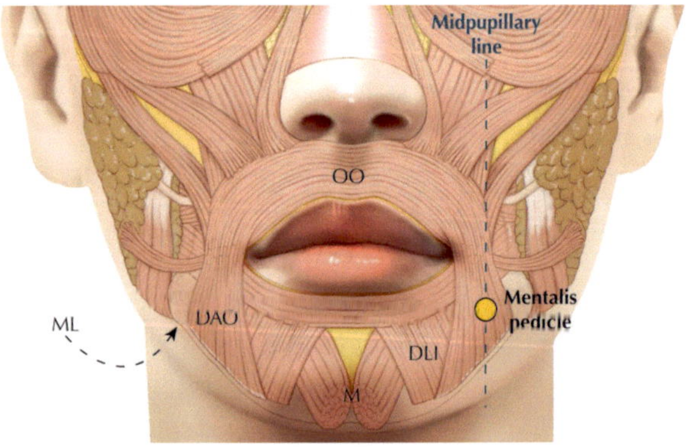

Figure 20.1 Pre-jowl anatomy. Different structures that should be considered during the treatment of the pre-jowl sulcus and marionette lines are *orbicularis oris* (OO) muscle, depressor *anguli orbis* (DAO) muscle, depressor *labii inferioris* (DLI) muscle, mentalis muscle (M), and mandibular ligament (ML).

20.3 ANATOMICAL DANGERS

Areas of caution are the mental artery, vein, and nerve. The mental foramen is located in the mid-pupillary line just under the first premolar. The facial artery remains at the posterior border of the DAO muscle (Figure 20.2) [5].

20.4 ASSESSMENT AND TREATMENT PLAN

A full-face assessment should be made on a static and also on a dynamic position, in both frontal and profile view. Injections should be performed from the top to the bottom for a better lifting effect. Cheek injections may reduce the ptotic jowl. Less product is then required in the pre-jowl area to achieve a natural result.

As the PJS deepens with the aging process, we can notice a triangular shaped "indentation" just past the central chin (Figure 20.3).

20.5 MARKING AND PHOTOGRAPHS

First, the treatment area should be marked, with the patient sitting upright, to consider the gravitational effect.

The loss of volume of the pre-jowl area appears as a triangle with an inferior base on the mandibular

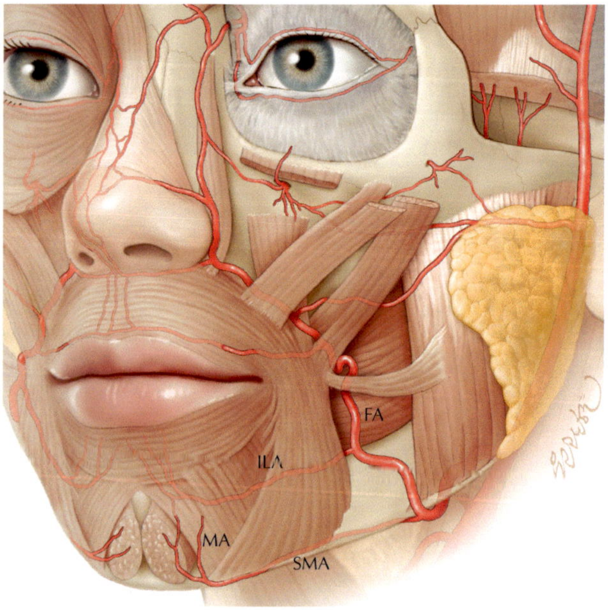

Figure 20.2 Arterial danger zones of the pre-jowl sulcus and marionette lines are: facial artery (FA), inferior labial artery (ILA), submental artery (SMA), and mental artery (MA).

DOI: 10.1201/9781003617129-20

border. The posterior border of the triangle may be precisely identified by pushing the jowl anteriorly. The anterior limit of the jowl corresponds to the skin insertion of the mandibular ligament. The apex of the triangle can be extended into the labial commissure.

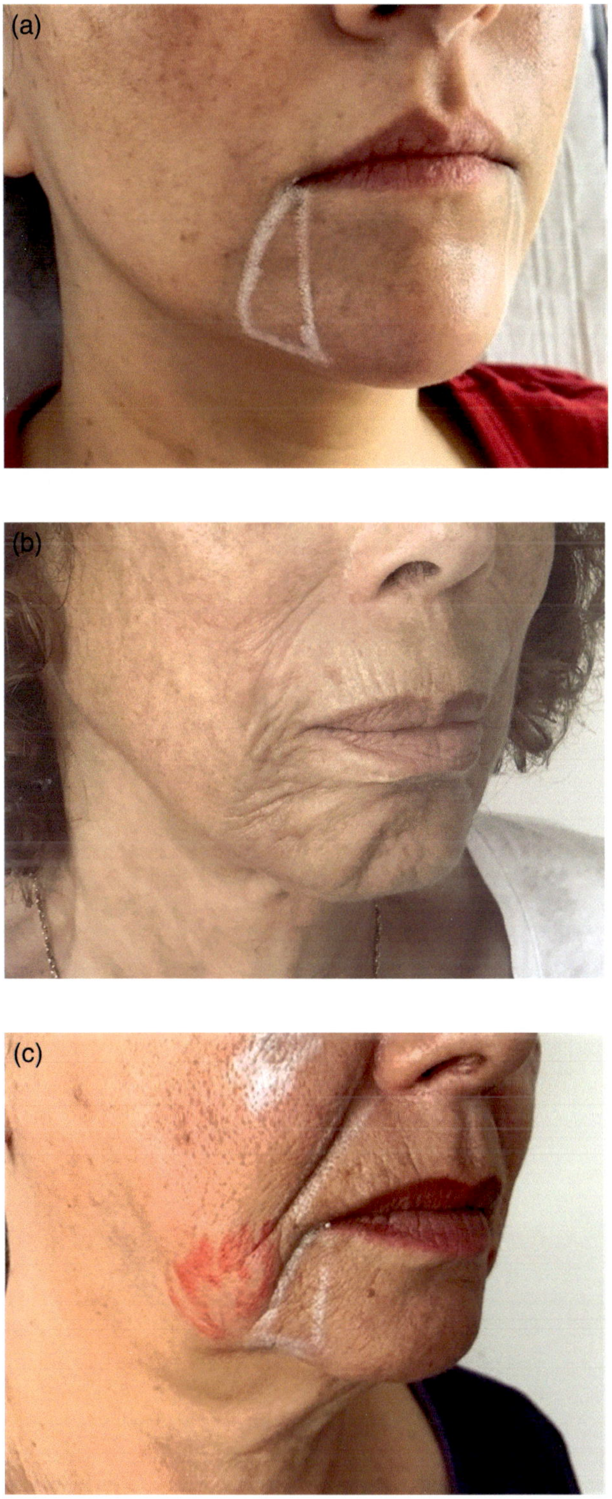

Figure 20.3 Different pre-jowl aspects caused by (a) a loss of volume of soft tissues in mid-aged patients, (b) skin laxity associated to a mandibular bone resorption, or (c) a combination of both factors.

Pretreatment photographs may be taken before and after the marking.

20.6 PRE-JOWL SULCUS CANNULA TECHNIQUE 1

For injection placement, see Figure 20.4.

20.6.1 Step-by-Step Technique

1. Identify and mark the PJS, creating a triangle extending to the oral commissure along the ML.
2. Mark the entry point at the lateral mentum (Figure 20.5).
3. Disinfect. Consider giving local anesthesia at the entry point.
4. Make a pre-hole with a 23G needle
5. Use nondiluted CaHA or standard dilution of CaHA (0.3 mL 1% lidocaine with adrenaline 1:200000 per 1.5 mL CaHA) and a 25G, 38 mm, or 50 mm cannula.
6. Point the cannula in the direction of the oral commissure.
7. Make sure no product is injected lateral to the ML and PJS during the whole treatment.
8. With the nondominant hand, stretch the skin in the direction of the cannula and advance the cannula in the dermal–subdermal plane to the oral commissure. Remain subcutaneous to avoid the mental pedicle and also to provide a lifting effect and skin stimulation (Figure 20.6).
9. Inject multiple retrograde linear threads of approximately 0.1 mL per retrograde in a fanning technique toward the mandible (Figure 20.7).
10. At the mandibular border, multiple passes might be necessary to reduce the PJS satisfactorily.
11. With thumb and index finger gently squeezing the tissue, the shape of the injectate can be improved to match the mandibular line.

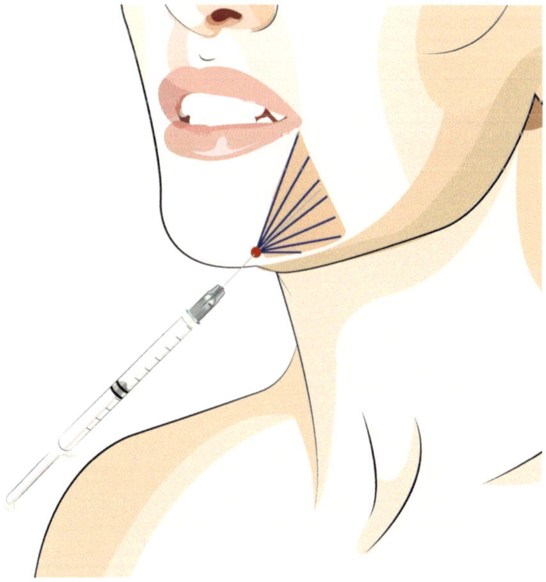

Figure 20.4 PJS cannula technique. Blue lines indicate subdermal placement of CaHA.

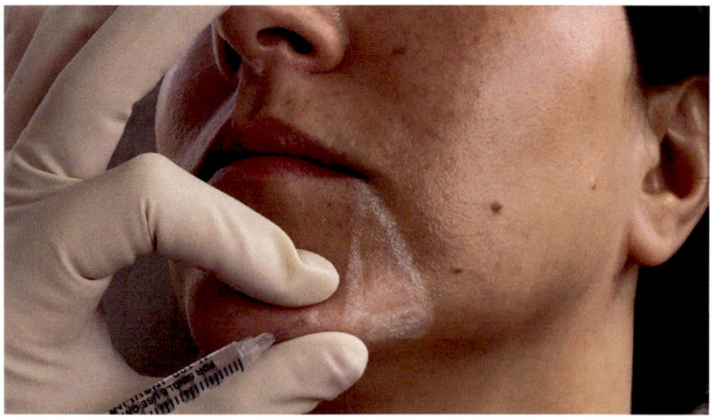

Figure 20.5 Determining the entry point at the lateral mentum.

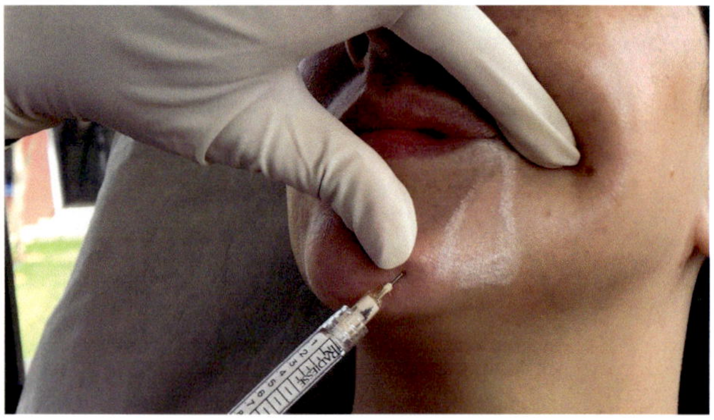

Figure 20.6 Stretching the skin will facilitate superficial subcutaneous injection.

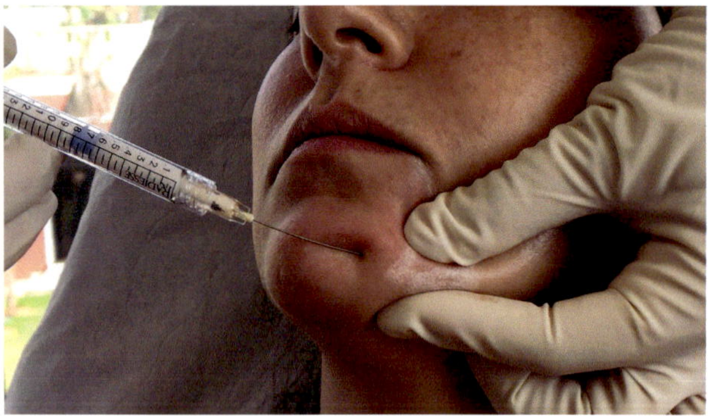

Figure 20.7 At the mandibular border, pressure of the fingers can aid in modulating the shape of the injected product.

12. When the bony resorption is important, multiple boluses of CaHA can be also added along the periosteum of the inferior mandible. This multilayer volumization gives a better contouring and a long-lasting result.
13. Do not overcorrect.
14. Even out with manual massage as needed.

20.7 PRE-JOWL SULCUS SHARP NEEDLE TECHNIQUE

For injection placement, see Figure 20.8.

20.7.1 Step-by-Step Technique

1. Identify and mark the PJS.
2. With one finger, check how deep the oral cavity extends behind the lower lip and mark the skin at that point (Figure 20.9).
3. Advance the needle from the middle of the PJS to the periosteum. Pull up the skin over the needle with the nondominant hand.
4. With the needle softly touching the periosteum, place two to three boluses on the periosteum of the mandible while making sure not to inject in the oral submucosa (Figure 20.10).
5. Retract the needle without exiting the skin and advance it in the subcutaneous plane cranially (even beyond the mark of the location of the deeper submucosa).
6. Stretch the skin in the length of the needle in order to have better control over the superficial placement of the needle.
7. Inject multiple retrograde linear threads in a fanning technique (Figure 20.11).
8. Mold as needed to even out.

20.8 PRE-JOWL SULCUS CANNULA TECHNIQUE 2

For injection placement, see Figure 20.12.

20.8.1 Step-by-Step Technique

1. Mark the PJS and ML. Disinfect.
2. Consider anesthesia with lidocaine containing adrenaline at the PJS entry point.
3. Make a pre-hole with a 23G needle.
4. Use non-diluted CaHA and a 25G, 38 mm cannula.
5. Advance the needle through the skin to the subcutis.

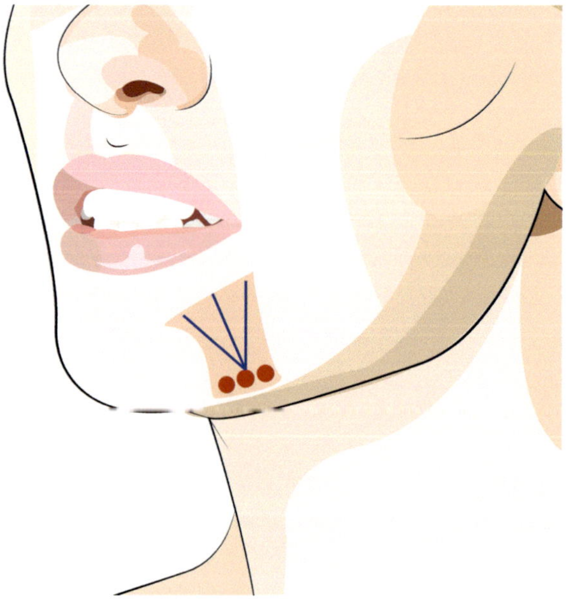

Figure 20.8 CaHA injection at the PSJ using sharp needle. Red dots indicate periosteal boluses; blue lines indicate subcutaneous retrograde injection.

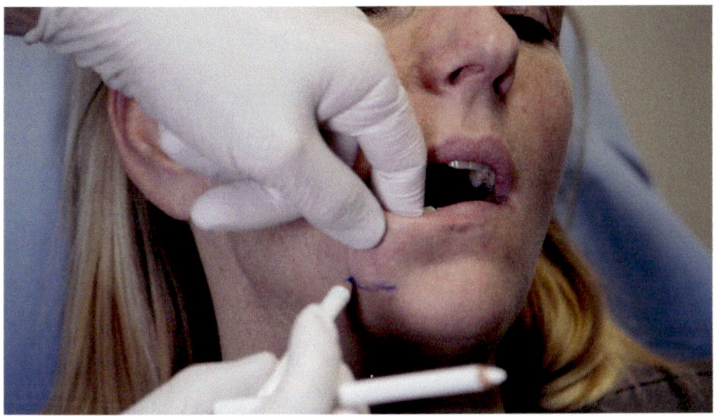

Figure 20.9 Determining the caudal extent of oral cavity.

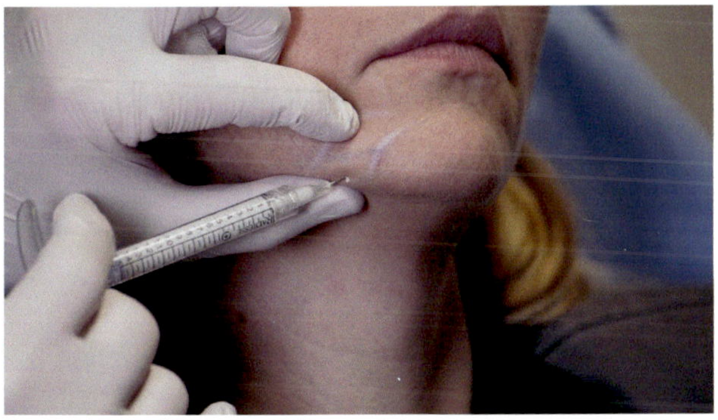

Figure 20.10 Periosteal boluses.

6. Advance the cannula past the PJS to the midline of the mentum (Figure 20.13).
7. Inject a thick retrograde linear thread of approximately 0.25 mL to the PJS.
8. Reorient and advance the cannula to the mental crease while staying in the subcutaneous plane (Figure 20.14).
9. Inject another retrograde linear thread toward the PJS.
10. Reorient and advance to the point of most depression and toward the ML while injecting retrograde linear threads (Figure 20.15).
11. Mold and massage.

See also Figure 20.16 and Videos 20.1–20.3 to visualize results and application techniques, respectively.

20.9 AFTERCARE

The procedure is followed by a gentle massage to achieve the desired contour. With one finger inside the mouth and the thumb on the skin, the product can easily be evened out. Swelling may be uneven but should subside in a day or two. Patients should be informed to sleep only on their back and to avoid dental procedures for one week. The follow-up is planned after 15 days to three months.

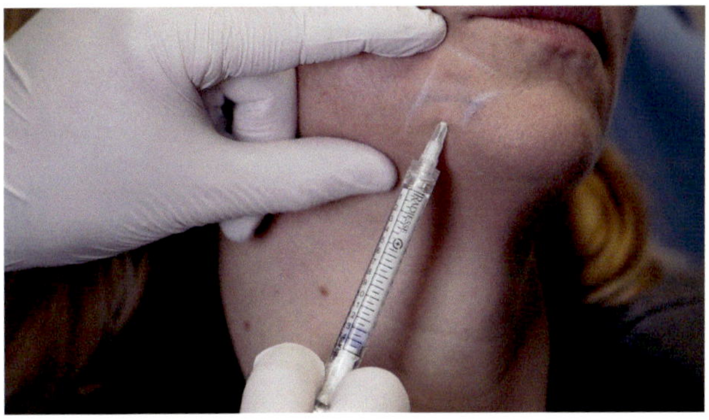

Figure 20.11 Subcutaneous fanning technique.

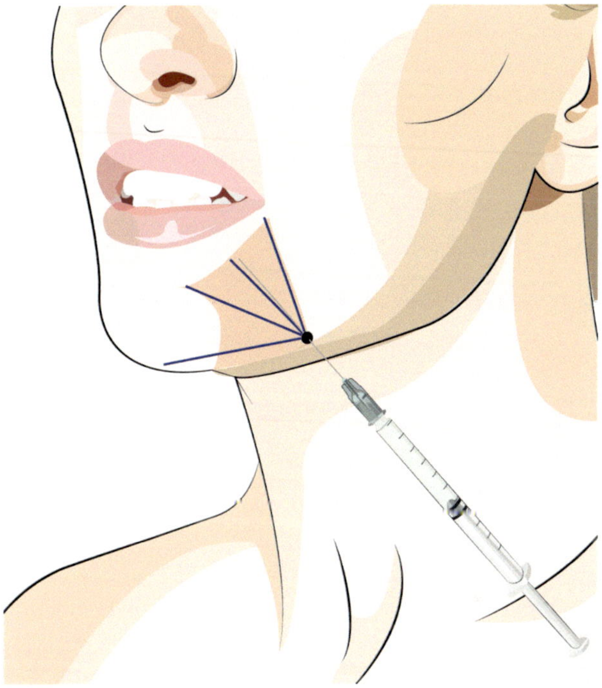

Figure 20.12 CaHA injection at the PSJ using cannula. Blue lines indicate subcutaneous retrograde injection.

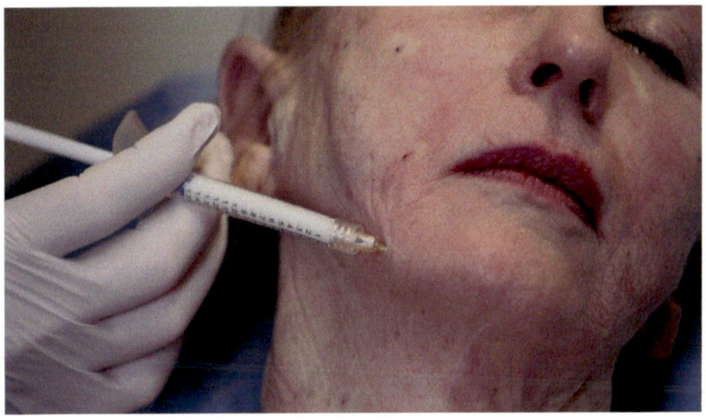

Figure 20.13 Subcutaneous injection to improve mandibular definition from the mentum to the PJS.

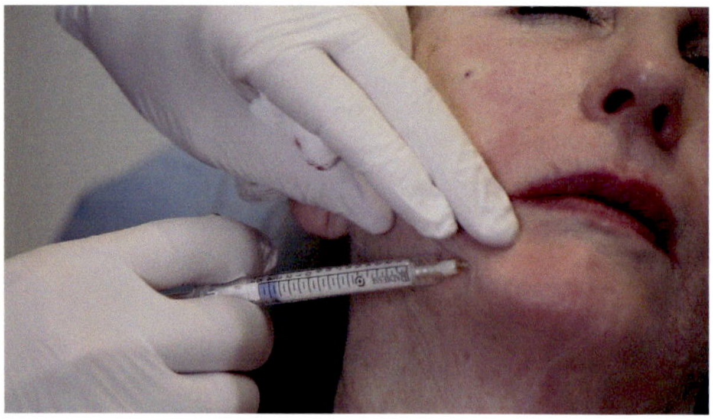

Figure 20.14 Subcutaneous injection from the mental crease to the PJS.

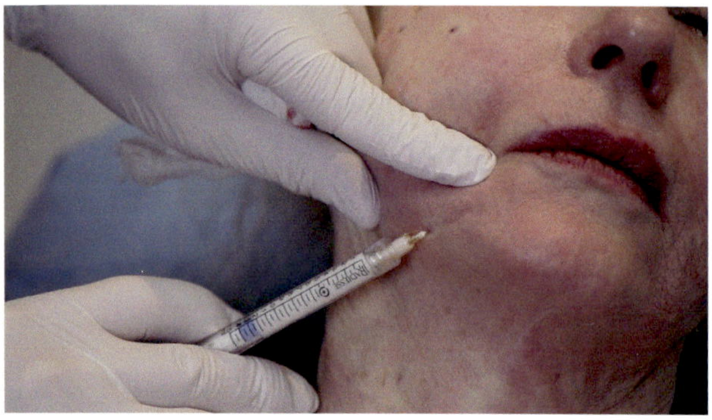

Figure 20.15 Subcutaneous injection from the ML to the PJS.

20.10 ADDITIONAL TREATMENTS FOR OPTIMAL RESULTS

Before addressing the PJS, a lifting technique, like cheek augmentation and mandibular angle augmentation, may be considered. Deep injection of CaHA or other volumizers to the cheek and CaHA to the mandible will usually reduce the PJS. Also, mentum augmentation will in many cases improve the aspect of the PJS. Improving skin quality and tightening the skin (e.g. by laser resurfacing, etc.) will aid in the reduction of the PJS. Last, fat-reducing therapy like (laser or injectable) lipolysis of the jowl fat may be of value.

Video 20.1 Pre-jowl sulcus and marionette lines: cannula technique 1.

Video 20.2 Pre-jowl sulcus needle technique 1.

Video 20.3 Pre-jowl sulcus needle technique 2.

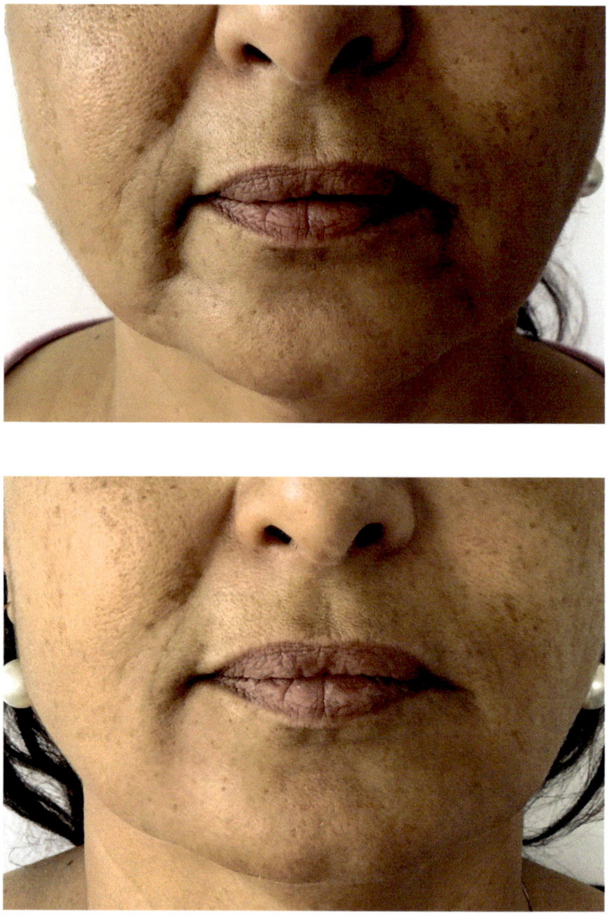

Figure 20.16 Pre-jowl and MLs injection with 1.5 mL CaHA. (Courtesy of Dr. Nabila Azib.)

REFERENCES

[1] R. B. Shaw et al., "Aging of the facial skeleton: Aesthetic implications and rejuvenation strategies," *Plast Reconstr Surg*, vol. 127, no. 1, pp. 374–383, 2011.

[2] M. H. Graivier et al., "Calcium hydroxylapatite (Radiesse) for correction of the mid- and lower face: Consensus recommendations," *Plast Reconstr Surg*, vol. 120, no. Suppl 6, 2007.

[3] H. Mittelman, "The anatomy of the aging mandible and its importance to facelift surgery," *Facial Plast Surg Clin North Am*, vol. 2, no. 3, pp. 301–309, 1994.

[4] T. Fattahi, "The prejowl sulcus: An important consideration in lower face rejuvenation," *J Oral Maxillofac Surg*, vol. 66, no. 2, pp. 355–358, 2008.

[5] T. K. Hamilton, "Skin augmentation and correction: The new generation of dermal fillers—a dermatologist's experience," *Clin Dermatol*, vol. 27, no. Suppl 3, 2009.

The Lower Third of the Face

Oral Commissures

21

JANI VAN LOGHEM

21.1 INTRODUCTION

The oral commissures can make the expression of the perioral area more negative. At the top of the marionette lines, the downward-pointing mouth corners suggest bitterness or dislike. Lifting the oral commissures with CaHA can dramatically impact the look in a positive way.

21.2 SAFETY CONSIDERATIONS

When injecting the oral commissures, care should be taken not to inject too deep, as the inferior labial artery usually runs in or below the orbicularis oris muscle (Figure 21.1).

21.3 ORAL COMMISSURES SHARP NEEDLE TECHNIQUE

For injection placement, see Figure 21.2.

21.3.1 Step-by-Step Technique

1. Check the location of the oral commissure and disinfect.
2. Use undiluted CaHA and a 27G needle.
3. Stretch the skin in the direction of the needle.
4. Advance the needle from the oral commissure to just below vermillion border of the lower lip.
5. Make sure the needle is not placed too superficially (the gray of the needle should not be seen through the skin).
6. Carefully place a retrograde linear thread or a fan of threads (Figure 21.3).
7. From the marionette line inferior to the commissure, enter the skin and advance the needle to the oral commissure.
8. Push the commissure slightly upward with needle while injecting product (Figure 21.4).
9. Place multiple threads if needed.
10. Even out with manual massage as needed.

21.4 ORAL COMMISSURES CANNULA TECHNIQUE

For injection placement, see Figure 21.5.

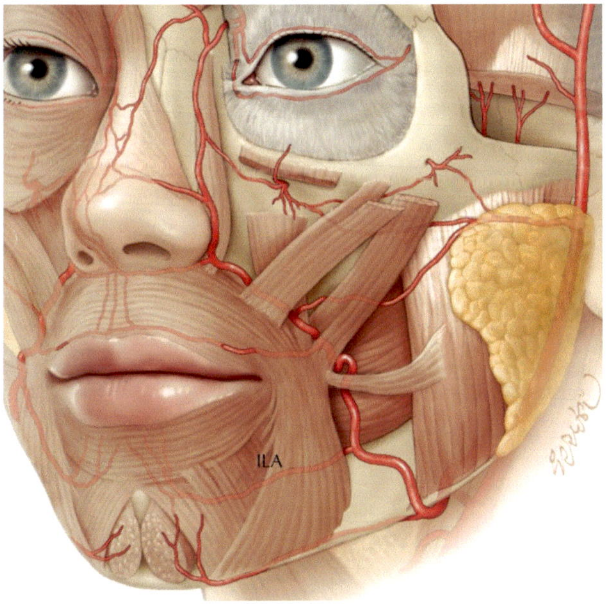

Figure 21.1 Arterial danger zone for the treatment of oral commissures is: inferior labial artery (ILA).

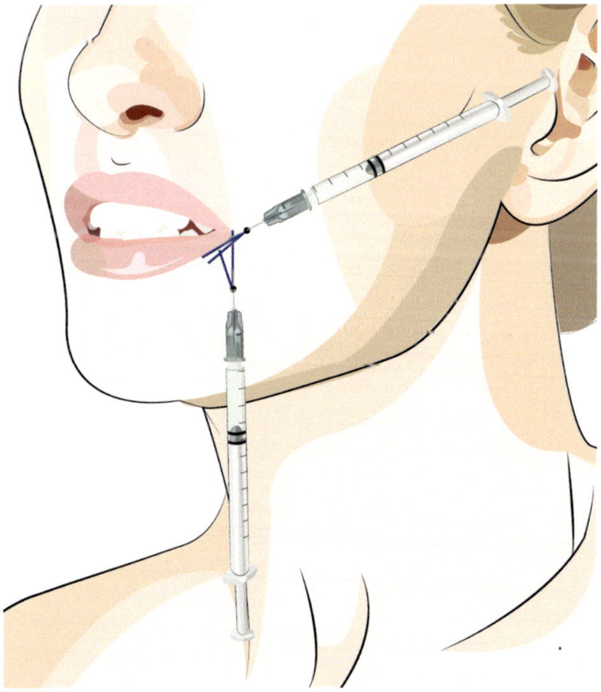

Figure 21.2 Treating the oral commissures with sharp needle. Vertical lines indicate direct retrograde dermal/subdermal injection.

DOI: 10.1201/9781003617129-21

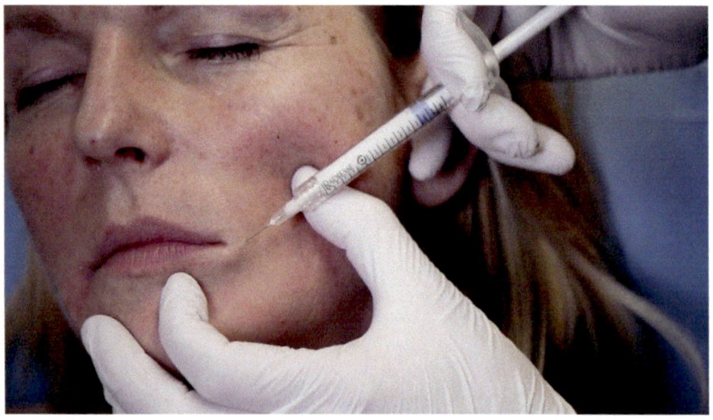

Figure 21.3 Horizontal retrograde.

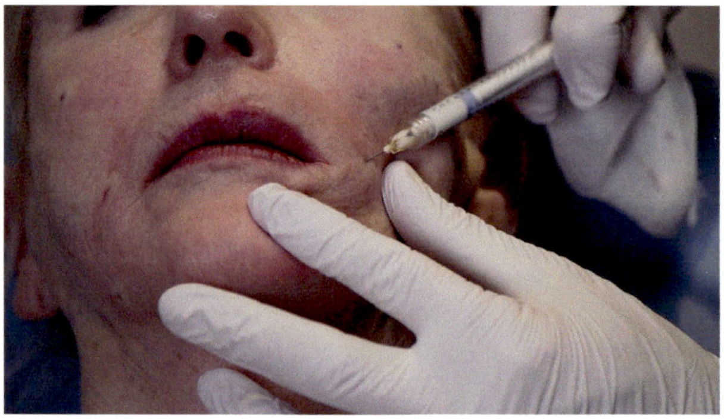

Figure 21.6 Horizontal retrograde.

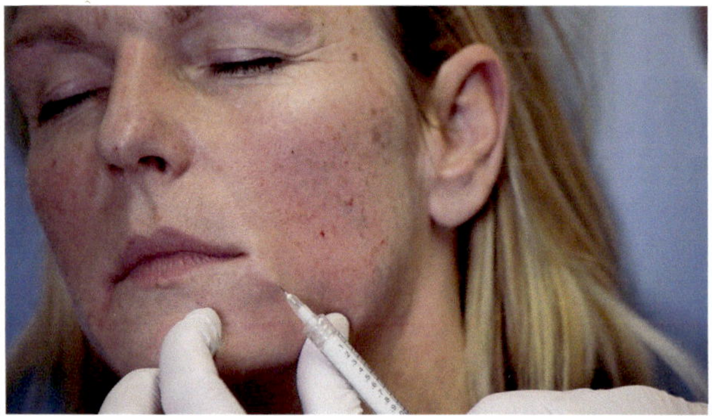

Figure 21.4 Vertical retrograde.

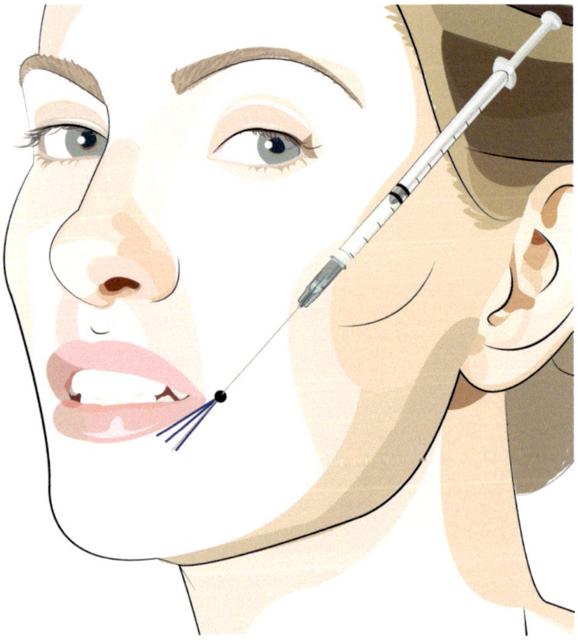

Figure 21.5 Treatment of the oral commissures with cannula. Blue lines indicate direct retrograde subdermal injection.

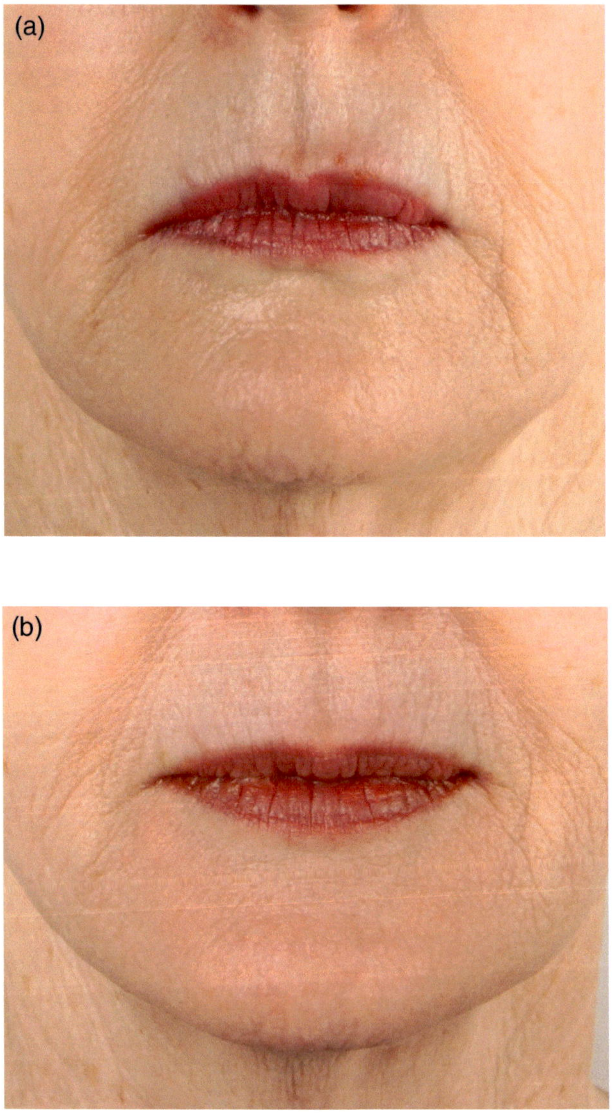

Figure 21.7 (a) Before treatment and (b) results after two months.

21.4.1 Step-by-Step Technique

1. Check the location of the oral commissure; disinfect.
2. Use undiluted CaHA and a 25G, 38 mm cannula.
3. Make a pre-hole with a 23G needle after local anesthesia.
4. Stretch the skin in the direction of the cannula.
5. Advance the cannula from the oral commissure to just below the vermillion border of the lower lip in the subcutaneous plane.
6. Carefully place multiple retrograde linear threads in a fanning technique (Figure 21.6).
7. Do not inject lateral to the marionette line (do not inject in the superior jowl fat compartment).
8. Place multiple threads if needed.
9. Even out with manual massage as needed.

See also Figure 21.7 and Videos 21.1–21.2 to visualize before and after results and application techniques, respectively.

21.5 AFTERCARE

If necessary, the area can be manually massaged to even out the product with one finger inside the mouth and one outside. Edema may be uneven but should subside in a day or two, and bruises can be observed, especially when using sharp needles.

21.6 ADDITIONAL TREATMENTS FOR OPTIMAL RESULTS

Before addressing the oral commissures, a lifting procedure should be considered (see the chapter on cheek augmentation) and treatment of pre-jowl sulcus and marionette lines (see separate chapter on that). Toxin treatment of the depressor anguli oris muscle may improve the oral commissure as well.

Video 21.1 Oral Commissures, sharp needle technique.

Video 21.2 Oral Commissures, cannula technique.

The Lower Third of the Face

22

Radial Lip Lines

JANI VAN LOGHEM

22.1 INTRODUCTION

Radial lip lines have both a muscular (dynamic) as well as a skin (non-dynamic) component. Due to reduction of skeletal platform and deep fat in the lips, the orbicularis oris muscle can become looser and thereby hyperactive, contributing to the dynamic component of radial lip lines. Maxillary and mandibular bone resorption can be corrected by placing non-diluted CaHA, or other volumizers, on the periosteum, as discussed in other chapters (nasolabial folds, pre-jowl sulcus, and marionette lines). CaHA for the correction of deep fat resorption of the lips is generally not recommended; as the CaHA product is white and as the deep fat is essentially the submucosa of the lips, the product may be visible when injected at that depth. The dermal component, however, is reduction of especially collagen and is a good indication for (hyper) diluted CaHA.

22.2 SAFETY CONSIDERATIONS

When injecting the radial lip lines, care should be taken not to inject too deep, as the superior and inferior labial arteries generally run below the *orbicularis oris* muscle (Figure 22.1).

22.3 RADIAL LIP LINE CANNULA TECHNIQUE

For injection placement, see Figure 22.2.

22.3.1 Step-by-Step Technique

1. Use preexisting pre-holes (nasolabial folds and pre-jowl sulcus) or determine entry points from where upper and lower cutaneous lips can be reached.
2. Use diluted CaHA (between 0.5–1.5 mL diluted lidocaine per 1.5 mL CaHA product) and a 25G, 38 mm, or 50 mm cannula.

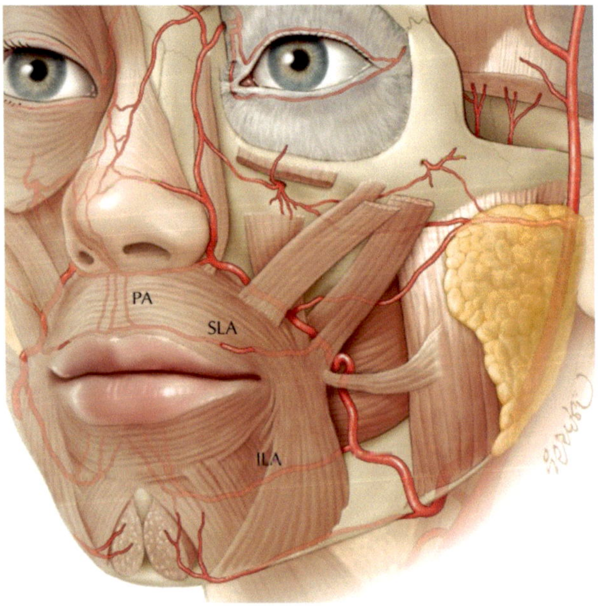

Figure 22.1 Arterial danger zones for the treatment of radial lip lines are: inferior labial artery (ILA), superior labial artery (SLA), and philtral artery (PA).

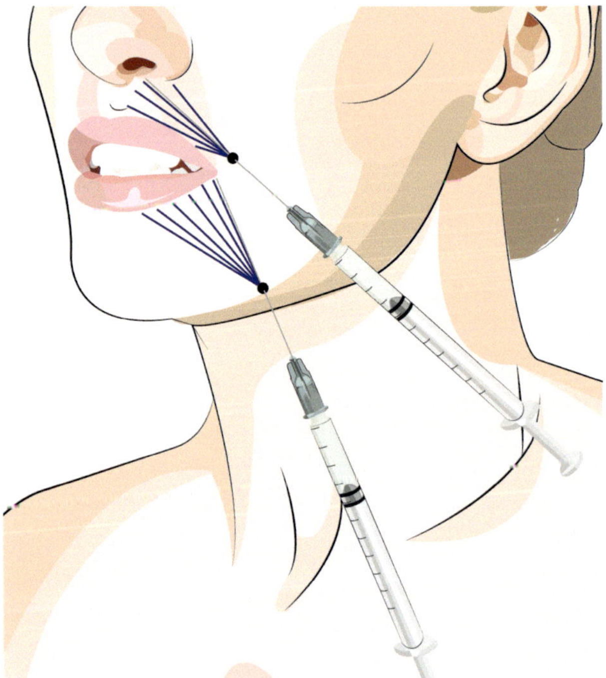

Figure 22.2 Treating the radial lip lines with cannula. Blue lines indicate direct retrograde subdermal injection.

DOI: 10.1201/9781003617129-22

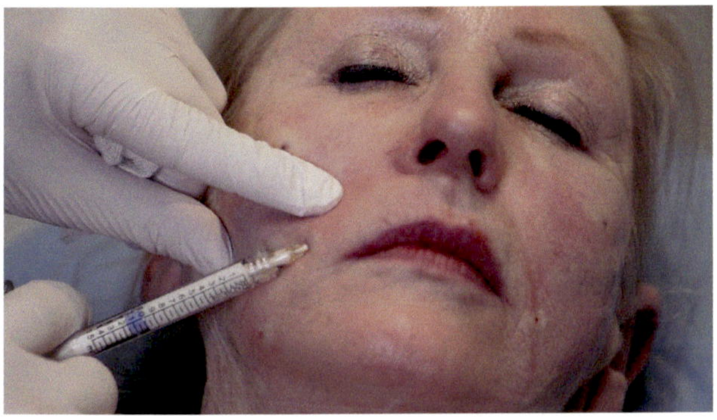

Figure 22.3 Horizontal retrograde linear threads in the upper lip at the dermal–subdermal junction.

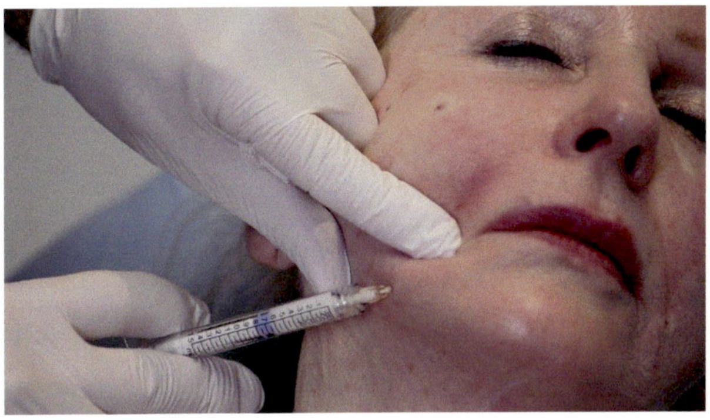

Figure 22.4 Retrograde linear threads in the infra-oral area at the dermal–subdermal junction.

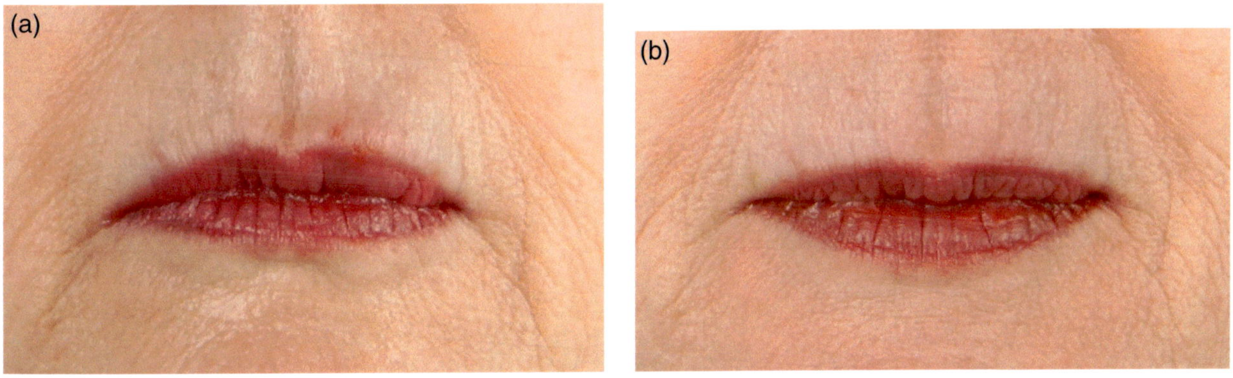

Figure 22.5 (a) Before and (b) results after two months.

3. Consider block anesthesia and make pre-holes with a 23G needle after local anesthesia.
4. Stretch the skin in the direction of the cannula.
5. Advance the cannula from lateral to the oral commissure to the philtrum.
6. Place multiple retrograde linear threads in a fanning technique (Figure 22.3).
7. Advance the cannula from the jowl entry point to the oral commissure.
8. Place multiple retrograde linear threads in a fanning technique towards the midline (Figure 22.4).
9. Even out with manual massage as needed.

See further Figure 22.5 and Video 22.1 for before and after results and application technique, respectively.

22.4 AFTERCARE

If necessary, the area can be manually massaged to even out the product with one finger inside the mouth and one outside. Edema may be uneven and should subside in a day or two, and bruises can be observed.

22.5 ADDITIONAL TREATMENTS FOR OPTIMAL RESULTS

Together with directly addressing the radial lip lines with (hyper)diluted CaHA, treatment of nasolabial folds, pre jowl sulcus, and marionette lines at the periosteal level (see Chapters 15 and 20) can be considered. Additional treatments may include botulinum toxin treatment to relax the orbicularis oris muscle and superficial dermal injection of a soft HA. Additional treatments to improve dermal strength and to reduce the radial lip lines include ablative lasers like fractional CO_2 and medium to deep chemical peels.

Video 22.1 Radial lip lines: cannula technique.

The Lower Third of the Face

23

Mentum Augmentation

JANI VAN LOGHEM

23.1 INTRODUCTION

Facial harmony can be defined as balance between the elements of the face. Augmentation of the chin is a powerful way of improving facial harmony, especially in patients who have a retruded chin. Retrognathia is a condition where the mandible is set further back than the maxilla, making it look like the person has a severe overbite. Surgically, this can be corrected with cutting the mandible and moving it forward. This is quite an invasive procedure with considerable risks and downtime. CaHA can be used with minimal risk, discomfort, and downtime for the patient and can produce a significant improvement in facial harmony.

23.2 AGE-RELATED ANATOMICAL CHANGES

Due to bone resorption, the mandible changes shape. The mandibular body height, the ramus height, and the mandibular body length all significantly decrease, resulting in a significant increase of mandibular angle. The bigonial distance (distance between the left and right mandibular angle) does not significantly change during ageing [1,2]. As discussed in the chapter on cheek augmentation, the inferior descent of the cheeks contributes significantly to the jowls. The mandibular angle moves medially due to bone resorption. Soft tissues attached to the bone are brought medially by this process. The mandibular retaining ligament stops the anterior descent and causes the jowls to prolapse over that ligament, adding significantly to jowling. At the same time, the mandible at the mentum shows bone resorption, reducing skeletal volume at the mentum. This process may add in deepening of the marionette lines and the pre-jowl sulcus. Volume replacement at the mentum may therefore aid in improving mandibular contour and reducing pre-jowl sulcus and marionette lines.

23.3 ANATOMICAL DANGERS

Both the inferior labial and the submental artery are branches of the facial artery and run deep in this area, although not in every patient, as these arteries may have loops or branches to the subcutaneous level as well. The mental nerve and artery arise from the mental foramen, located in approximately the mid-pupillary line, just above the mandibular prominence (Figure 23.1).

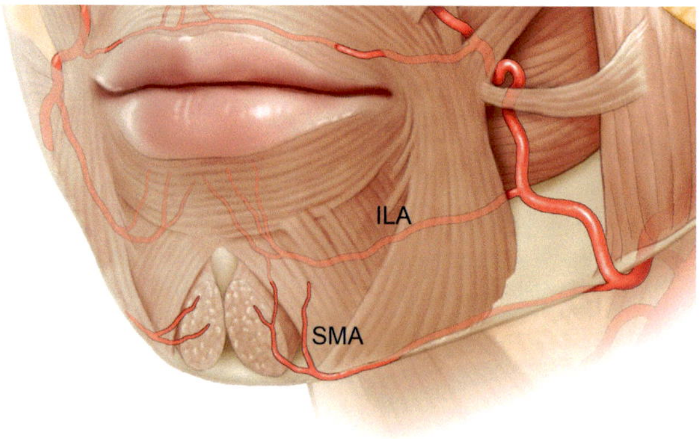

Figure 23.1 Arterial danger zones for the treatment of mentum augmentation: inferior labial artery (ILA), submental artery (SA), and mental artery (MA not shown).

Injecting into the jowl fat compartments themselves should be avoided, as this can lead to aesthetically displeasing worsened jowling.

In Western cultures, the ideal width of the female chin is approximately the same width as the intercanthal distance, or the distance from the columella to the vermillion border of the lower lip. The ideal length of the chin is approximately the intercanthal distance from the vermillion border of the lower lip. For males, the ideal width of the chin is the same as the width of the mouth.

In Asian cultures, the chin is ideally less wide and pointier, accentuating the "heart shape" of the face.

23.4 CANNULA TECHNIQUE 1 (ANTERIOR PROJECTION)

For injection placement, see Figure 23.2.

23.4.1 Step-by-Step Technique

1. Consider giving a mentalis nerve block and local anesthesia in the skin in the midline at the submental crease.
2. Disinfect and mark the width and vertical position of maximum projection, taking the Steiner's line into consideration.

DOI: 10.1201/9781003617129-23

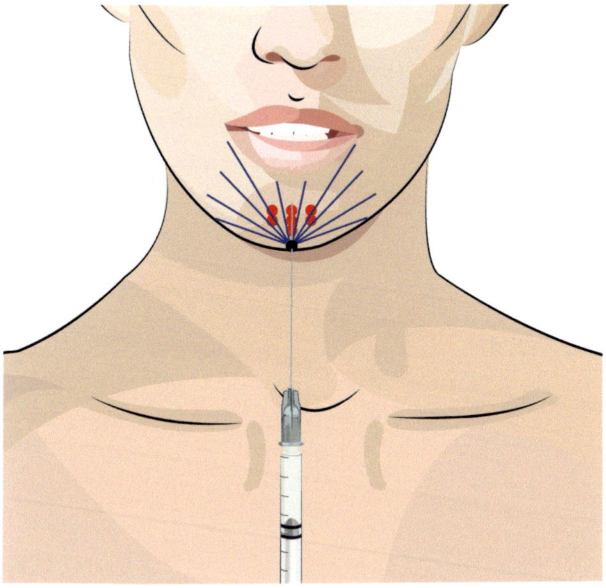

Figure 23.2 Product injection for mentum augmentation using cannula from a central entry point. Red dots indicate supraperiosteal boluses; blue lines represent subcutaneous retrograde linear threads.

3. Make a pre-hole with a 23G needle in the midline at the submental crease.
4. Use undiluted CaHA and a 25G, 38 mm cannula.
5. With the nondominant hand, lift up the mentalis muscle and advance the cannula to the periosteum to the space between the two bellies of the mentalis muscles (Figure 23.3).
6. Make sure that the cannula tip is not visible in the oral mucosa.
7. Inject multiple boluses of approximately 0.1 mL per bolus on the periosteum.
8. Avoid injecting too close to the entry point to avoid superficial accumulation of product.
9. If necessary, more lateral deposits can also be injected under the mentalis, depressor *labii inferioris*, and depressor *anguli oris* muscles from this entry point (Figure 23.4).
10. Additionally, subcutaneous retrograde linear threads can be injected from this entry point to smooth out the result, to define the mandibular contour, and to reduce pre-jowl sulcus and marionette lines.
11. Check for symmetry.
12. Mold into the desired shape.

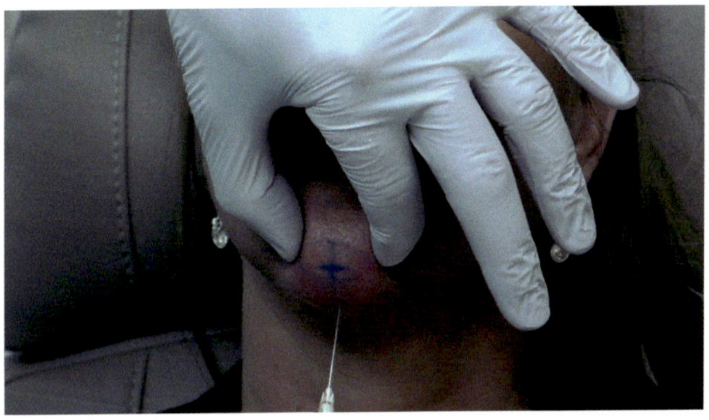

Figure 23.3 Lifting the muscle to advance the cannula to the periosteum.

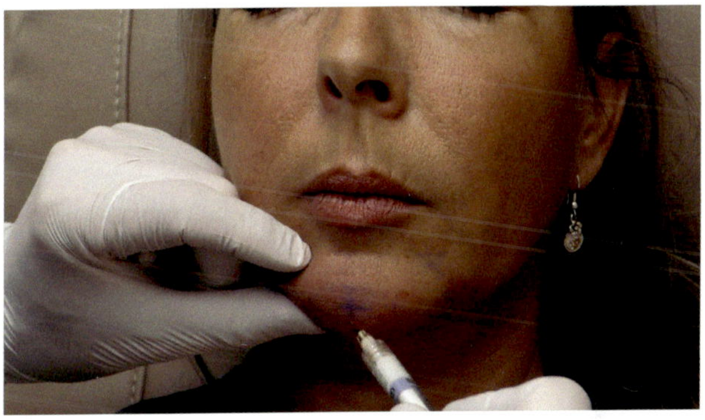

Figure 23.4 Injecting boluses sub-muscularly.

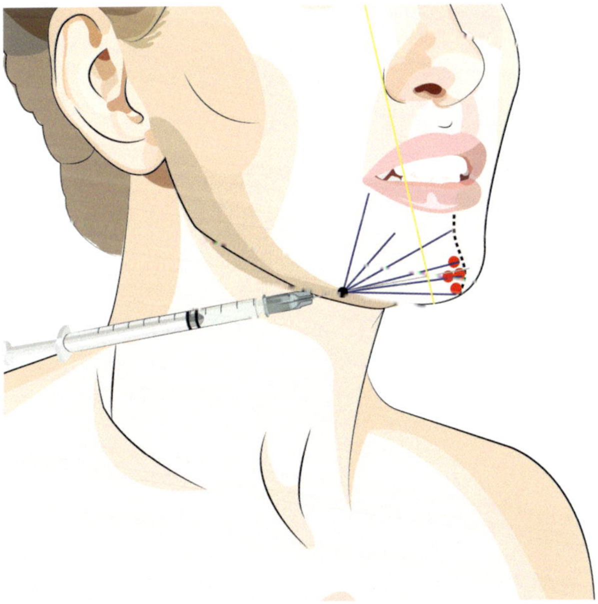

Figure 23.5 Product injection for mentum augmentation using cannula. The dotted line represents the midline. The yellow line represents a vertical line from the inner canthus along the lateral ala to indicate maximum width of the female chin. Red dots indicate supraperiosteal boluses; blue lines represent subcutaneous retrograde linear threads.

23.5 CANNULA TECHNIQUE 2 (ANTERIOR PROJECTION, LENGTHENING, AND CONTOURING)

For injection placement, see Figure 23.5.

23.5.1 Step-by-Step Technique

1. Consider a mentalis nerve block and local anesthesia in the skin in the midline at the pre-jowl sulcus.

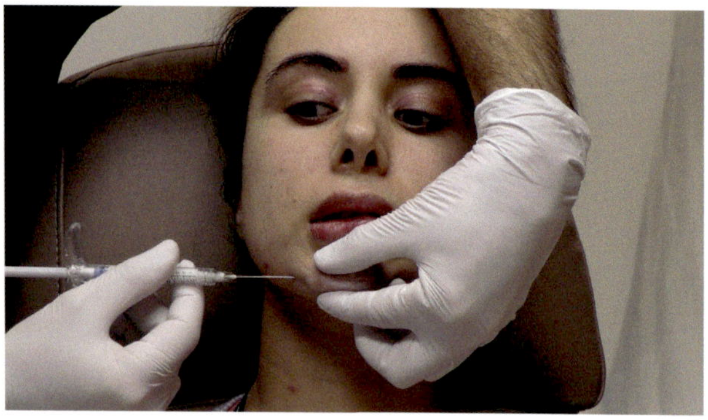

Figure 23.6 Lifting the muscle to advance the cannula to the periosteum.

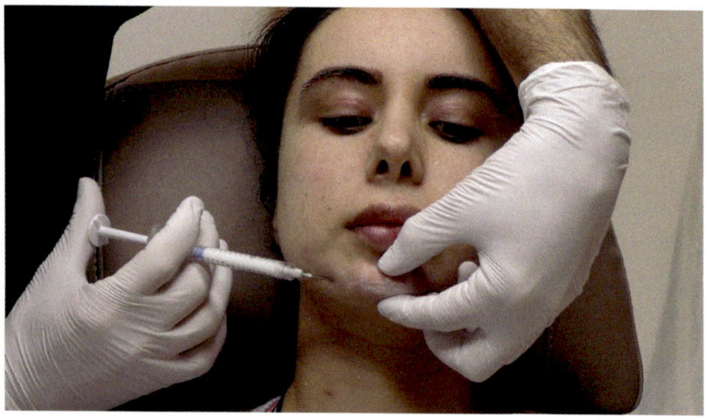

Figure 23.7 Injecting boluses sub-muscularly.

2. Disinfect and mark the width and vertical position of maximum projection, taking the Steiner's line into consideration.
3. Make a pre-hole at the pre-jowl sulcus with a 21G needle.
4. Use undiluted CaHA and a 22G, 50 mm cannula.
5. Lift up the mentalis muscle with the nondominant hand (Figure 23.6).
6. Enter through skin and maneuver the cannula to the periosteum under the mentalis muscle and advance to the midline.
7. Place multiple boluses at the periosteal level until desired anterior projection of the mentum is achieved (Figure 23.7).
8. Retract toward the entry point and readvance in the subcutaneous plane.
9. For contouring of the mandible and lengthening of the mentum, place multiple retrograde linear threads along the mandibular border, keeping the ideal width of the chin in mind (Figure 23.8).
10. If necessary, also the pre-jowl sulcus and marionette lines can be treated from here.
11. Check for symmetry.
12. Mold into the desired shape.

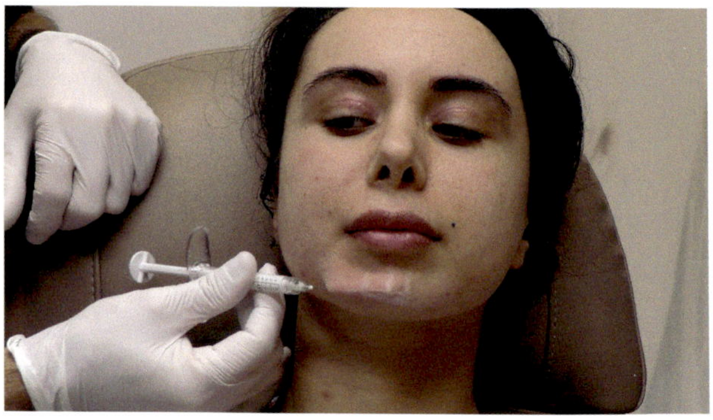

Figure 23.8 Injecting subcutaneous retrograde linear.

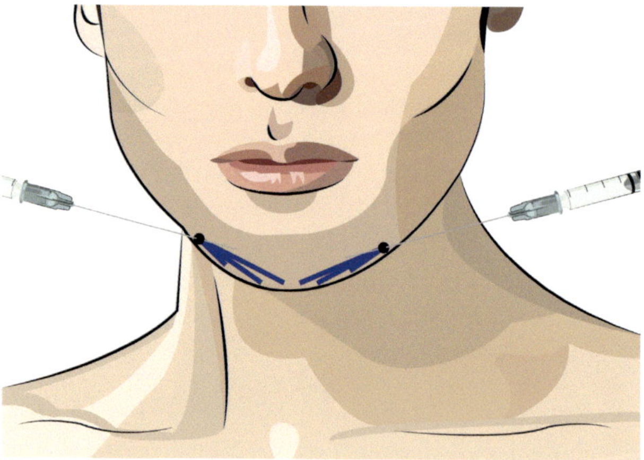

Figure 23.9 Mentum augmentation in male patients.

23.6 CANNULA TECHNIQUE FOR MENTUM AUGMENTATION IN MALES

For injection placement, see Figure 23.9.

23.6.1 Step-by-Step Technique

1. Consider a mentalis nerve block.
2. Disinfect and mark the width (same as the width of the mouth) and vertical position of maximum projection, taking the Steiner's line into consideration.
3. Use undiluted CaHA and a 25G, 38 mm cannula.
4. Mark the entry points just medial to the pre-jowl sulcus.
5. Advance cannula along the mandibular border (Figure 23.10).
6. Inject thick retrograde linear threads totaling approximately 0.5 mL at the mandibular border (Figure 23.11).
7. Check for symmetry.
8. Mold into the desired shape.

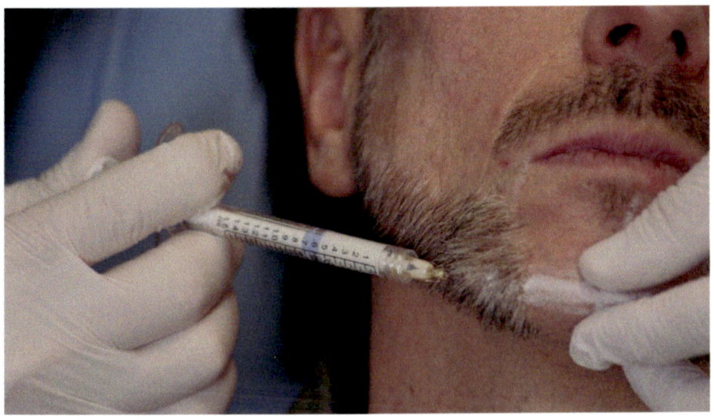

Figure 23.10 Advance the cannula along the mandibular border.

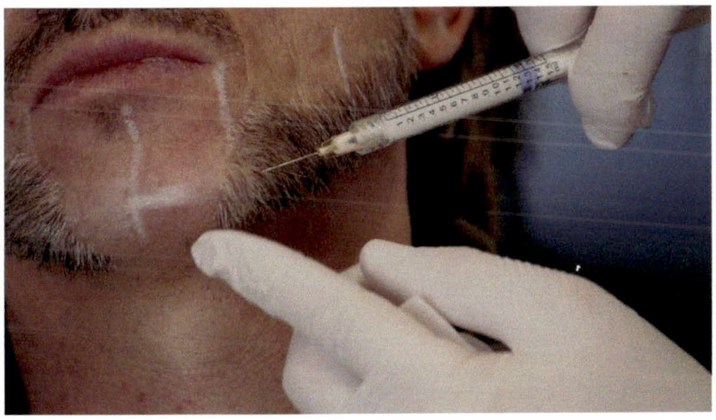

Figure 23.11 Inject thick deposits to increase width of the mentum.

23.7 NEEDLE TECHNIQUE

For injection placement, see Figure 23.12.

23.7.1 Step-by-Step Technique

1. Consider a mentalis nerve block.
2. Disinfect and mark the width and vertical position of maximum projection, taking the Steiner's line into consideration (Figure 23.13).
3. Use undiluted CaHA and a 27G needle.
4. At the point of maximum projection, choose the entry site for the needle.
5. With the nondominant hand, lift up the mentalis muscle and advance the needle straight to the periosteum to the space between the two bellies of the mentalis muscles.
6. Inject multiple boluses of approximately 0.1 mL per bolus on the periosteum (the product will be placed in multiple anatomical layers) (Figure 23.14).
7. For increased projection, retrograde linear threads may also be injected from the periosteum toward the skin.

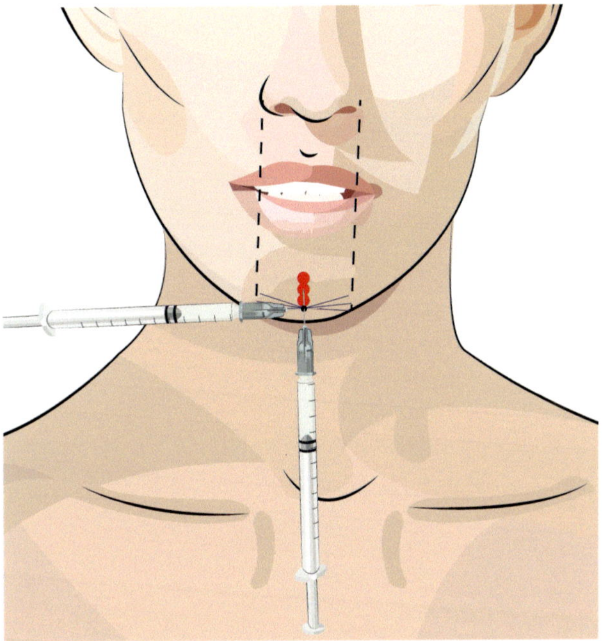

Figure 23.12 Product injection for mentum augmentation with a sharp needle. Black dotted line: alar width (ideal width of the chin in Western cultures); red dots: periosteal deposits of 0.1 mL CaHA; blue lines: subcutaneous linear threads of CaHA.

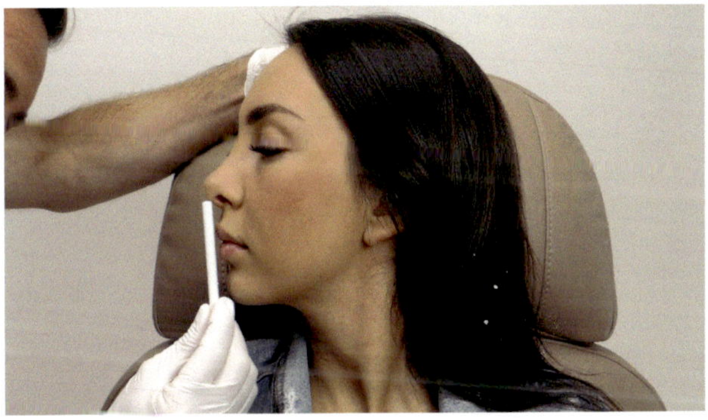

Figure 23.13 Determining the point and desired amount of anterior projection of the pogonion.

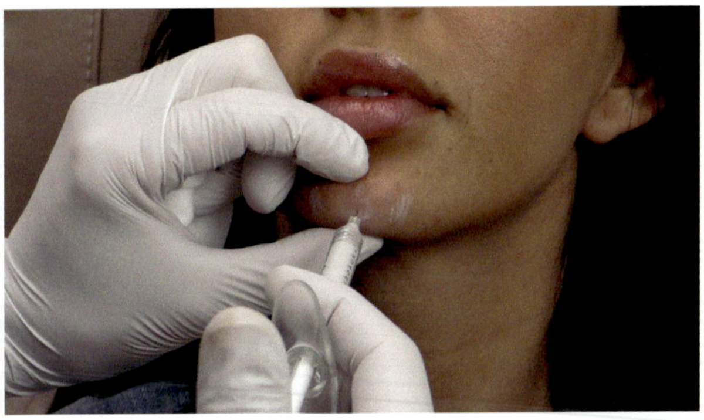

Figure 23.14 Periosteal boluses of 0.1 mL each in the midline for anterior projection of the pogonion.

8. As a secondary option to create a less pointy projection, from the same entry point, the needle may be advanced laterally in the subcutaneous fat for several retrograde linear threads as needed (Figure 23.15).
9. Last, to create a smooth transition from the lower cheek to the pogonion and to reduce the pointy chin effect, subcutaneous retrogrades can be placed in the marionette to mental crease area.
10. Check for symmetry.
11. Mold into the desired shape.

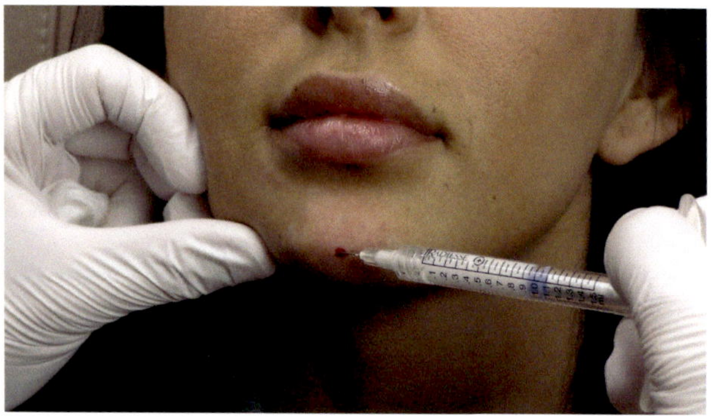

Figure 23.15 Retrograde linear threads of subcutaneous CaHA for shaping of the mentum.

See further Figure 23.16 and Videos 23.1–23.4 for before and after results and application techniques, respectively.

Video 23.1 Mentum augmentation: cannula technique 1.

Video 23.2 Mentum augmentation: cannula technique 2 (anterior projection).

Video 23.3 Mentum augmentation: cannula technique 3 (males).

Video 23.4 Mentum augmentation: needle technique.

23.8 AFTERCARE

If necessary, the area can be manually massaged to even out the product.

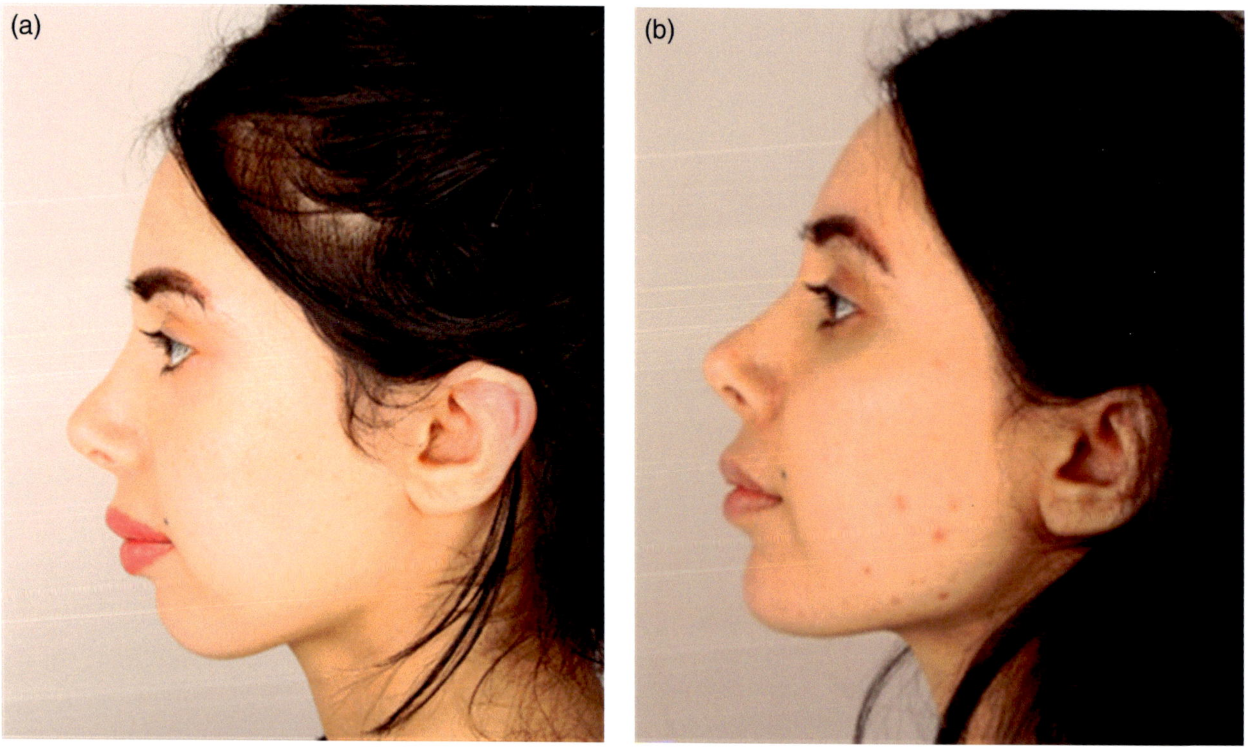

Figure 23.16 (a) Before and (b) one-month post-treatment with CaHA.

23.9 ADDITIONAL TREATMENTS FOR OPTIMAL RESULTS

The mentalis muscle may be treated with botulinum toxin to reduce dimpling and anterior projection. The treatment can be done prior to the CaHA application in order to reduce risk of muscular contraction associated migration of the CaHA product. After projecting the chin, the entire infraoral area should be assessed and potentially adjusted by injecting additional CaHA or other fillers in the mental crease, pre-jowl sulcus, and/or marionette lines.

REFERENCES

[1] R. B. Shaw et al., "Aging of the facial skeleton: Aesthetic implications and rejuvenation strategies," *Plast Reconstr Surg*, vol. 127, no. 1, pp. 374–383, 2011.

[2] B. Mendelson, C. H. Wong, "Changes in the facial skeleton with aging: Implications and clinical applications in facial rejuvenation," *Aesthetic Plast Surg*, vol. 36, no. 4, pp. 753–760, 2012.

The Lower Third of the Face

Mental Crease

24

JANI VAN LOGHEM

24.1 INTRODUCTION

The mental crease is a horizontal crease between the lower lip and the mentalis muscle. It has both a dynamic and a static component.

24.2 ANATOMICAL DANGERS

The inferior labial artery runs deep in this area, although not in every patient, as this artery may have loops or branches to the subcutaneous level. If CaHA is injected too deeply, visible yellowish deposits can be seen in the mucosa of the lower lip. Pay attention also to the submental and mental arteries (Figure 24.1).

24.3 CANNULA TECHNIQUE

For injection placement, see Figure 24.2.

24.3.1 Step-by-Step Technique

1. Consider giving local anesthesia in the skin lateral to the mental crease.
2. Disinfect and make a pre-hole with a 23G needle.
3. Use undiluted CaHA and a 25G, 38 mm cannula, or CaHA with standard dilution.
4. With the nondominant hand, stretch the skin in order to remain superficial and advance the cannula in the subcutaneous level along the mental crease.
5. Make sure that the cannula is not visible in the oral mucosa to avoid mucosal injection (Figure 24.3).
6. Inject multiple retrograde linear threads of 0.05–0.1 mL (Figure 24.4).
7. Repeat on contralateral side.

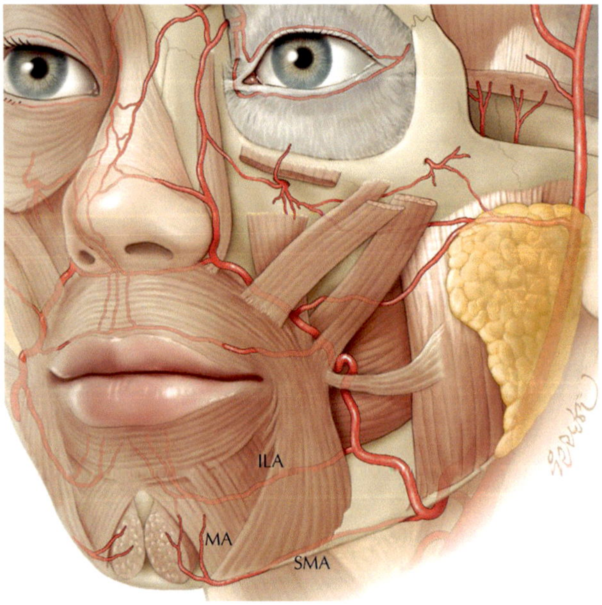

Figure 24.1 Arterial danger zones for the treatment of the mentum crease: inferior labial artery (ILA), submental artery (SMA), and mental artery (MA).

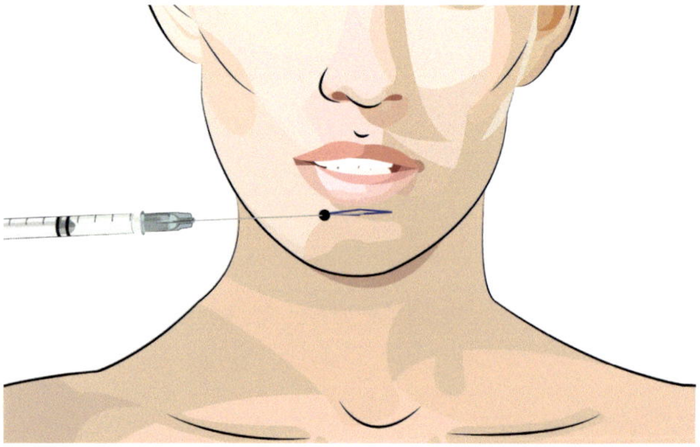

Figure 24.2 Product injection in the mental crease. Blue lines represent subcutaneous retrograde linear threads.

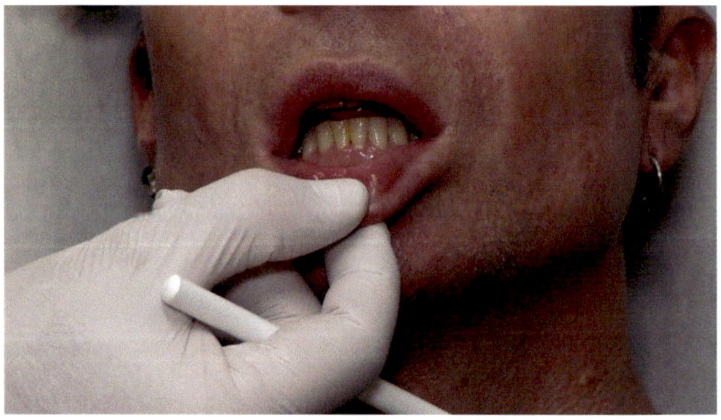

Figure 24.3 Examination to avoid placement of the cannula in the oral mucosa.

DOI: 10.1201/9781003617129-24

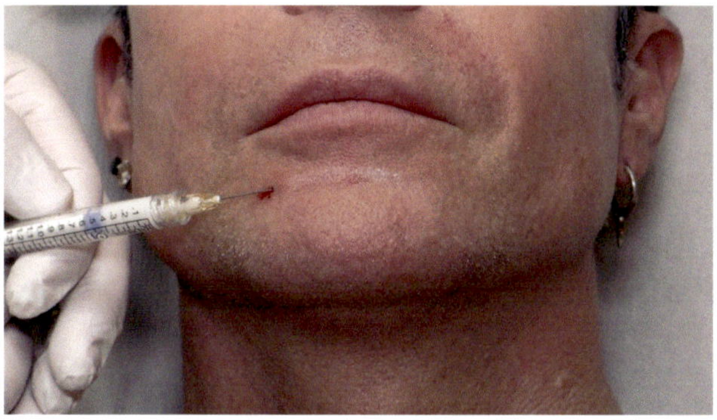

Figure 24.4 Retrograde linear thread with cannula. A finger may be used intraorally to guide the injection.

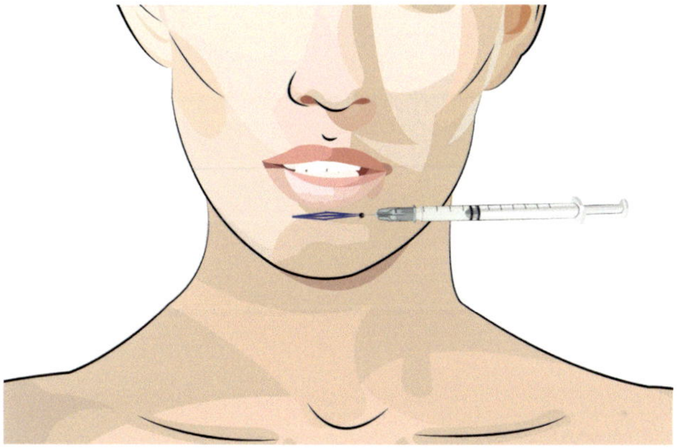

Figure 24.5 Product injection in the mental crease using sharp needle. Blue lines represent deep dermal or subcutaneous retrograde linear threads.

8. Mold to even out the product.

24.4 NEEDLE TECHNIQUE

For injection placement, see Figure 24.5.

24.4.1 Step-by-Step Technique

1. Use undiluted CaHA or CaHA with standard dilution and a 27 or 28G needle.
2. Choose the entry point at the lateral limit of the mental crease.
3. Insert the needle and remain superficial: at the deep dermal level or in the subcutaneous level.

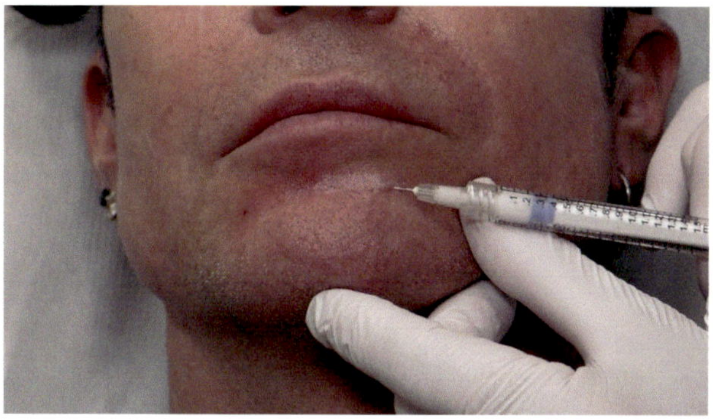

Figure 24.6 Retrograde linear thread with sharp needle.

4. Avoid advancing the needle to the submucosa, as product may be visible then.
5. Inject multiple retrograde linear threads in a tight fanning shape (Figure 24.6).
6. Mold to even out the product.

See further Videos 24.1–24.2 to visualize different application techniques.

24.5 AFTERCARE

If necessary, the area can be manually massaged to even out the product. The area may be swollen up to a day or two. Sometimes the patient may report palpable product with the tongue or the feeling of presence of product. Massaging can help reduce palpability. When the product is placed too deeply, it might be visible in the oral mucosa. Expressing the product after making an incision with an 18G needle is indicated.

24.6 ADDITIONAL TREATMENTS FOR OPTIMAL RESULTS

As the mental crease has a dynamic component, injection of botulinum toxin in the mentalis muscle will improve results. It will also help prevention of displacement of product, especially when injected prior to injection of CaHA.

Video 24.1 Mental crease: cannula technique.

Video 24.2 Mental crease: sharp needle technique.

The Lower Third of the Face

The Mandibular Angle and Jawline

25

JANI VAN LOGHEM, SHINO BAY AGUILERA, AND LUIS SORO

25.1 INTRODUCTION

A nicely defined jawline is a sign of youth and is considered a beauty trait for women in western culture. For men in Western countries, a strong mandibular profile is considered attractive (also discussed in Chapters 22 and 23). In Asian cultures, jawline definition is not generally seen as a beauty trait, so cultural differences will influence the direction the physician should take toward the ideal treatment outcome. Independent from sex and culture, the ageing process will result in jowling. When patients present with jowling, the preferred order is to start with lifting the midface before proceeding to the lower face, as treating the midface will influence the position of the jowls in the lower face (as well as the nasolabial folds and tear troughs).

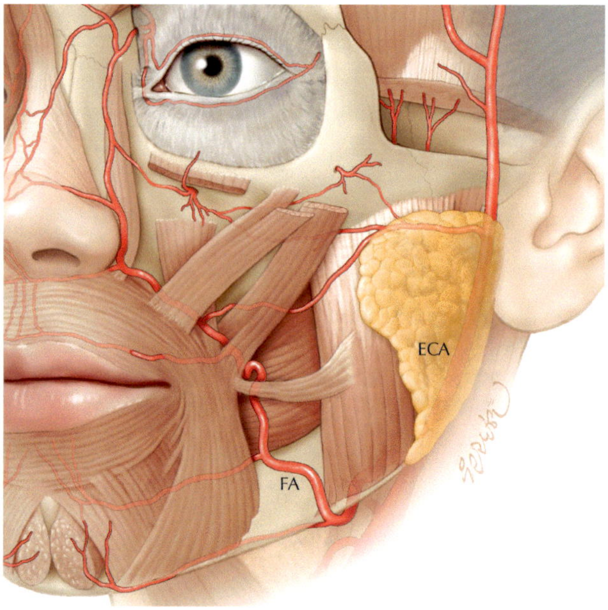

Figure 25.1 Arterial danger zones for the treatment of the mandibular angle and jawline include the facial artery (FA) and the external carotid artery (ECA).

25.2 AGE-RELATED ANATOMICAL CHANGES

The anatomical changes of the lower third of the face, from the mandibular angle and jawline down to the mentum, are closely related. Therefore, further discussion of age-related anatomical changes can be found in Chapter 23.

25.3 ANATOMICAL DANGERS

Both the facial and the external carotid arteries run deep in this area. The facial artery runs over the periosteum, just anterior of the masseter muscle. Dorsal to the ramus, the external carotid artery runs deep into the mandible.

The parotid gland is located sub-SMAS and lies over the masseter muscle. Injection of CaHA in this salivary gland should be avoided, as it can lead to stasis and accumulation of saliva by blocking salivary ducts, and therefore possibly stone formation and parotitis (Figure 25.1).

Injecting into the jowl fat compartments themselves should be avoided, as this can lead to aesthetically displeasing worsened jowling.

25.4 JOWL CORRECTION

For injection placement, see Figure 25.2.

25.4.1 Step-by-Step Technique

1. Identify and outline the jowl, which resembles a "U" shape.
2. Mark the recommended insertion points at both the pre-jowl sulcus and the mandibular angle. The pre-jowl sulcus is found anterior to the U-shaped deformity or by extending a vertical line down from the outer alar rim (Figure 25.3).
3. Use 0.1–0.2 mL boluses supraperiosteally to recreate the contour of the jawline (Figure 25.4).
4. Use a retrograde linear threading technique at the dermal–subcutaneous junction with the aid of a cannula (Figure 25.5).
5. In patients with severe jowl formation, create an insertion point just inferior to the zygoma directed toward the U-shaped deformity.
6. Use a blunt-tip cannula to perform a retrograde fanning technique, further enhancing the jawline and lifting the lower face.

25.5 DEFINING THE JAWLINE CANNULA TECHNIQUE 1

For injection placement, see Figure 25.6.

DOI: 10.1201/9781003617129-25

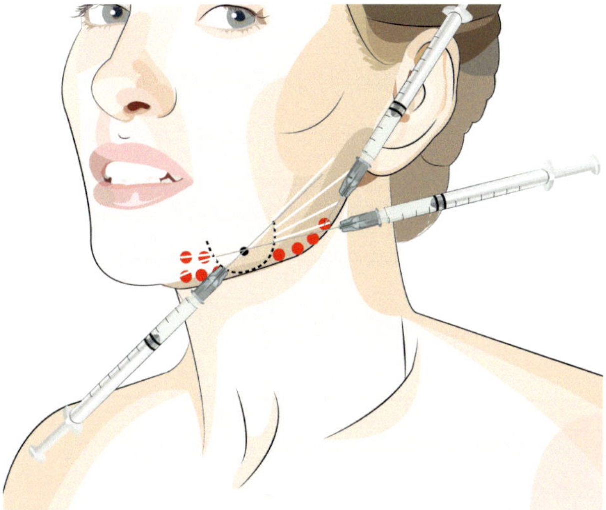

Figure 25.2 Product injection for jowl correction. The red dots represent supraperiosteal boluses of approximately 0.1 mL each injected with a sharp needle. The white lines represent retrograde linear threads at the dermal–subdermal junction injected with a blunt cannula and the dashed line the location of the jowl.

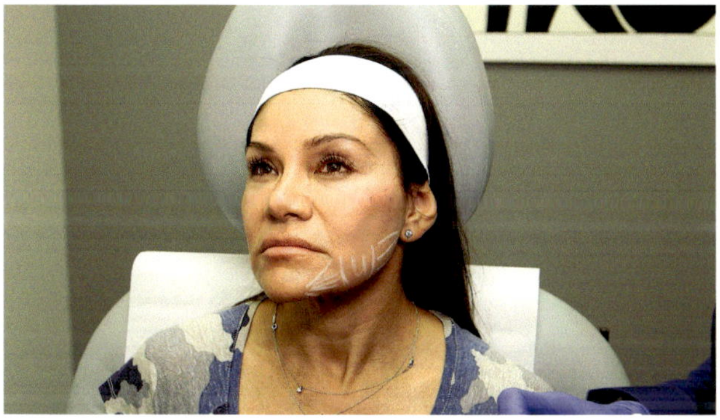

Figure 25.3 Mapping the U-shape of the jowl area.

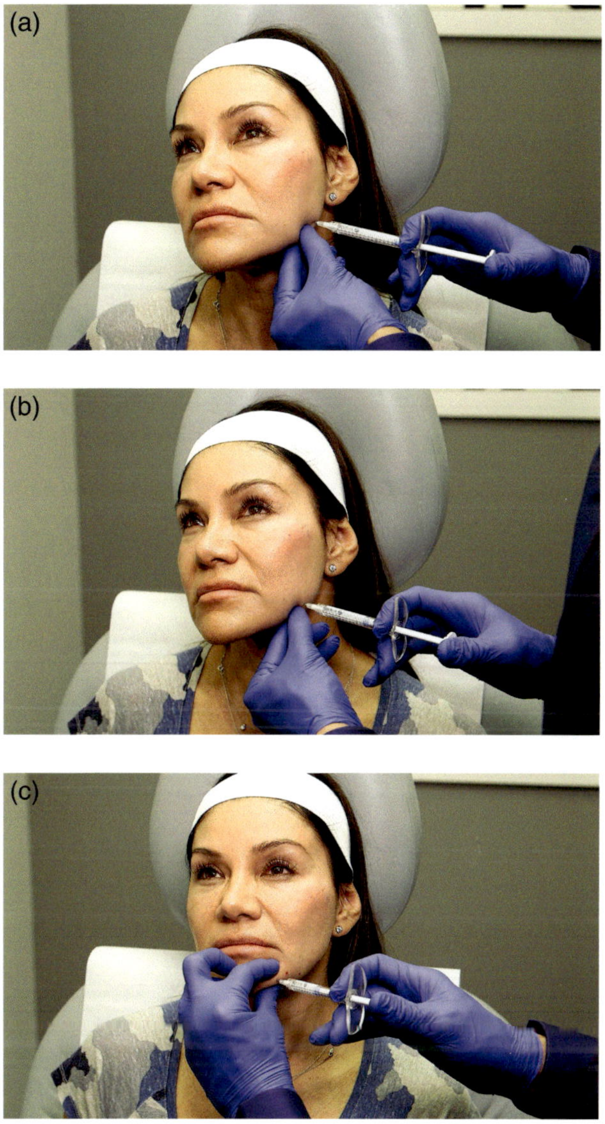

Figure 25.4 Use 0.1–0.2 mL supraperiosteally along the mandible to recreate the contour of the jawline at the level of the (a) mandibular angle, (b) the post-jowl sulcus, and (c) the pre-jowl sulcus.

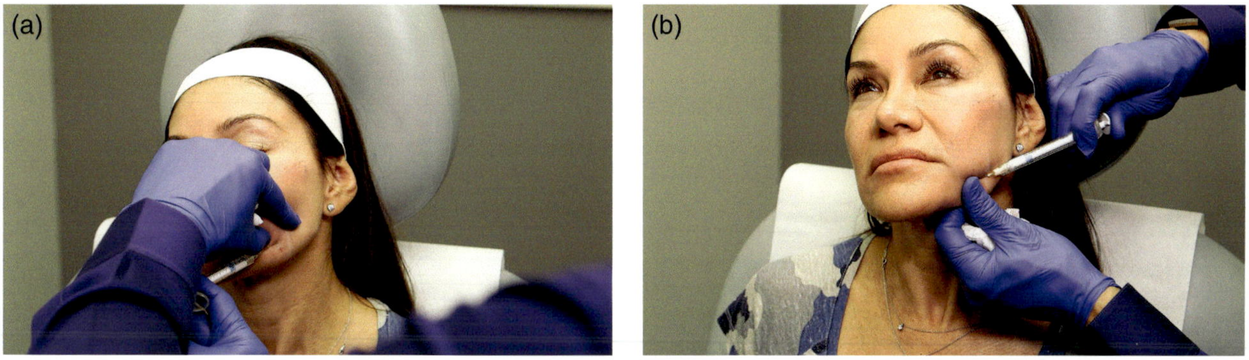

Figure 25.5 Use a 25G, 50.8 mm blunt-tip cannula to perform a retrograde fanning technique, further enhancing the jawline and lifting the lower face: (a) from the jowl to the mandibular angle and (b) from the jowl to the mentum.

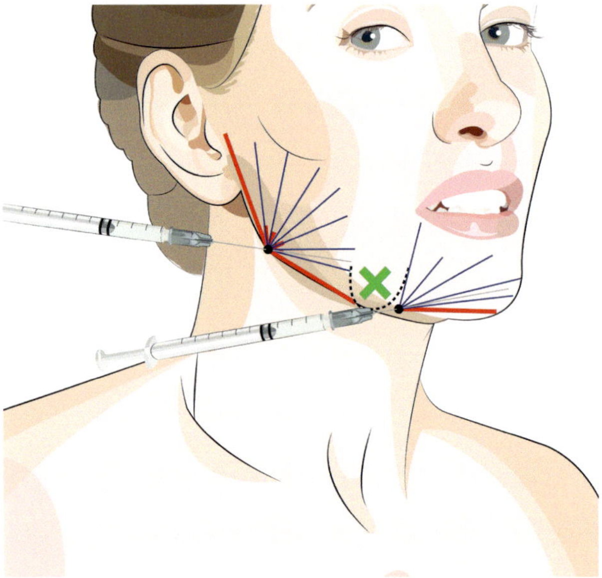

Figure 25.6 Schematic drawing of CaHA injection at the mandibular area using cannula. Red lines indicate tick retrograde linear threads of undiluted CaHA. Blue lines indicate retrograde linear threads of diluted CaHA at the dermal–subdermal junction. The U-shaped dashed line and green cross indicate the jowl.

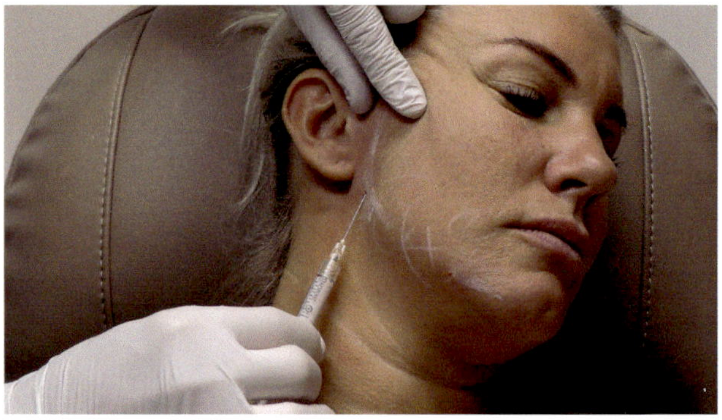

Figure 25.7 Mandibular definition from mandibular angle to the preauricular area.

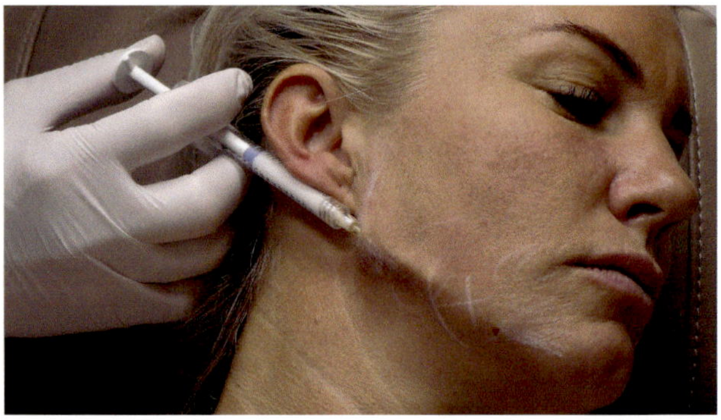

Figure 25.8 Mandibular definition from mandibular angle toward the post-jowl sulcus.

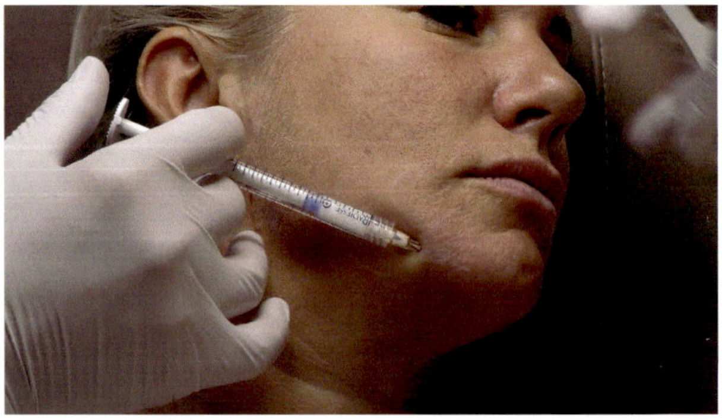

Figure 25.9 Mandibular definition from the pre-jowl sulcus to the mentum.

25.5.1 Step-by-Step Technique

1. Mark the jowl, determine the position of the mandibular angle, and disinfect.
2. Determine entry points at or just superolateral to the mandibular angle and at the pre-jowl sulcus.
3. Consider local anesthesia and make pre-holes with 23G needle.
4. Use undiluted CaHA and a 25G, 38 mm cannula for contouring and diluted CaHA for skin quality improvement and smoothing out the effect of undiluted CaHA.
5. With the nondominant hand, lift the lower cheek vertically upward.
6. Advance the cannula from the mandibular angle entry point to the preauricular area and place a thick retrograde linear thread of approximately 0.2–0.3 mL subcutaneously (Figure 25.7).
7. With the same undiluted CaHA, make a small fan at the angle, toward the lower border of the mandible.
8. At the lower border of the mandible, advance the cannula toward the post-jowl sulcus.
9. Inject a retrograde linear thread of about 0.3 mL at the mandibular border. With the nondominant hand, pinching the skin, the retrograde can be guided and the product can be injected in a sharp line (Figure 25.8).
10. From the pre-jowl sulcus entry point, advance the cannula toward the mentum midline along the mandibular border.
11. Inject a retrograde of about 0.2 mL (Figure 25.9).
12. Now switch to diluted CaHA (depending on skin thickness but usually about 0.5 to 1.5 mL lidocaine per 1.5 mL syringe of CaHA) and a 25G, 50 mm cannula.

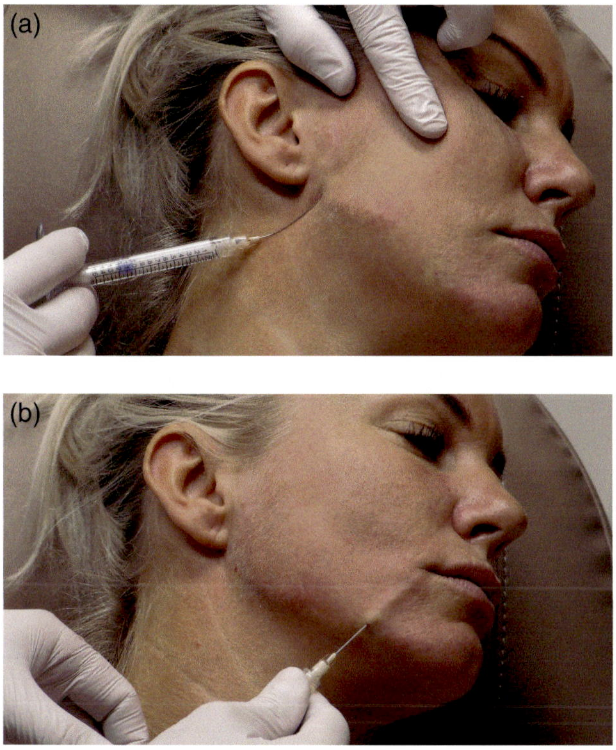

Figure 25.10 Smoothing out mandibular definition and improving skin quality from (a) mandibular entry point and (b) pre-jowl sulcus entry point with diluted CaHA. Stretching the skin and pushing down the syringe will aid in keeping the cannula tip from scraping against the dermal–subdermal junction.

13. Inject retrograde linear threads in a fanning technique in between the initial contouring CaHA injections (Figure 25.10).
14. From the pre-jowl sulcus entry point, inject retrograde linear threads in a fanning pattern from the marionette line down to the mandibular border.
15. Even out with massage if needed.

25.6 DEFINING THE JAWLINE CANNULA TECHNIQUE 2

For injection placement, see Figure 25.11.

25.6.1 Step-by-Step Technique

1. Mark the jowl and disinfect.
2. Determine entry points at mentum and post-jowl sulcus.
3. Consider local anesthesia and make pre-holes with 23G needle.
4. Use undiluted CaHA and a 25G, 38 mm cannula.
5. Advance the cannula from the mentum to the pre-jowl sulcus and place a thick retrograde linear thread of approximately 0.2–0.3 mL subcutaneously (Figure 25.12).

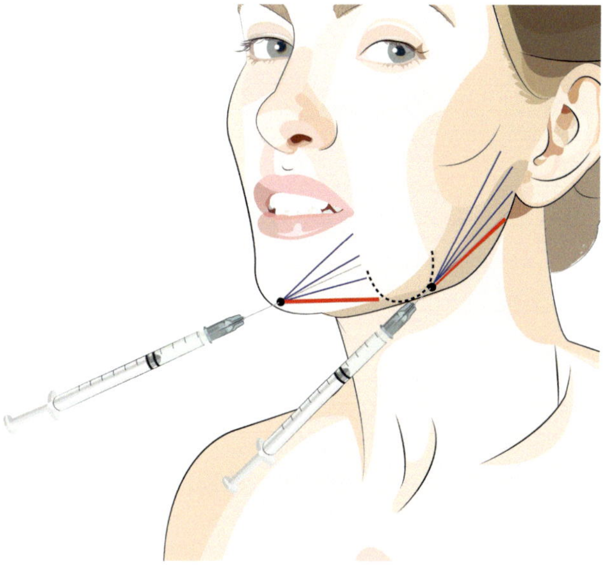

Figure 25.11 CaHA injection at the mandibular area using cannula. Red lines indicate tick retrograde linear threads of undiluted CaHA, blue lines indicate retrograde linear threads of diluted CaHA, at the dermal–subdermal junction, and the dashed line the jowl area.

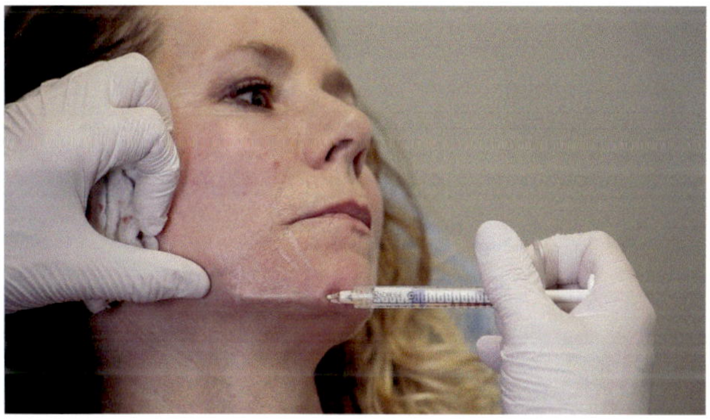

Figure 25.12 Mandibular definition from mentum to pre-jowl sulcus.

6. From the post-jowl sulcus entry point, advance the cannula to the lobule of the ear and place another thick retrograde linear thread of approximately 0.2–0.3 mL subcutaneously (Figure 25.13).
7. Now switch to diluted CaHA (depending on skin thickness but usually about 0.5–0.8 mL lidocaine per 1.5 mL syringe of CaHA) and a 25G, 50 mm cannula.
8. Inject retrograde linear threads in a fanning technique cranial to the first lines (Figure 25.14).
9. Even out with massage if needed.

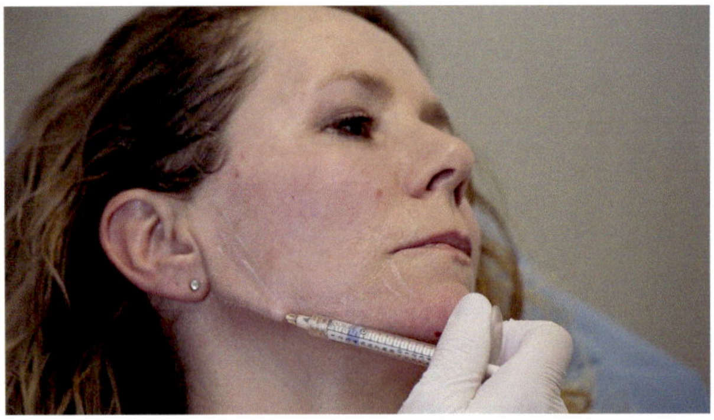

Figure 25.13 Mandibular definition from post-jowl sulcus toward the lobule of the ear.

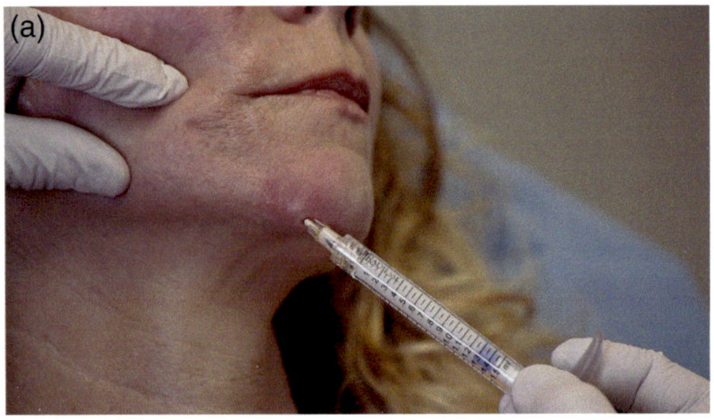

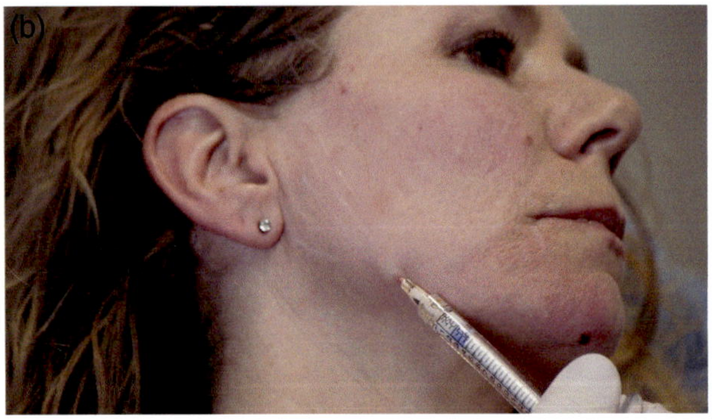

Figure 25.14 Smoothing out mandibular definition and improving skin quality from (a) mentum entry point and (b) post-jowl sulcus entry point with diluted CaHA.

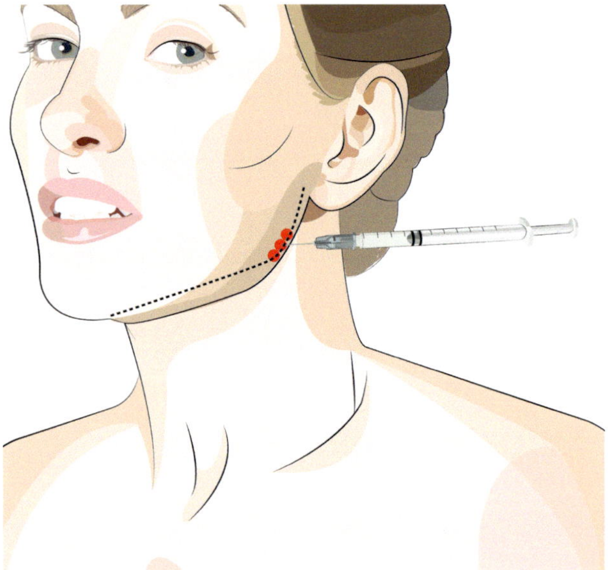

Figure 25.15 CaHA injection at the mandibular angle using a sharp needle. The red dots indicate periosteal boluses of undiluted CaHA, and the dashed line indicates the border of the mandible.

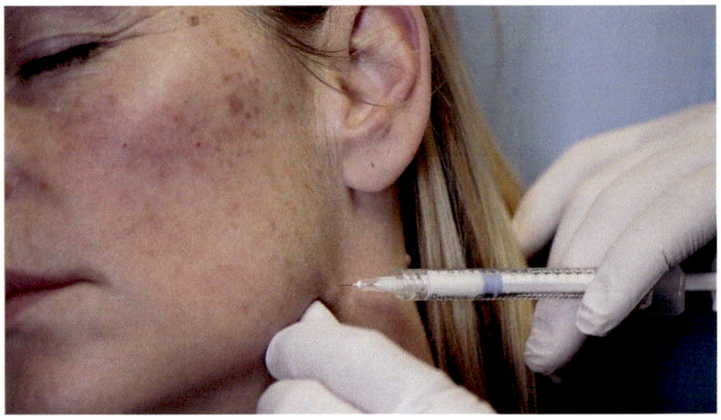

Figure 25.16 Mandibular angle periosteal boluses injected at the dorsal side.

25.7 MANDIBULAR ANGLE SHARP NEEDLE PERIOSTEAL BOLUS TECHNIQUE

For injection placement, see Figure 25.15.

25.7.1 Step-by-Step Technique

1. Mark the mandibular angle and disinfect.
2. Consider local anesthesia from the skin to the periosteum.
3. Use undiluted CaHA and the 27G needle supplied with the product.
4. Advance the needle from the dorsal side of the mandibular angle to the periosteum (Figure 25.16).
5. Place a periosteal bolus.
6. Partially retract, reorient, and readvance the needle and inject additional boluses around the mandibular angle.
7. As product may flow back through the tunnel created by the needle, massaging may be indicated to mold the product into the desired shape.

See also Figure 25.17 and Videos 25.1–25.4 for end-result and application techniques visualization, respectively.

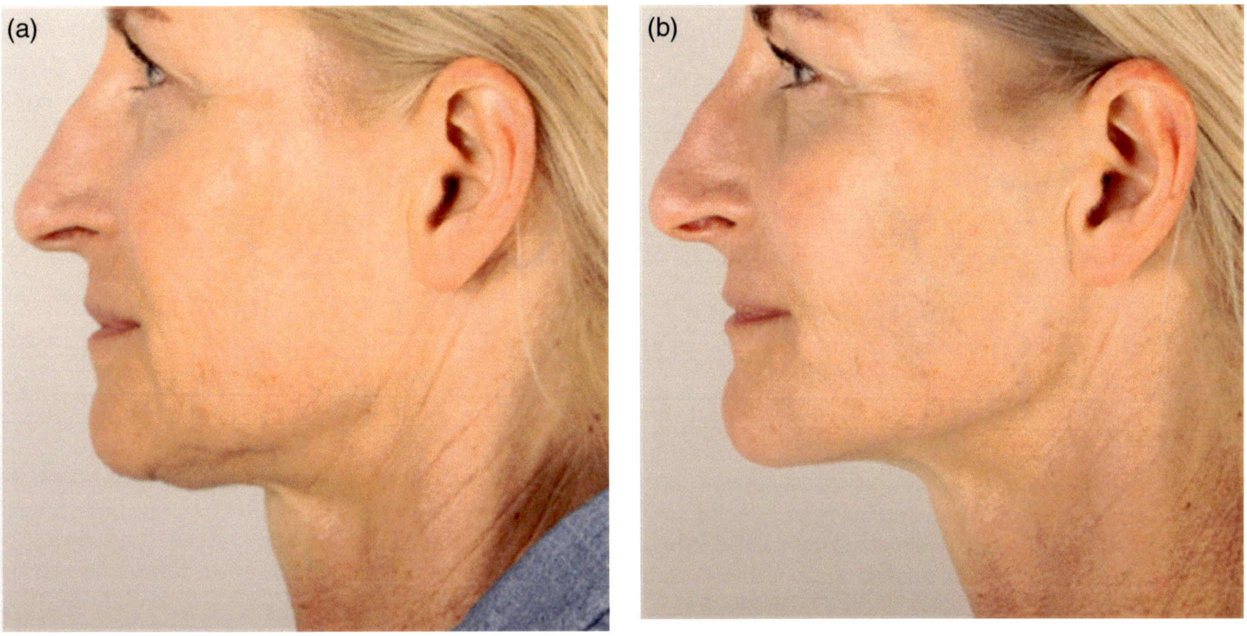

Figure 25.17 (a) Before and (b) after treatment of the jawline with CaHA.

25.8 AFTERCARE

If necessary, the area can be manually massaged to even out the product. If injected on the periosteum at the mandibular angle, part of the product may end up intramuscularly, especially when injecting with a sharp needle. This might lead to pain or sensitivity on mastication. This is a temporary problem and should resolve in approximately three days. Subcutaneous palpable depositions at the mandibular angle or the mandibular border can be disturbing to some patients. Patients should be informed of this possibility prior to treatment. Usually, this problem subsides after the gel part of the product has been partially resorbed after approximately one month.

25.9 ADDITIONAL TREATMENTS FOR OPTIMAL RESULTS

Before addressing the jawline, cheek augmentation may be considered, as deep injection of CaHA or other volumizers to the cheek will usually reduce the jowls. Any other lifting procedure of the midface may benefit the jawline as well. Besides lifting the cheek, augmentation of the mentum, pre-jowl sulcus, and marionette lines can significantly improve the mandibular contour and reduce jowling.

For male augmentation and additional mandibular treatments, please see Chapters 20, 23, and 26.

Video 25.1 Jowl correction.

Video 25.2 Mandibular angle: cannula technique 1 (left).

Video 25.3 Mandibular angle: cannula technique 1 (right).

Video 25.4 Mandibular angle: cannula technique 2.

Video 25.5 Mandibular angle: sharp needle technique.

The Lower Third of the Face

Masseter Augmentation in Men

26

JANI VAN LOGHEM

26.1 INTRODUCTION

Male attractiveness can be improved by accentuating male facial characteristics. As high testosterone levels will increase muscular volume, a well-developed masseter muscle is associated with masculinity and male attractiveness. The masseter can be augmented in different anatomical layers: subcutaneous, as discussed in the chapter on mandibular angle and jawline, and on the periosteum of the mandible. When injecting at the periosteum with a sharp needle perpendicular to the bone, the product will be positioned intramuscularly due to product backflow. A cannula technique will result in product positioning mainly on the periosteum [1]. Due to bone resorption, the mandible changes shape and becomes smaller [2]. In order to create a strong mandibular profile, the mandible can be accentuated.

26.2 ANATOMICAL DANGERS

The anatomical dangers of the masseter augmentation procedure (Figure 26.1) share commonalities with both the mandibular angle and jawline treatments discussed in Chapter 25.

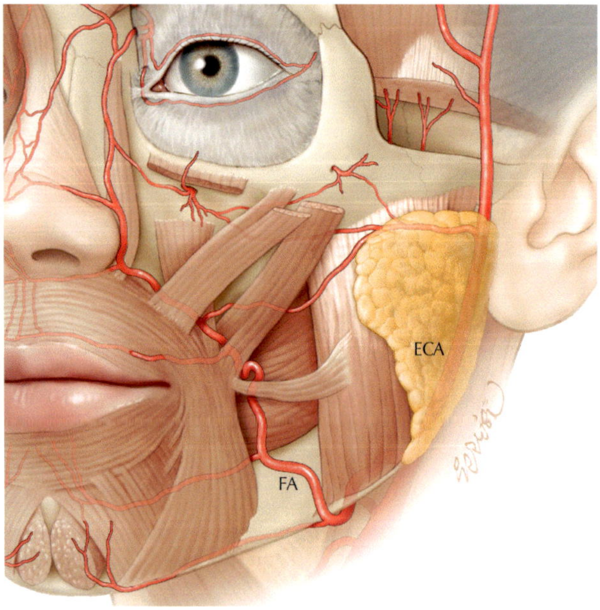

Figure 26.1 Arterial danger zones for the treatment of masseter augmentation in men include the facial artery (FA) and the external carotid artery (ECA).

In short, both the facial and the external carotid arteries run over and through the mandibular periosteum where the masseter muscle inserts. Moreover, the parotid gland and its salivary ducts lie over the muscle. A sharp needle procedure on the periosteum will result in backflow of product through the needle trajectory, and limited amounts of CaHA should be injected to minimize the risk of intravascular and intraglandular injection. Injecting in the superficial muscular compartment of the masseter should be avoided, as nodules may also form.

26.3 MASSETER AUGMENTATION WITH THE CANNULA TECHNIQUE

For injection placement, see Figure 26.2.

26.3.1 Step-by-Step Technique

1. Identify the mandibular angle.
2. Inject anesthesia containing adrenaline at the skin entry site and continue to inject toward the bone at the mandibular angle (Figure 26.3).
3. Make a pre-hole.
4. Use a 22G, 50 mm or a 25G, 38 mm cannula and non-diluted CaHA.
5. Advance the cannula through the skin.

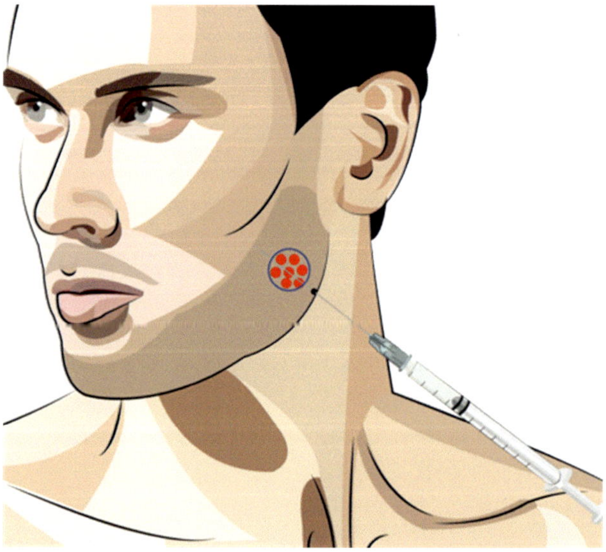

Figure 26.2 Masseter augmentation with the cannula technique. The red dots indicate the injection sites.

DOI: 10.1201/9781003617129-26

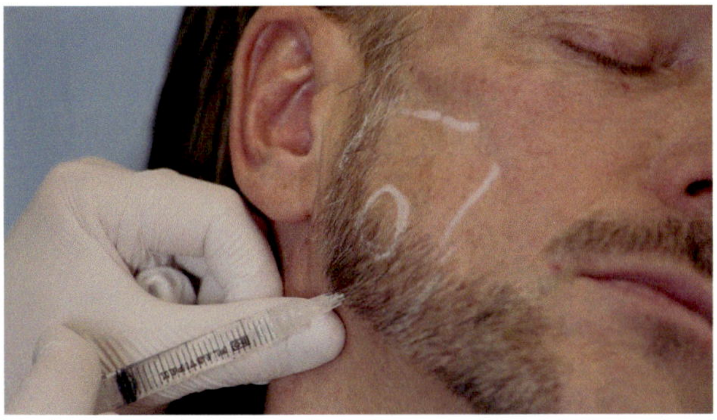

Figure 26.3 Anesthesia from the skin to the periosteum.

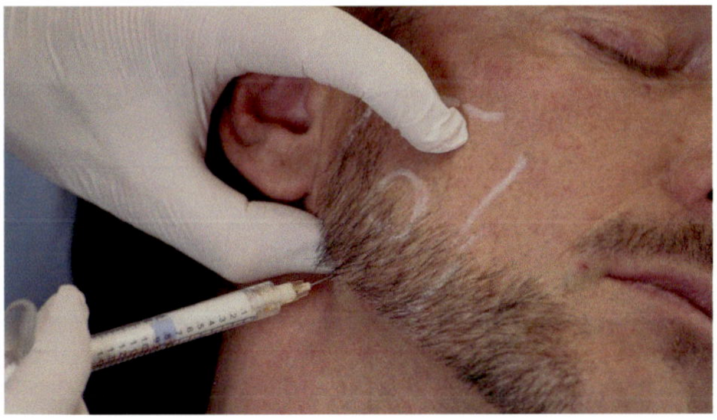

Figure 26.4 Guide the cannula through the adhesions and inject 0.1–0.2 mL boluses below the masseter belly supraperiosteally.

6. Place the thumb of the nondominant hand below the mandibular border to avoid advancing the cannula behind the mandible.
7. Inject a bolus of 0.1–0.2 mL, position the cannula a few millimeters away and inject another bolus of 0.1–0.2 mL.
8. Repeat injecting below the muscle belly until the desired result has been achieved.
9. While rotating, use adequate force to pass the resistance of the SMAS and the adhesions of the masseter muscle to the mandible (Figure 26.4).
10. Advance the cannula over the periosteum to the level of the marked point of maximum projection at the belly of the masseter.

26.4 MASSETER AUGMENTATION WITH THE NEEDLE TECHNIQUE

For injection placement, see Figure 26.5.

26.4.1 Step-by-Step Technique

1. Identify the belly of the masseter muscle, mark, and disinfect (Figure 26.6).
2. Use non-diluted CaHA and a 27G, 20 mm needle.
3. Advance the needle through the skin just lateral from the central masseter belly toward the periosteum.

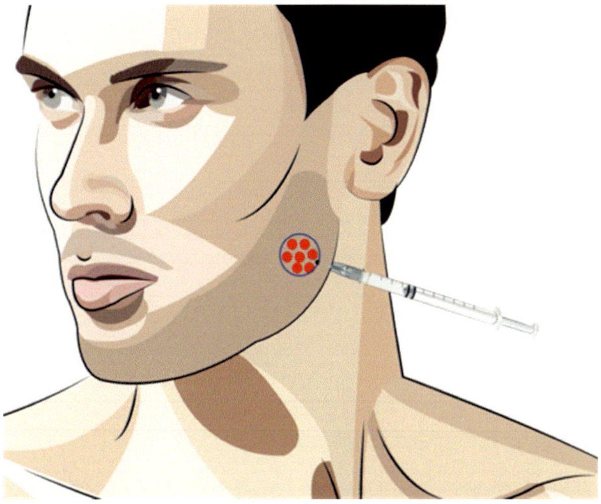

Figure 26.5 Masseter augmentation with sharp needle.

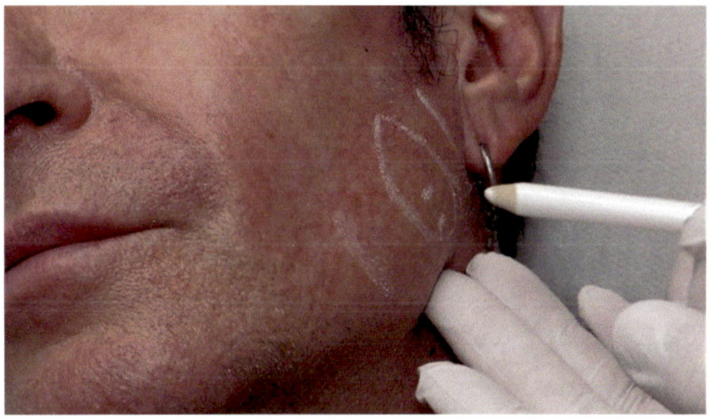

Figure 26.6 Marking the masseter.

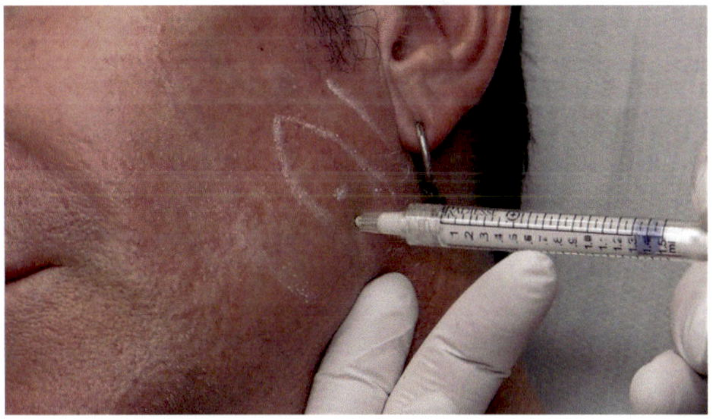

Figure 26.7 Needle positioned on periosteum below the masseter muscle. Note the angle of the needle being not perpendicular but at approximately 45°.

4. Place the needle with soft touch to the periosteum with the bevel down and with an angle of approximately 45°. This will reduce risk backflow to more superficial areas of the muscle (Figure 26.7).
5. Inject a bolus of 0.1–0.2 mL at the periosteum.
6. Partially retract, reorient and re-advance to the periosteum.

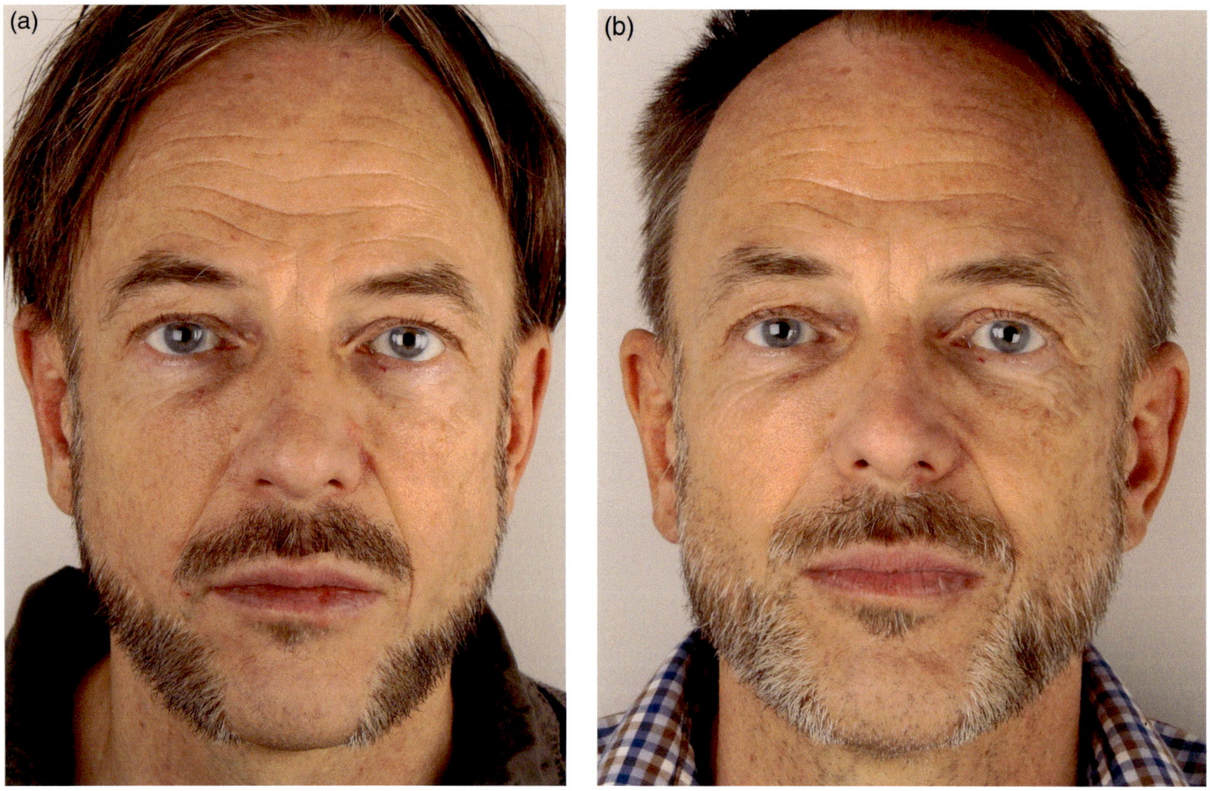

Figure 26.8 (a) Before and (b) after masseter augmentation employing the submuscular cannula technique. Results are 5 weeks after treatment of 1.5 mL non-diluted CaHA divided over both sides.

7. Inject multiple boluses of 0.1–0.2 mL under the central belly of the muscle, a few millimeters apart at the periosteal level.
8. Repeat injecting below the muscle belly until the desired result has been achieved.

See also Figure 26.8 and Videos 26.1–26.2 for before and after results and application techniques, respectively.

> **Video 26.1** Masseter augmentation: submuscular cannula technique.

> **Video 26.2** Masseter augmentation: sharp needle technique.

26.5 AFTERCARE

If necessary, the area can be manually massaged to even out the product. Product injected on the periosteum may end up intramuscularly, especially when injecting with a sharp needle. This might lead to pain or sensitivity on mastication. This is a temporary problem and should resolve in approximately three days.

26.6 ADDITIONAL TREATMENTS FOR OPTIMAL RESULTS

Besides addressing the masseter, mentum augmentation may be considered to enhance the male appearance.

REFERENCES

[1] J. A. J. van Loghem et al., "Cannula versus sharp needle for placement of soft tissue fillers: An observational cadaver study," *Aesthet Surg J*, vol. 38, no. 1, pp. 73 88, 2017.
[2] R. B. Shaw et al., "Aging of the facial skeleton: Aesthetic implications and rejuvenation strategies," *Plast Reconstr Surg*, vol. 127, no. 1, pp. 374–383, 2011.

Neck, Chest, and Abdomen

27

Neck Rejuvenation

JANI VAN LOGHEM

27.1 INTRODUCTION

The neck is an increasingly popular area for rejuvenation. To avoid contrast with the rejuvenated face, patients often inquire about possibilities for reducing signs of ageing. Especially the fine vertical laxity wrinkles in the midline, horizontal necklines, and sagging submental area can be of concern to patients. A full-face and neck assessment should be made on a static and on a dynamic position, in both frontal and profile view. As a general approach, the jawline can be treated first. CaHA can be used to treat laxity of the skin of the neck. For additional technique, please refer to Chapter 32 on mesoCaHA.

27.2 ANATOMY

The skin is thin in the neck, and hyperdiluted CaHA should be used. The submental fat compartment is relatively thick compared to the almost absent subcutaneous fat in the lower neck where the platysma is almost directly attached to the skin. Very dilute CaHA can therefore be used, as the risk of losing the particles to deeper subcutaneous fat is low.

27.3 ANATOMICAL DANGERS

Areas of caution are the jugular vein and the much more deeply located carotid arteries.

27.4 NECK REJUVENATION CANNULA TECHNIQUE

For injection placement, see Figure 27.1.

27.4.1 Step-by-Step Technique

1. Identify and mark the vertical line from the mandibular angles, the vertical midline, and vertical lines in between.
2. At the horizontal neck lines, mark the entry points. Mark an entry point at the submental crease.
3. Disinfect. Consider giving local anesthesia at the entry points.
4. Make pre-holes with a 23G needle.
5. Use hyperdiluted CaHA at a 1:2 or 1:3 dilution (1:3 is 0.5 mL 1% lidocaine with adrenaline and 4 mL of saline per 1.5 mL CaHA) and a 25G, 50 mm cannula (Figure 27.2).
6. Make sure the cannula stays at the dermal–subdermal junction throughout the treatment.

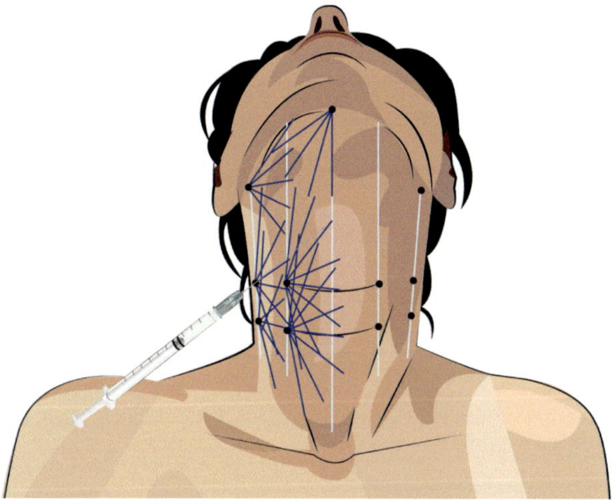

Figure 27.1 The neck rejuvenation cannula technique. Blue lines indicate subdermal placement of CaHA. The five parallel light blue lines indicate the vertical midline, a line from the mandibular angle, and one line in between. Note that the entry points are on the horizontal neck lines.

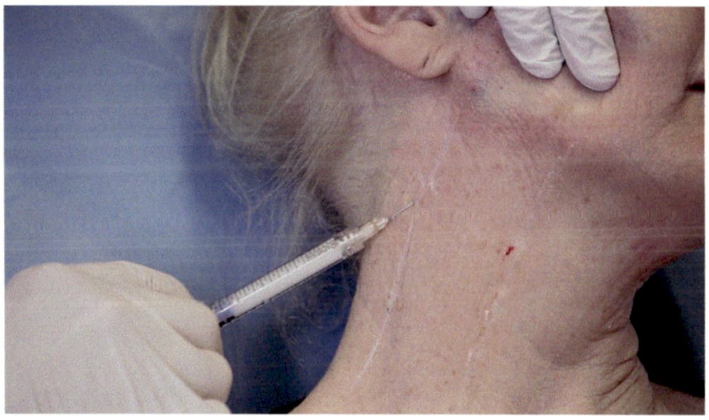

Figure 27.2 Stretch the skin on advancing the cannula to remain superficial.

7. With the nondominant hand, stretch the skin in the direction of the cannula and advance the cannula in the dermal–subdermal plane (Figure 27.3).
8. Inject multiple retrograde linear threads of approximately 0.1 mL per retrograde in a fanning technique (Figure 27.4).

DOI: 10.1201/9781003617129-27

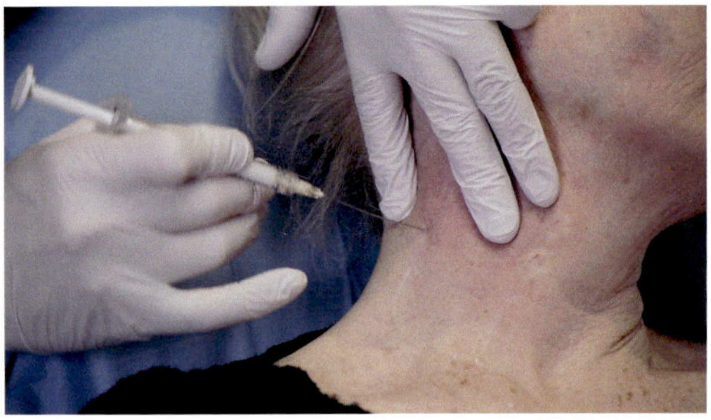

Figure 27.3 Stretching the skin will facilitate superficial subcutaneous injection.

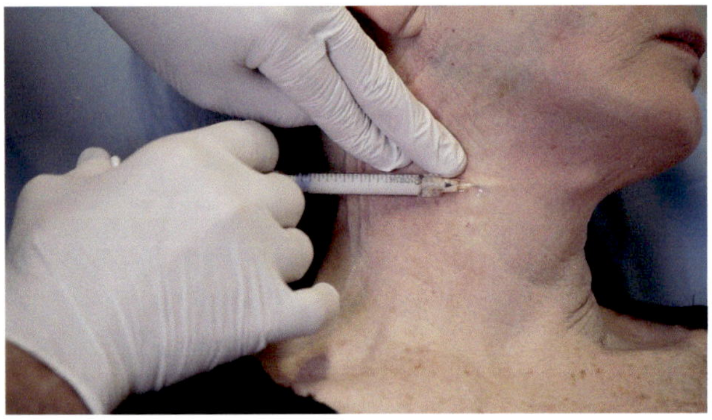

Figure 27.4 As we have a total of five entry points per side, calculate the amount of product to be injected per entry point.

9. Cross-hatching should be done to improve homogeneous distribution of the diluted product in the superficial plane.
10. Do not overcorrect.
11. Even out with manual massage as needed.

See Figure 27.5 for the end-results of neck treatment with CaHA.

27.5 AFTERCARE

The procedure may be followed by a gentle massage to achieve homogeneous distribution but is not necessary with the proper technique of low-dose retrograde linear threads of hyperdiluted CaHA. Swelling may be uneven and should subside in a day or two; ecchymosis usually occurs even with the use of cannulas. The follow-up is planned after three to six months.

27.6 ADDITIONAL TREATMENTS FOR OPTIMAL RESULTS

Combination therapy with botulinum toxin type-A in both platysma bands and horizontal neck lines, as well as treating the horizontal neck lines with either CaHA (see chapter on horizontal neck lines in this book) or soft hyaluronic acid with superficial dermal injection in a blanching technique. Other modalities like laser, peels, and topical creams can benefit this area as well.

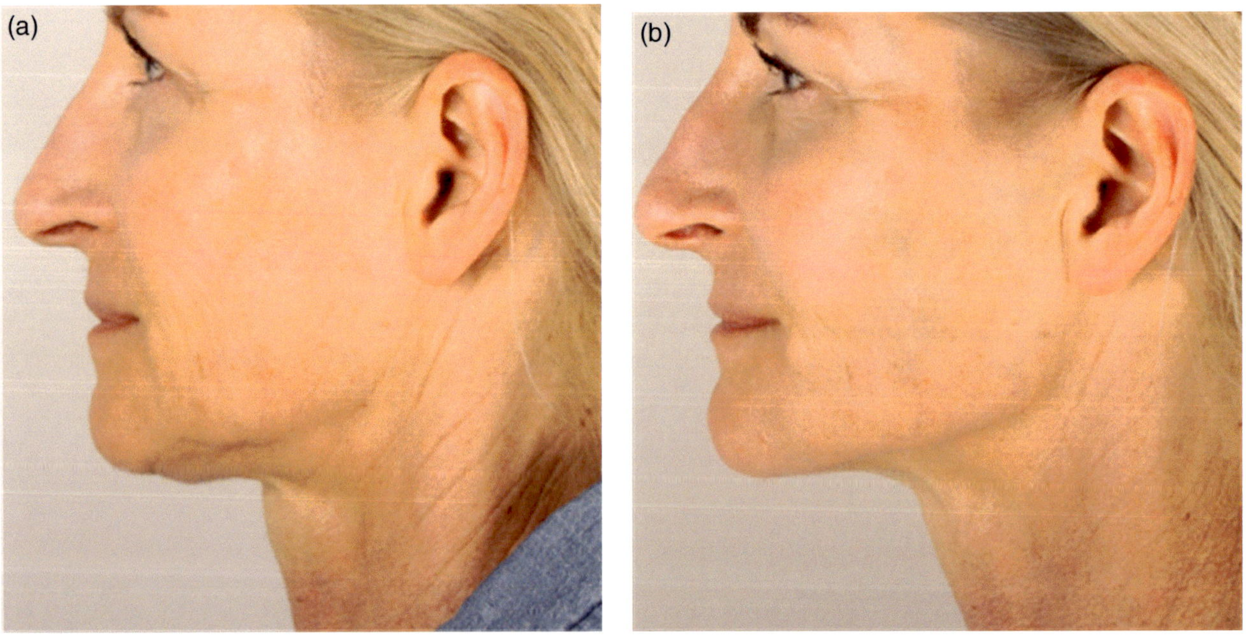

Figure 27.5 Before (a) and after (b) treatment with diluted CaHA in the neck.

Neck, Chest, and Abdomen

28

Horizontal Neck Lines

YATES YEN-YU CHAO AND JANI VAN LOGHEM

28.1 INTRODUCTION

The application of injectable filler in the neck area is uncommon. Most of these treatments have been focused on the aging symptoms of skin laxity using injectables as biostimulators, such as hyperdiluted CaHA to induce collagen formation. However, long before CaHA was used in diluted form for skin quality, it had been published as a treatment for the correction of horizontal neck lines.

Horizontal neck lines are multiple linear indentations of the neck skin along the curve of the neck and are distributed horizontally. The percentage of people who have neck lines is quite high. The lines can be visible at an early age and therefore it is not necessarily a senile change; however, with sagging of the soft tissue due to aging, horizontal neck lines look more prominent. Surface skin photoaging can also worsen the problem with additional fine wrinkles and deepened original lines. That is why the horizontal lines are often interpreted as a sign of age and disliked by most of the people who have them. In addition to weakening of the skin, soft tissue, and fascia of the neck, fat accumulation can also make the horizontal lines worse by contrasting the grooves and bulging fat compartments next to the folds.

Treatment of these horizontal lines, albeit limited, has been not easy. Surgical neck lifting and platysma plication or fixation can tighten the skin and improve the contour but seem ineffective for these lines. Energy-based tissue tightening, like radiofrequency or microfocused ultrasound, can improve skin quality and firm it up but usually give little help to diminish these lines. The reason for this is that the mechanism of neckline formation is not only related to tissue laxity.

The grooves of these horizontal neck lines are usually very shallow, except in patients with fat accumulation or more advanced aging. The author has found that most of these horizontal lines are less than 1 mm wide and 1 mm deep. With shallow grooves like the horizontal neck lines, the skin indentation is found above the muscle (platysma), with some subcutaneous tethering to the underlying structure comparable to the linear marks on the wrist and facial static wrinkles.

Facial wrinkle treatments, laser resurfacing, or fractional treatments usually improve these fine lines; however, they are not so effective for the deeper lines. Correction of the static wrinkles of the face can be more effective, using both deep and shallow injections of injectable fillers. Considering the very thin skin and highly mobile character of our necks, the filler used in this area should have no colloid light scattering (also known as the Tyndall effect) and little tendency to migrate or be dislocated after repeated movements. As the volume deficit of these linear grooves is very tiny, the volume to be filled underlying the skin should be very small. Fillers that are too soft in character or with less lifting capacity cannot fill the gap precisely. A filler that is too soft or with more spreading tendency when filling these lines can possibly augment the neighboring skin as well and can result in unnatural elevated loops.

The author has been trying many different materials and has found diluted or hyperdiluted CaHA to be very suitable for this indication. In fact, diluted CaHA has many advantages over other choices. First, injectable CaHA has a very high lifting capacity, high elasticity, and high viscosity. Even if the CaHA filler is diluted with lidocaine, the property of elasticity can be well preserved despite losing some of its viscosity. The less viscous diluted CaHA can be used easily in minimal amounts for filling and can be molded properly. The retained elasticity of the diluted filler will not reduce the filling and lifting effect of these grooves. After the disappearance of the water content of the diluted mixture, the CaHA filler will behave more like the original and have less tendency to spread or to deform.

The CaHA product is whitish in color, not transparent, and will not produce the undesirable effects of light scattering. The filler particles of CaHA are very small (25–45 μm in diameter) and thus should not cause a beading appearance. CaHA has been proven to induce collagen and elastin formation and can be beneficial for rejuvenating the aging anatomy while maintaining the exact position of injection [1]. However, deploying these minimal amounts of diluted CaHA is not so easy. Most doctors report that controlling a steady flow and injecting in a very superficial plane while staying consistently in the same injection plane is quite challenging. Because the flow must be very limited and the injection level is very superficial, only sharp needle instruments can accomplish this. When using a 27G needle as the usual needle for CaHA injection, the diluted filler can still be elastic and easily extruded out of the needle. This makes it difficult to push the plunger with steady control. The injection level, according to the experience of the author, is in the superficial subcutaneous layer. Because a scanty

DOI: 10.1201/9781003617129-28

amount of fat is distributed above the platysma muscle, the injection could possibly be at the level just above the muscle in patients with very thin subcutaneous fat. The level of injection should be at about 1–1.5 mm in depth [2]. Because the neck is a structure with a circular surface, the precision of this 1–1.5 mm depth must be controlled by the other hand stretching the skin flat, with the injecting hand inserting the needle parallel to the skin surface. For a better control of depth, 12.7 mm needles are preferable to the longer ones. Usually, the dilution of CaHA would be most effective in a one-to-one concentration with lidocaine, but for Caucasians—or for patients with thinner skin—one portion of CaHA to two portions of lidocaine might be better suited to the skin condition of the horizontal neck lines.

The danger zones to take into consideration during horizontal neck lines rejuvenation are the jugular veins and carotid artery.

28.2 NEEDLE TECHNIQUE FOR HORIZONTAL NECK LINE CORRECTION USING DILUTED AND HYPERDILUTED CAHA

For injection placement, see Figure 28.1.

28.2.1 Step-by-Step Technique

1. Disinfect the neck and mark the horizontal neck lines. Note the position of the superficial jugular veins.
2. Use hyperdiluted CaHA (1.5 mL CaHA diluted with 1.5′3 mL of diluted lidocaine) and a sharp 27G, 1.8 cm needle.

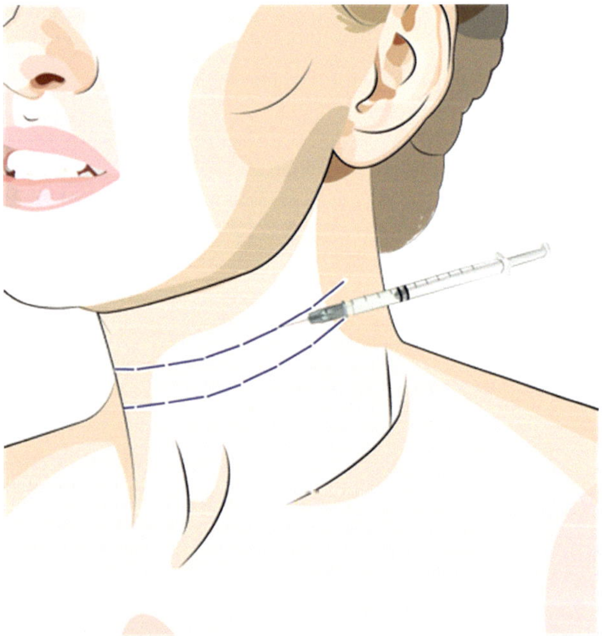

Figure 28.1 A diluted CaHA injection at the horizontal neck lines using a sharp needle technique. The white lines indicate horizontal neck lines, and the blue lines indicate retrograde linear threads of diluted CaHA at the dermal–subdermal junction.

3. Use a horizontal approach with the needle bevel upward.
4. Stretch the skin in the direction of the needle (Figure 28.2).
5. Insert the needle with its full length in the deep dermis, approximately 1–1.5 mm deep.
6. While retracting, slowly inject approximately 0.05 mL in a retrograde linear thread.
7. Repeat until all lines have been corrected.
8. Mold as needed, with the skin rolling between two fingers (Figure 28.3).

28.3 CANNULA TECHNIQUE FOR HORIZONTAL NECK LINE CORRECTION USING DILUTED AND HYPERDILUTED CAHA

For injection placement, see Figure 28.4.

28.3.1 Step-by-Step Technique

1. Disinfect the neck and mark the horizontal neck lines. Note the position of the superficial jugular veins.
2. Use local anesthetics for the entry points.
3. Make a pre-hole with a 23G needle. Work from the most lateral point of the horizontal neckline towards the midline. A new entry point should be made where the previous injections with CaHA ended (Figure 28.5).

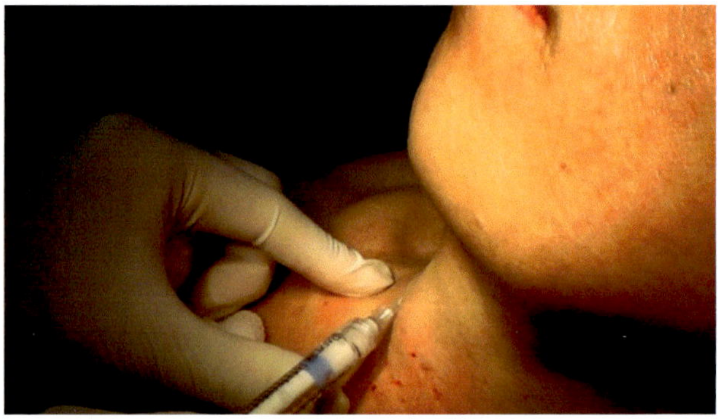

Figure 28.2 Stretching the skin is essential for controlling the correct depth of the needle.

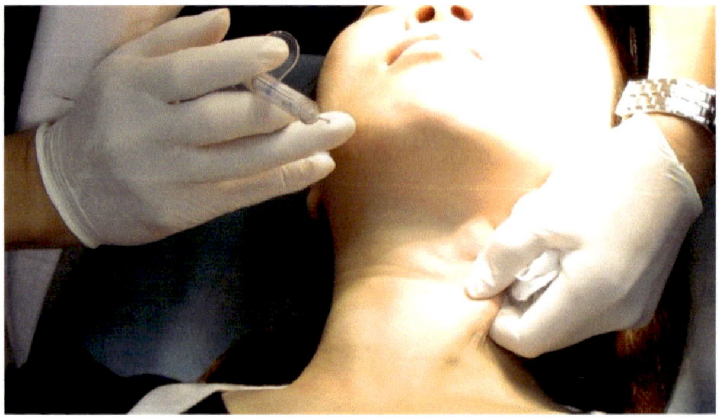

Figure 28.3 Molding after injection ensures an even result.

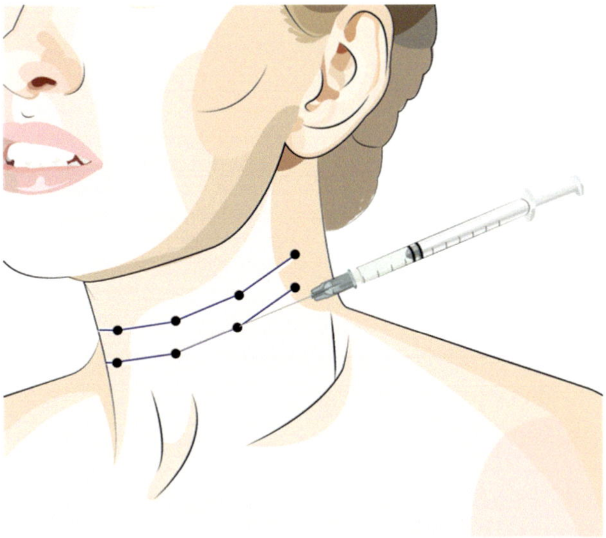

Figure 28.4 A diluted CaHA injection at the horizontal neck lines using the cannula technique. The white lines indicate horizontal neck lines, and the blue lines indicate retrograde linear threads of diluted CaHA at the dermal–subdermal junction. The black dots indicate entry points.

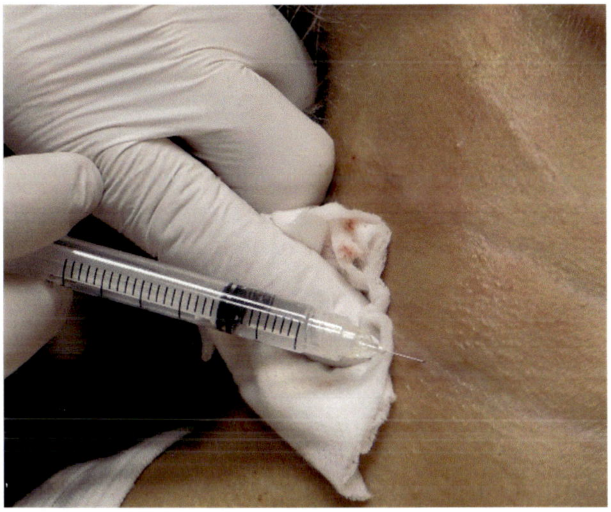

Figure 28.5 Local anesthesia for the next entry point. Inject at the border of treated and untreated area.

4. Use hyperdiluted CaHA (1.5 mL of CaHA diluted with 0.5 mL of lidocaine) with a 25G, 38 mm cannula.
5. Stay superficial in the dermal–subdermal junction. To avoid depositions, it is important not to go too superficial (Figure 28.6).
6. Stretch the skin and advance the cannula inside the wrinkle. Inject small deposits in a fanning technique with the bevel directed upwards. Correct the line until it is filled completely. Do not overcorrect it (Figure 28.7).
7. Repeat until all lines are corrected.

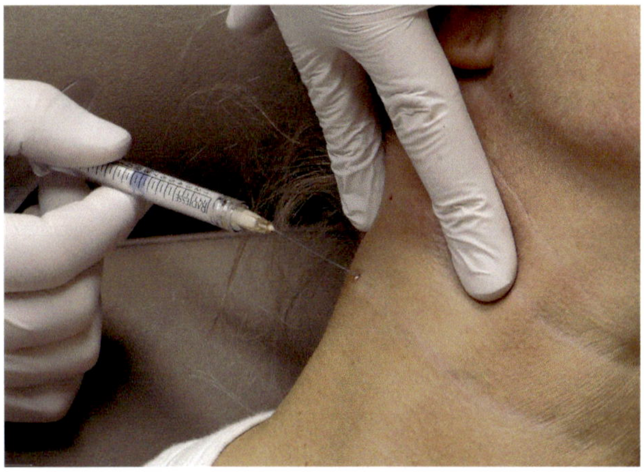

Figure 28.6 Stretching the skin is essential for controlling the correct depth of the needle.

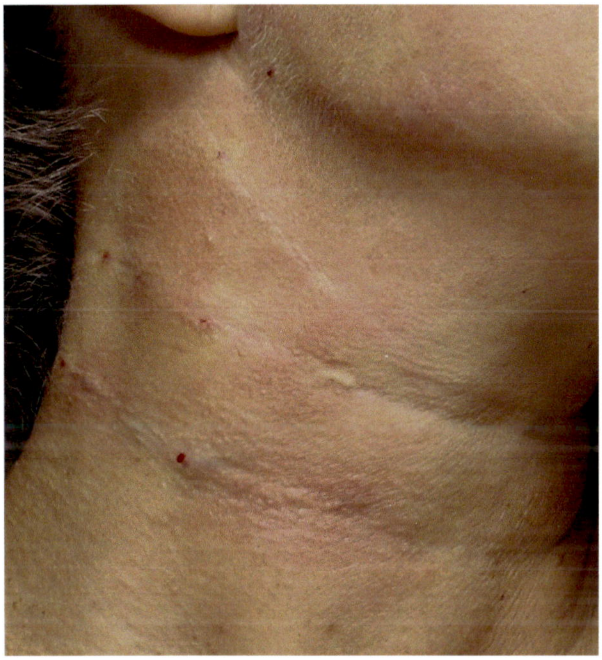

Figure 28.7 Do not overcorrect the wrinkle, but stop when the wrinkle is filled completely.

See further Video 28.1 for application technique.

28.4 AFTERCARE

Extensive massage immediately after each threading and after the whole procedure is extremely important to make sure all filling material has been evenly placed without focal accumulation. The patient should be advised that any swelling is to be expected and is temporary but can last up to five days. Because the area is very well vascularized, bruising can also be expected. Sun protection is advised in this case.

Massaging at home is not necessary, but if the patient wishes to do so, the advice is to limit to gentle massaging twice a day with a skincare product.

28.5 ADDITIONAL TREATMENTS FOR OPTIMAL RESULTS

As the horizontal neck lines are part of the neck, a more general approach to neck rejuvenation may be considered. Energy-based tissue tightening, like radiofrequency or microfocused ultrasound, can improve the skin quality and firm it up, just like chemical peels. Please see the chapter on neck rejuvenation in this book for more details on using diluted CaHA for this indication. As a touchup treatment, a soft hyaluronic acid (HA) can be considered a few months after the CaHA injection, using a blanching technique to further smooth out the horizontal neck lines.

Video 28.1 Horizontal neck lines: cannula technique.

References

[1] Y. A. Yutskovskaya, E. A. Kogan, "Improved neocollagenesis and skin mechanical properties after injection of diluted calcium hydroxylapatite in the neck and décolletage: A pilot study," *J Drugs Dermatol*, vol. 16, no. 1, pp. 68–74, 2017.

[2] Y. Y. Chao et al., "A novel injection technique for horizontal neck lines correction using calcium hydroxylapatite," *Dermatol Surg*, vol. 37, no. 10, pp. 1542–1545, 2011.

Neck, Chest, and Abdomen

Skin Rejuvenation of the Décolletage

29

PIETER SIEBENGA AND JANI VAN LOGHEM

29.1 INTRODUCTION

The décolletage is a part of the body that is particularly prone to solar damage. The skin around the décolletage is more susceptible to aging due to UVB exposure because the skin is thinner compared with the skin of the face or arms and has reduced adipose tissue and fewer sebaceous glands [1]. Apart from pigmentation spots or telangiectasias, damaged collagen fibers can lead to increased wrinkling. Especially in women with relatively large breasts or breast implants, wrinkles can run from the sternum between the breasts toward the clavicle in a widening pattern, also referred to as the devil's fountain. CaHA can be used to tighten the skin in the décolletage area. Improvement of the collagen architecture, skin thickness, and elasticity translates into a more aesthetically pleasing look. As with the other diluted indications, one 1.5 mL syringe should be used per surface area of approximately 100 cm^2. Dilution should be 1:1 to 1:3, depending on the severity of laxity (the thinner the skin, the higher the dilution).

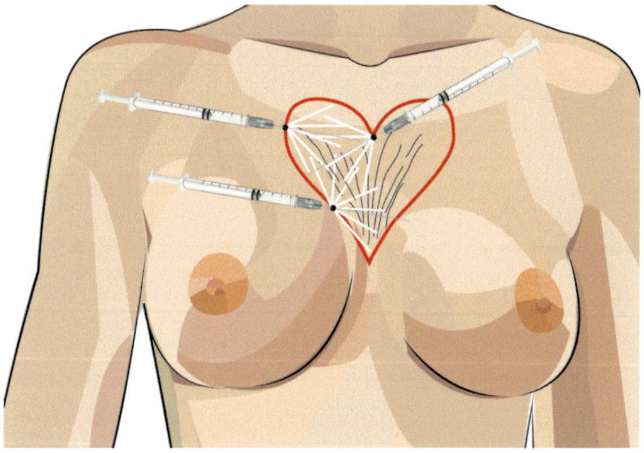

Figure 29.1 Diluted CaHA at the décolletage using the needle technique. The white lines indicate retrograde linear threads of diluted CaHA at the dermal–subdermal junction.

29.2 ANATOMICAL DANGERS

Injection should be done as close to the dermis as possible, at the dermal–subdermal junction. When careful technique is used, it is safe to treat, as the real danger zones are located within the rib cage. The risk of damaging mammary tissue is also negligible, as the mammary glands are located underneath the superficial fascia of the breast, which should be beyond the reach of a cannula or needle.

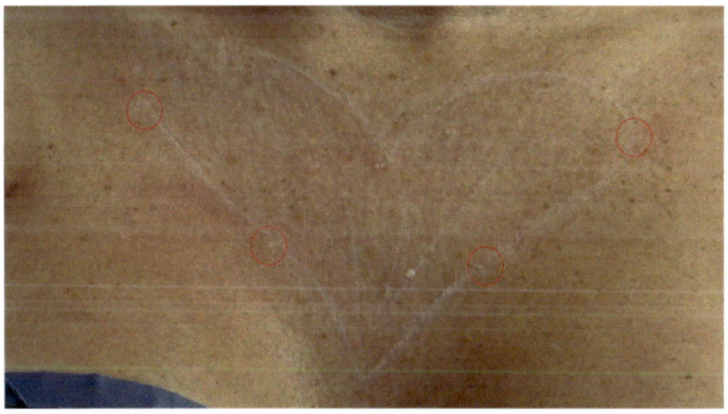

Figure 29.2 Markings of the area to be treated. The red circles indicate where the entry points will be.

29.3 DÉCOLLETAGE CANNULA TECHNIQUE

For injection placement, see Figure 29.1.

29.3.1 Step-by-Step Technique

1. Disinfect the chest.
2. Mark the area that needs to be treated. Usually this is a heart-shaped area, but the shape may be altered depending on the extent of skin laxity and décolletage wrinkles (Figure 29.2).
3. Avoid making a pre-hole in the midline at the bottom of the heart, as the breasts will be interfering with freely handling the syringe on injection.
4. Depending on the thickness of the skin, use hyperdiluted CaHA between 1:1 and 1:3 and a 22G, 70 mm cannula or a 25G, 50 mm cannula.
5. Start at the inferior entry point. Consider bending the cannula for ease of handling the syringe.
6. Stretch the skin in the direction of injection to control the correct depth of the cannula. Make sure the cannula is at the dermal–subdermal junction (Figure 29.3).
7. Slowly inject approximately 0.05–0.1 mL per retrograde injection in a fanning pattern.
8. Cross the midline with the cannula to ensure bilateral crosshatching of the medial part that has the most severe wrinkles (Figure 29.4).

DOI: 10.1201/9781003617129-29

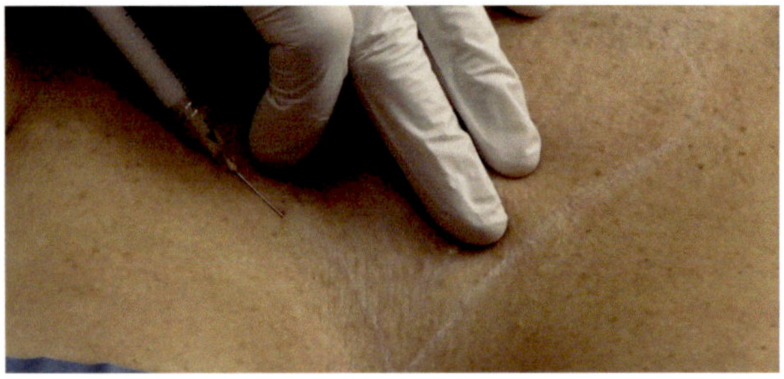

Figure 29.3 Stretch the skin in the direction of the cannula and inject retrogrades in a fanning pattern immediately underneath the dermis.

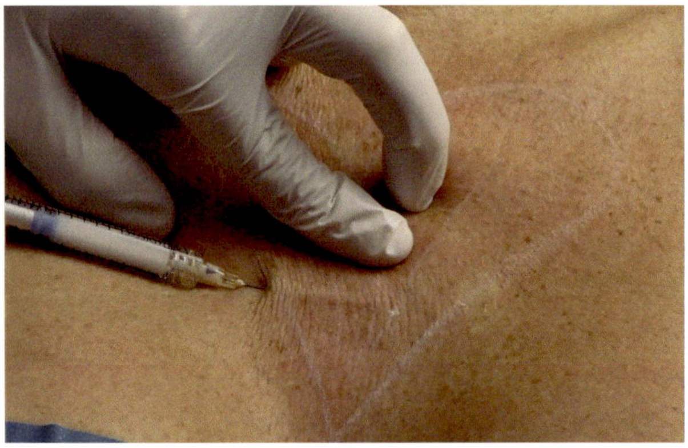

Figure 29.4 Passing the midline with the cannula for crosshatching.

29.4 DÉCOLLETAGE NEEDLE TECHNIQUE

1. Disinfect the chest.
2. Evaluate the chest for wrinkles. Usually, they run in a V-shape over the chest. Mark the area around it for treatment.
3. Examine the thickness of the skin. Thicker skin, or skin with a low laxity, can be injected with a 1:1 hyperdiluted CaHA. Thinner skin, or skin with more laxity, needs a higher hyperdilution to avoid the risk of visible depositions.
4. Bend the 27G needle slightly (15–20°) with the bevel up.
5. Inject retrograde linear lines in the wrinkle of about 0.05 mL. Pinch the skin for better visualization of the wrinkles (Figure 29.5).
6. The correct anatomical layer is subcutaneous, just below the dermis.
7. Once all lines have been filled, crosshatch. Inject retrograde linear lines of about 0.025 per line with <1 cm between each line. Always stay perpendicular to the wrinkles (Figure 29.6).
8. After treatment, check for palpable depositions. If present, massage them out.

See further Video 29.1 for application technique.

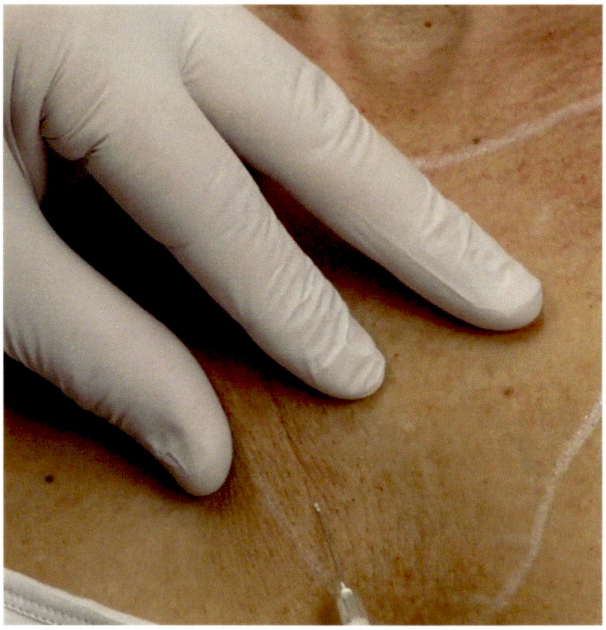

Figure 29.5 Pinch the wrinkle for optimal visualization. Inject CaHA in the direction of the line.

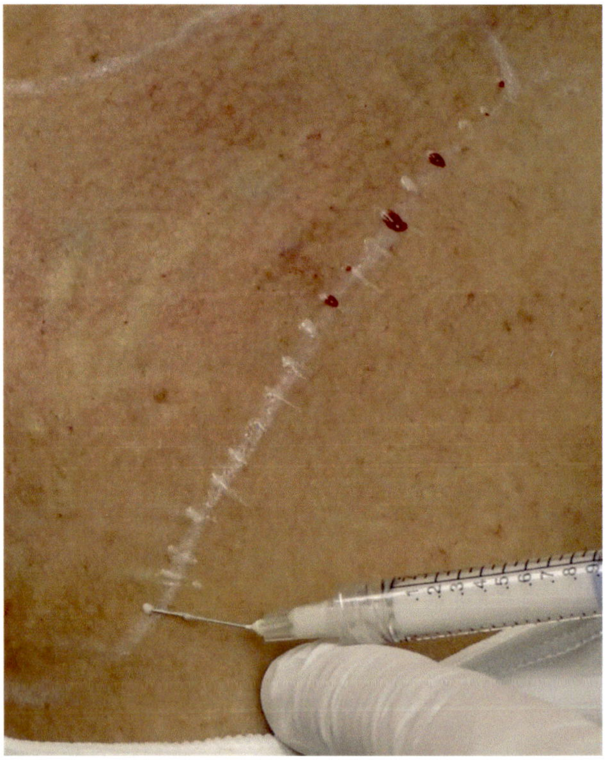

Figure 29.6 A direction perpendicular to the wrinkles combined with crosshatching.

29.5 AFTERCARE

The procedure may be followed by a gentle massage to achieve homogeneous distribution but is not necessary with the proper technique of low dose retrograde linear threads of hyperdiluted CaHA. Advise the patient to avoid the sun, since bruising will usually occur with the needle technique.

After three to four months, the results should be evaluated. If necessary, additional treatment can be suggested then.

29.6 ADDITIONAL TREATMENTS FOR OPTIMAL RESULTS

Additional intradermal cohesive HA injection, directly into the wrinkles, may be considered using the blanching technique [2]. Reduction of pigmentation spots may contribute significantly to the aesthetic situation of the décolletage. IPL or chemical peels are good candidates for this indication. Diluted CaHA can be used in combination with medical devices, such as microfocused ultrasound with visualization (Ultherapy), for skin improvement [3].

Video 29.1 Decolletage: cannula technique.

REFERENCES

[1] J. Uitto, "The role of elastin and collagen in cutaneous aging: Intrinsic aging versus photoexposure," *J Drugs Dermatol*, no. Suppl 2, pp. s12–s16, 2008.

[2] A. Alessandrini, K. Tretyakova, "The rejuvenating effect and tolerability of an auto-cross-linked hyaluronic acid on décolletage: A pilot prospective study," *Aesthetic Plast Surg*, vol. 42, no. 2, pp. 520–529, 2018.

[3] G. Casabona, G. Pereira, "Microfocused ultrasound with visualization and calcium hydroxylapatite for improving skin laxity and cellulite appearance," *Plast Reconstr Surg Glob Open*, vol. 5, no. 7, 2017.

Neck, Chest, and Abdomen

30

Skin Rejuvenation of the Breast

PIETER SIEBENGA AND JANI VAN LOGHEM

30.1 INTRODUCTION

The use of injectable fillers in the breast is uncommon, but hyperdiluted CaHA can be used to treat age-related changes of the skin of the breasts. Age-related changes of the breast have important implications, since the breast is supported anatomically by the overlying skin and the fascia within the breast [1,2]. Changes in the function and appearance of the skin are related to a loss of collagen, elastin, and hydration [3,4] and lead to sagging of the breast [5–7]. Besides, due to menopausal changes, the composition of the breast also changes (e.g. regression of the breast parenchyma and loss of glandular epithelium [8]), affecting the shape of the breast and, with that, the appearance of the skin. Treatment of the skin with hyperdiluted CaHA will result in a rejuvenation of the skin due to the neocollagenesis, neoelastogenesis, and neoangiogenesis described earlier [9], which will lead to firming and lifting of the skin; more projection of the upper pole; and contraction of the lower pole, glands, and fat.

30.2 ANATOMICAL DANGERS

Injection should be done in the subcutaneous plane. Care should be taken to avoid intraglandular injection or into the neurovascular bundle supplying the nipple (Figure 30.1).

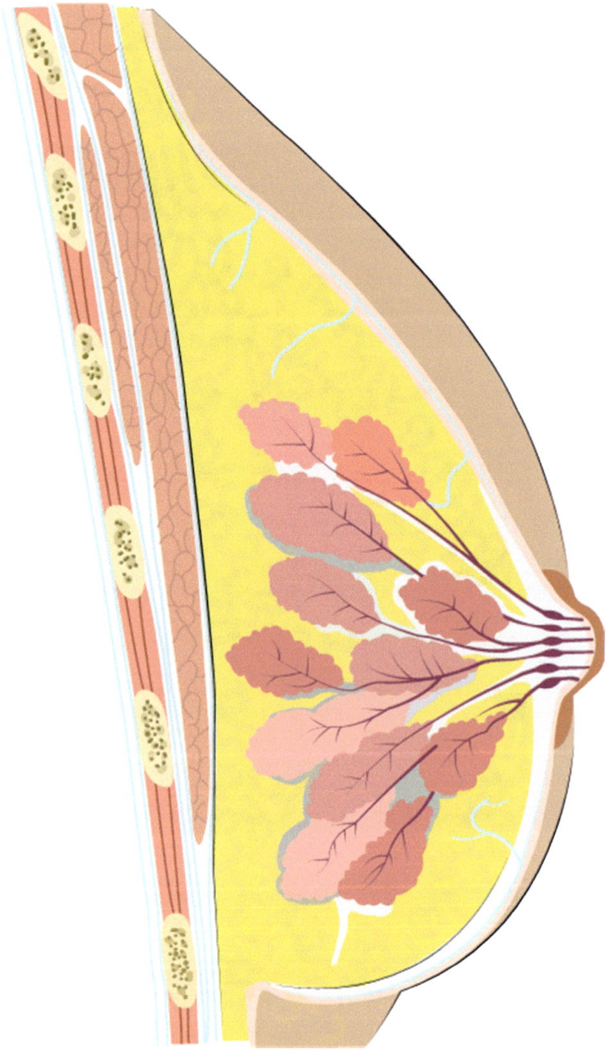

Figure 30.1 Danger zones for the skin rejuvenation of the breast includes the mammary gland and the neurovascular bundle supplying the nipple (neurovascular bundle not shown).

30.3 SKIN REJUVENATION NEEDLE TECHNIQUE

30.3.1 Step-by-Step Technique

For injection placement, see Figure 30.2.

1. Disinfect the breasts.
2. Mark the upper pole of the breast with a vertical line from midclavicular to the areola and expand to a pattern for a multiple retrograde fanning technique approach (Figure 30.3).
3. Directly inferior of the areola, draw three spokes dividing the lower pole into equal parts and mark for the fanning technique.
4. Use a 1:1 to 1:3 hyperdiluted CaHA and a 27G, 50.8 mm sharp needle.
5. Start at the midclavicular point.
6. Stretch the skin in the direction of injection to control the correct depth of the needle (Figure 30.4).
7. Insert the needle and advance it until the full needle is in the subcutaneous plane. Make sure the needle stays anterior from the superficial fascia that envelops the breast, and stay outside the areole during treatment (Figure 30.5).
8. Slowly inject approximately 0.05–0.1 mL per retrograde injection.
9. Repeat until both breasts are treated. Use approximately 1.5 mL of hyperdiluted CaHA per 10 cm^2 area.

DOI: 10.1201/9781003617129-30

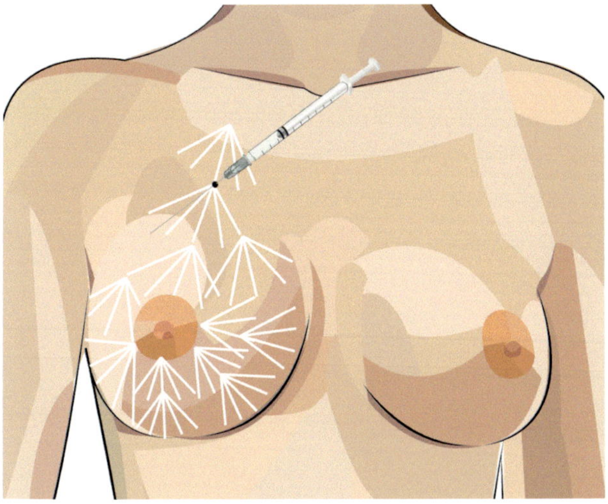

Figure 30.2 Diluted CaHA at the breast using the sharp needle technique. The white lines indicate retrograde linear threads of diluted CaHA at the subdermal level.

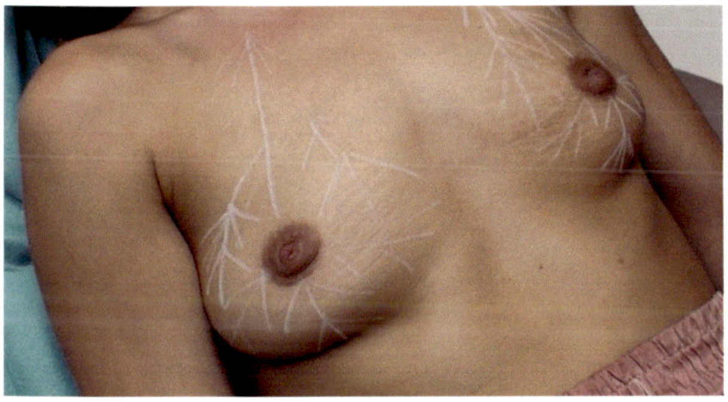

Figure 30.3 Markings on the upper and lower pole of the breast for a multiple retrograde fanning technique approach.

See also Figure 30.6 and Video 30.1 for before and after results and application techniques, respectively.

30.4 AFTERCARE

The procedure may be followed by a gentle massage to achieve homogeneous distribution but is not necessary with the proper technique of low dose retrograde linear threads of hyperdiluted CaHA.

After three to four months, the results should be evaluated. If necessary, additional treatment can be suggested then. As a general guideline, two to three syringes of 1.5 mL CaHA product each should be injected per breast.

30.5 ADDITIONAL TREATMENTS FOR OPTIMAL RESULTS

Dermal filler injection in the breast is uncommon. Women who wish for a breast lift (mastopexy) or breast augmentation are looking to surgery, which requires the placement of an implant or autologous fat transplantation. Even though it is very unlikely that CaHA treatment can have anything to do with developing breast cancer, some physicians suggest making a mammogram or ultrasound prior to treatment for legal reasons.

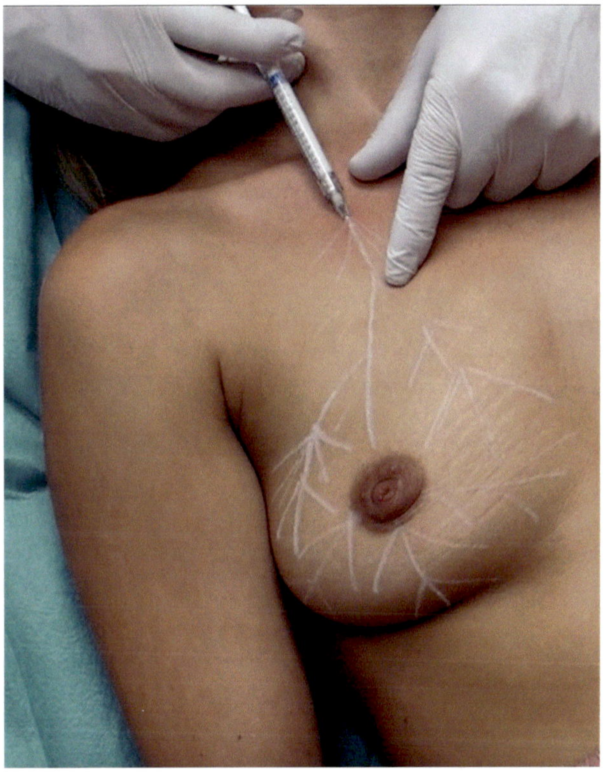

Figure 30.4 Stretch the skin in the direction of the needle.

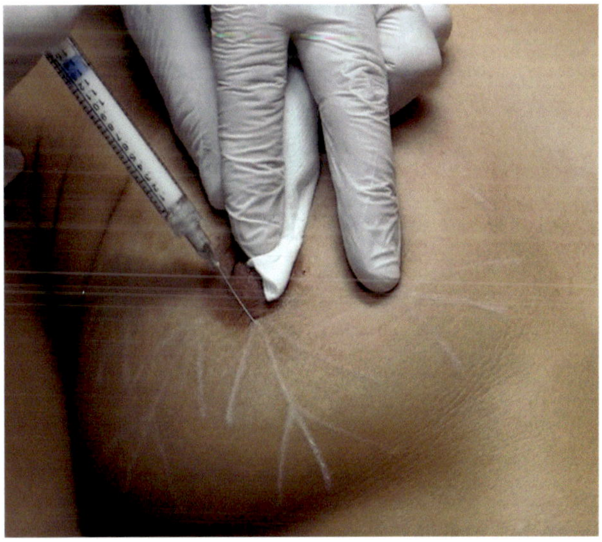

Figure 30.5 Stay outside the areola when treating the lower pole of the breast.

Video 30.1 Skin rejuvenation of the breast.

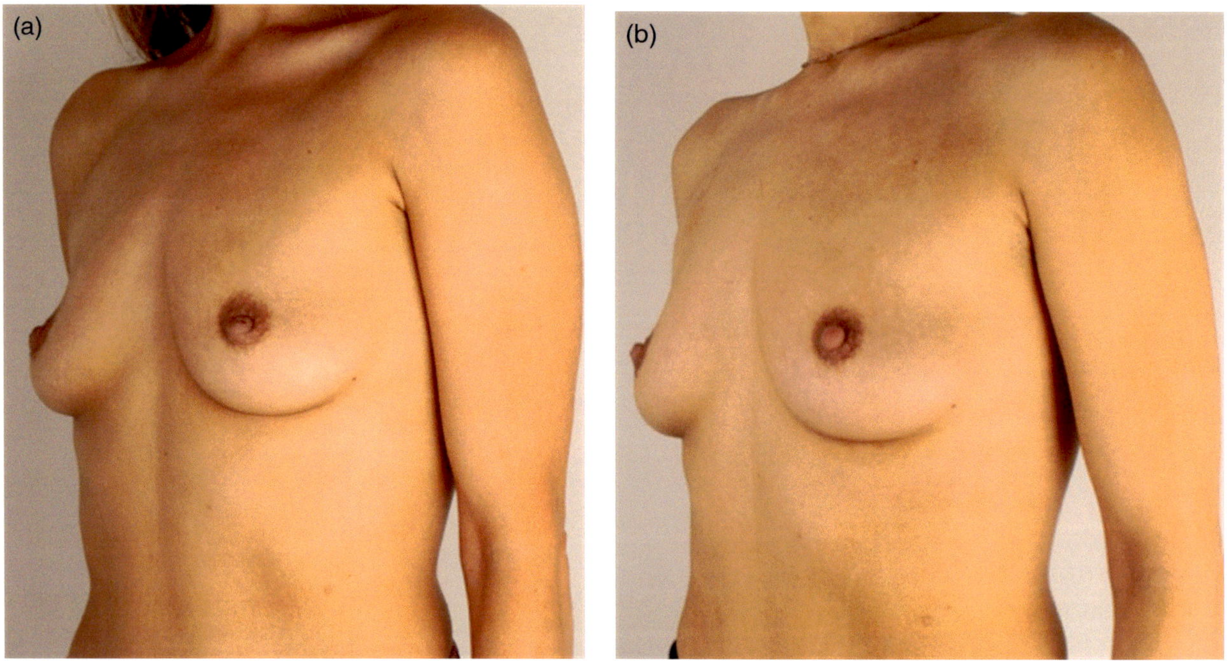

Figure 30.6 Before (a) and two months after treatment (b) with CaHA. The treatment consisted of one session of two syringes per breast.

REFERENCES

[1] J. R. Steele et al., *Sports Bra Fitness*. Wollongong: Breast Research Australia, Biomechanics Research Laboratory, University of Wollongong, 2008.
[2] A. Gefen, B. Dilmoney, "Mechanics of the normal woman's breast," *Technol Health Care*, vol. 15, no. 4, pp. 259–271, 2007.
[3] J. Uitto, "The role of elastin and collagen in cutaneous aging: Intrinsic aging versus photoexposure," *J Drugs Dermatol*, no. Suppl 2, pp. s12–s16, 2008.
[4] C. Escoffier et al., "Age-related mechanical properties of human skin: An in vivo study," *J Investig Dermatol*, vol. 93, no. 3, pp. 353–357, 1989.
[5] Y. Machida, M. Nakadate, "Breast shape change associated with aging: A study using prone breast magnetic resonance imaging," *Plast Reconstr Surg Glob Open*, vol. 3, no. 6, p. e413, 2015.
[6] N. I. Elsahy, "Correction of abnormally high nipples after reduction mammaplasty," *Aesthetic Plast Surg*, vol. 14, no. 1, pp. 21–26, 1990.
[7] D. E. McGhee, J. R. Steele, "How do respiratory state and measurement method affect bra size calculations?," *Br J Sports Med*, vol. 40, no. 12, pp. 970–974, 2006.
[8] R. G. Abramson et al., "Age-related structural and functional changes in the breast: Multimodality correlation with digital mammography, computed tomography, magnetic resonance imaging, and positron emission tomography," *Semin Nucl Med*, vol. 37, no. 3, pp. 146–153, 2007.
[9] Y. A. Yutskovskaya, E. A. Kogan, "Improved neocollagenesis and skin mechanical properties after injection of diluted calcium hydroxylapatite in the neck and décolletage: A pilot study," *J Drugs Dermatol*, vol. 16, no. 1, pp. 68–74, 2017.

Neck, Chest, and Abdomen

31

Rejuvenation of the Abdominal Skin

PIETER SIEBENGA AND JANI VAN LOGHEM

31.1 INTRODUCTION

The abdominal skin can be permanently stretched, resulting in stretch marks, laxity, and thinning of the dermis, especially after pregnancies or major weight loss. Given the risks of complications, significant downtime, and the significant costs, a surgical approach (e.g. abdominoplasty or "tummy tuck") has too much impact for most patients. Because of this, non- or minimally invasive procedures are becoming increasingly popular. Diluted CaHA can be used in the treatment of abdominal skin laxity. It is a safer, more affordable way to improve skin quality without downtime.

31.2 ANATOMICAL DANGERS

Injection should be performed as close to the dermis as possible (dermal–subdermal junction). The patient should be examined for umbilical herniation, and care should be taken to avoid entering a hernia with a cannula or needle. Superficial and perforating veins may pose a risk of ecchymosis but do not pose a risk of serious adverse events.

31.3 ABDOMEN CANNULA TECHNIQUE

For injection placement, see Figure 31.1.

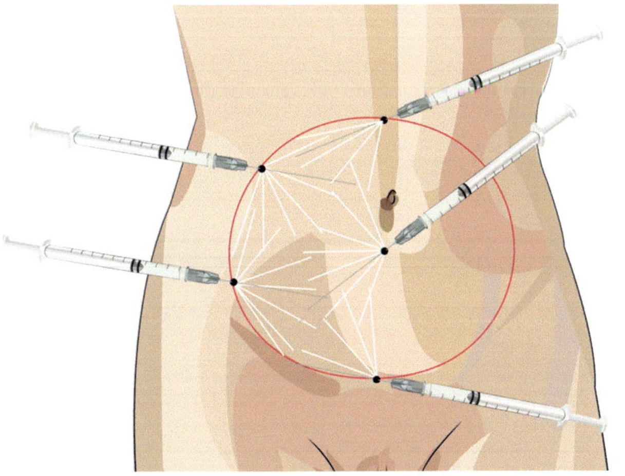

Figure 31.1 Diluted CaHA at the abdomen using the cannula technique. The white lines indicate retrograde linear threads of diluted CaHA at the dermal-subdermal junction.

31.3.1 Step-by-Step Technique

1. Disinfect the abdomen.
2. Mark the area that needs to be treated. Usually this is a periumbilical oval area (Figure 31.2).
3. Use 1.5 mL CaHA per 100 cm^2 surface area. The surface area of an oval is width (cm) × length (cm) × $\pi/4$. In the schematic example shown here, the width of the oval is ~20 cm; the height is ~15 cm, so the surface area is about 20 × 15 × 3.14/4 = 236 cm^2. So approximately two to three syringes of 1.5 mL will be necessary to treat the abdomen in this example.
4. Dilute CaHA between 1:1 and 1:3 (depending on severity of laxity) and use a 25G, 50 mm cannula or a 22G, 70 mm cannula.
5. Start at the inferior entry point. Consider bending the cannula for ease of handling the syringe.
6. Stretch the skin in the direction of injection to control the correct depth of the cannula. Make sure the cannula is at the dermal-subdermal junction (Figure 31.3).
7. Slowly inject 0.05–0.1 mL per retrograde injection in a fanning pattern with the bevel directed upwards.
8. Repeat until all of the marked skin has a thin layer of diluted CaHA.

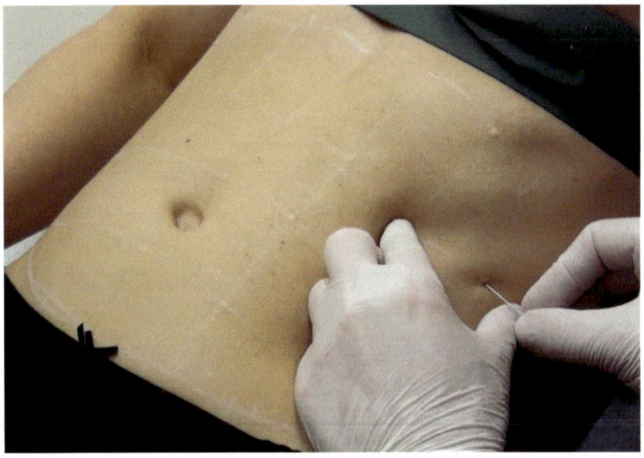

Figure 31.2 Markings of the area to be treated and the pre-holes.

DOI: 10.1201/9781003617129-31

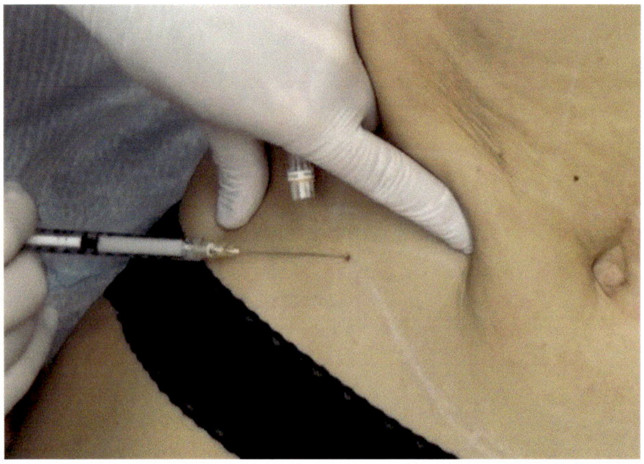

Figure 31.3 Stretch the skin in the direction of the cannula and inject retrograde.

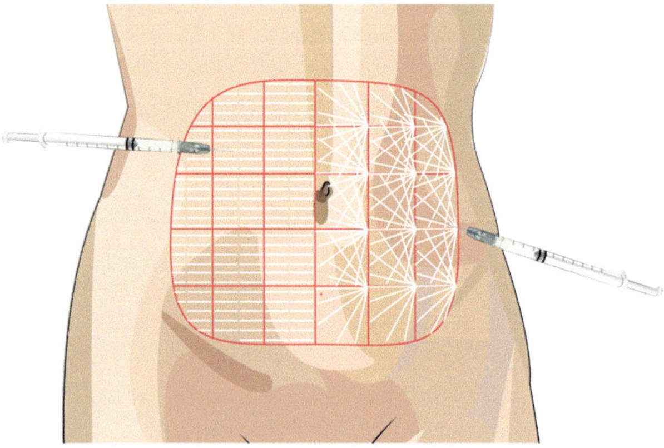

Figure 31.4 Diluted CaHA at the abdomen using the sharp needle technique. The white lines indicate retrograde linear threads of diluted CaHA at the dermal-subdermal junction. On the right side of the patient, the short needle (19 mm) technique is shown. On the left side, the long needle (40 mm) technique is presented using squares of approximately 15–16 cm^2.

31.4 ABDOMEN NEEDLE TECHNIQUE

For injection placement, see Figure 31.4; for evaluation of the abdomen, see Figure 31.5.

31.4.1 Step-by-Step Technique

1. Disinfect the abdomen.
2. Mark the area that needs to be treated (Figure 31.6).
3. Use 1.5 mL CaHA per 100 cm^2 surface area. In the schematic example shown, approximately 13–14 squares of 4 × 4 cm are used per side, equaling 208–224 cm^2. This means that a total of approximately two to three syringes is necessary to treat the abdomen in this example.
4. Dilute CaHA between 1:1 and 1:3 (depending on severity of laxity) and use a 27G, 19 mm needle or a 27G, 40 mm needle.

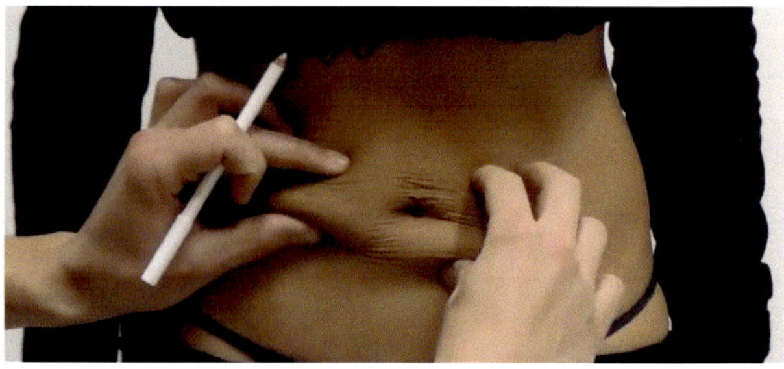

Figure 31.5 Evaluation of the abdomen shows mild laxity of the skin, which is accentuated when the patient is asked to bend forward.

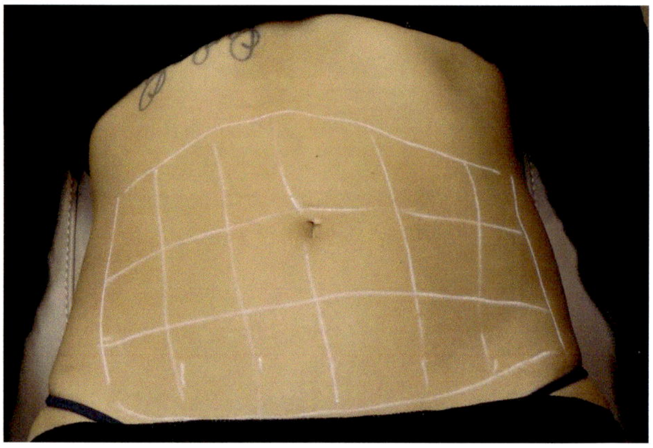

Figure 31.6 Markings on the patient before treatment. Landmarks are the lower border of the ribcage, the lateral sides of the abdomen, and the bikini line. Then mark squares of 4 × 4 cm.

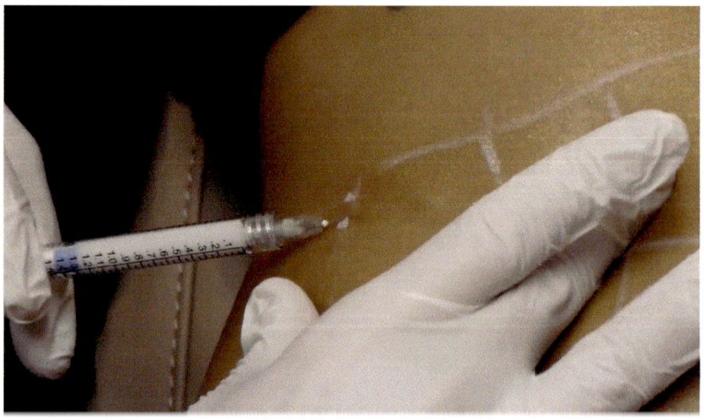

Figure 31.7 Stretch the skin in the direction of the needle and inject in a retrograde manner.

5. Work from lateral to medial.
6. Stretch the skin in the direction of injection to control the correct depth of the needle. Make sure the needle is at the dermal-subdermal junction (Figure 31.7).
7. Slowly inject approximately 0.05 mL per retrograde injection. Use either the fanning technique (left side

of patient in Figure 31.4) or retrograde linear threads (right side of patient in Figure 31.4).
8. Repeat until all the marked skin has a thin layer of diluted CaHA.

See also Videos 31.1–31.2 to visualize application techniques.

31.5 AFTERCARE

The procedure may be followed by a gentle massage to achieve homogeneous distribution but is not necessary with the proper technique of low dose retrograde linear threads of hyperdiluted CaHA. After three to four months, the results should be evaluated. If necessary, additional treatment can be suggested then.

31.6 ADDITIONAL TREATMENTS FOR OPTIMAL RESULTS

Reduction of subcutaneous fat may be beneficial in some patients. Additional neocollagenesis stimulating techniques will improve outcome (microfocused ultrasound, radiofrequency, lasers, peels, needling, etc.).

Video 31.1 Abdomen: cannula technique.

Video 31.2 Abdomen: needle fanning technique.

Neck, Chest, and Abdomen

32 MesoCaHA for Cheeks, Neck, and Décolletage

YANA A. YUTSKOVSKAYA AND ANNA DANIILOVNA LOKASTOVA

32.1 INTRODUCTION

When correcting age-related changes in the skin of the face, neck, and décolletage—manifested by thinning skin, reduced turgor and elasticity, and the presence of sagging, CaHA is used by the authors of this chapter in dilution with 0.9% NaCl (saline). The technique consists of maintaining the product in the form of a gel-sol on the border of the dermis and hypodermis. The purpose of this procedure is the stimulation of neocollagenesis and tissue lifting. This chapter presents several options for markup and methods of administering the diluted product with a needle and cannula. The recommended dilutions of the product are:

- Face 1:1
- Submental area, neck, and décolletage 1:2

Aging of the skin occurs mainly due to atrophic changes in the dermis and hypodermis. Here, we will highlight some of the main actors involved in skin aging, starting with glycosaminoglycans (GAGs). GAGs (hyaluronic acid among them) are molecules from the ECM that have hydrating and space-filling functions. They can be complexed through glycosylation to core proteins, forming proteoglycans (PGs) like versican, known to be involved in elastogenesis [1,2]. Moreover, the skin also contains glycoproteins, in particular fibronectin, that play a role in the interaction of fibroblasts with collagen fibers. In fact, fibronectin is the first matrix assembled by fibroblasts in wound healing, replacing the provisional fibrin clot [3]. Eventually, fibroblasts deposit a composite of fibronectin and collagen that contributes to the structural integrity of the matrix during the formation of the granulation tissue [4]. In aging, there is a thinning in collagen fibers from the superficial dermis, which the deep dermis attempts to thicken as a compensatory mechanism, adding temporary density. In a later stage, fragmentation and lysis of the collagen fibers become evident, with a tendency to separate [5]. The dermal elastic networks, composed of fibrillin and elastin, are also affected by (photoinduced-)aging. In intrinsic aging, a depletion of elastic skin is visible [6]. In contrast, in photoaged skin, the fibers are degraded and degenerated, gradually accumulating (solar elastosis) [7]. In both cases, the hypodermis plays a major role, since it participates in the formation of granulation tissue during wound repair, together with fibroblasts—a pivotal morphofunctional element of the regenerative process.

CaHA dermal filler in dilution with saline is an effective and well-tolerated remedy for the correction of age-related skin changes, clinically manifested by a decrease in skin thickness, a decrease in turgor and elasticity, sagging, and solar elastosis [8]. This technique consists in administering the product not in the form of a gel (in the original concentration) but in the form of a gel-sol (diluted with saline) subdermally—at the border of the dermis and hypodermis. The purpose of this procedure is to stimulate the synthetic activity of fibroblasts.

Researchers have shown in animal models that stimulation of collagen in the skin occurs as early as four weeks [9]. In humans, three to four months later, maximum stimulation of collagen types I and III and elastin is observed [10], and nine months after injection, the processes stabilize and the collagen type I and III deposition ratio observed is 3:1, respectively [11]. Moreover, treatment improvements have been registered for up to 30 months [12]. In the authors' opinion, this technique is recommended for patients under 40 years of age in order to treat skin dermatoporosis and a clinical sign of flaccidity of the skin one time in nine months. For patients older than 40 years, once in four months is recommended. In general, there is no age limit for this treatment, since the stimulation of collagen is a genetically determined process.

32.2 THE MESOCAHA TECHNIQUE

For injection placement, see Figure 32.1.

32.2.1 Step-by-Step Technique

1. For a comfortable procedure, it is advisable to use topical anesthesia (1–2% lidocaine). Exposure time is 40 minutes under occlusion.
2. Mark the area of the middle, lower third of the face, neck, and décolletage (Figure 32.1). In this case, there are several options for injection techniques. When using a needle, injections are done along the skin tension lines (Langer lines). When using a cannula, the preferred technique is the fanning technique.

DOI: 10.1201/9781003617129-32

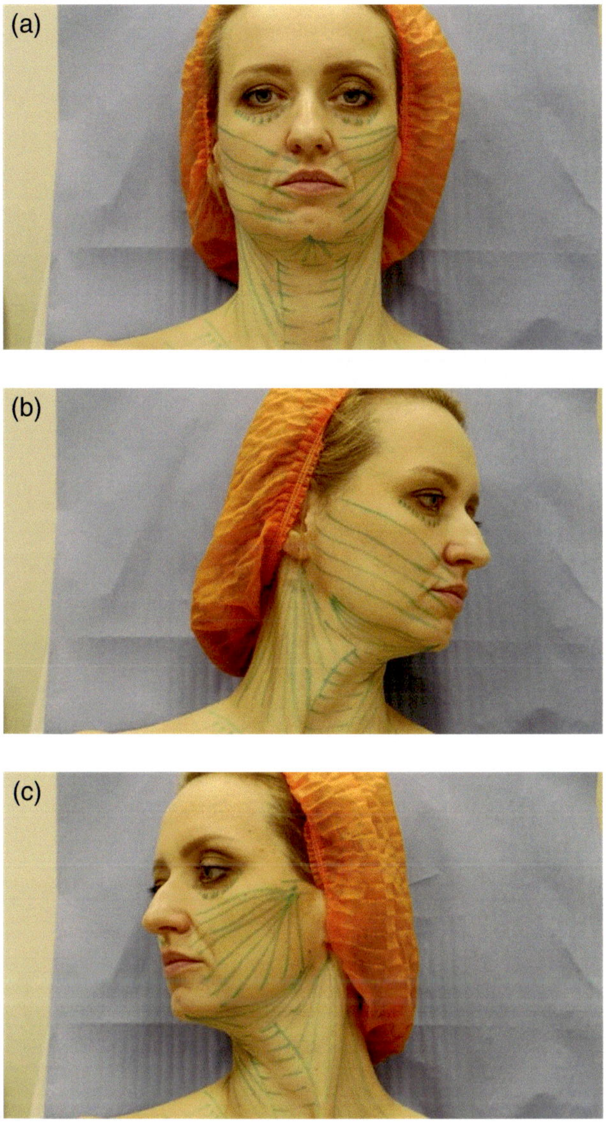

Figure 32.1 (a) Anterior, (b) right, and (c) left markings on the patient to conduct the MesoCAHA technique. On the cheeks, a needle on the right side and a cannula on the left were used. For submental application, a cannula was used. In the lateral of the neck, a cannula was used and in the medial region, a needle instead.

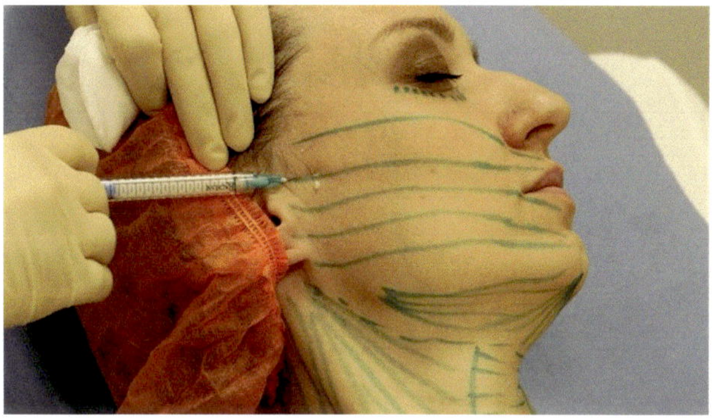

Figure 32.2 Using a sharp needle, a total of 1.5 mL are injected per side (diluted 1:1) at the dermal-subdermal junction using serial retrograde linear threads in the direction of the lines.

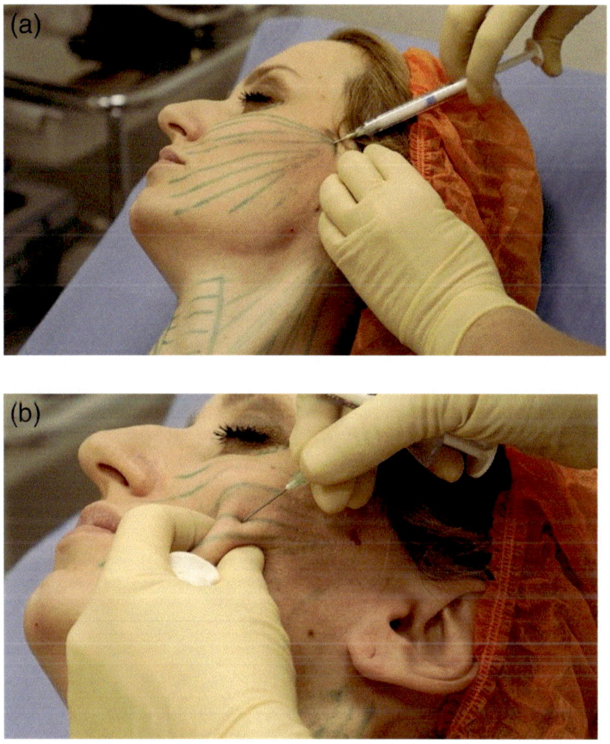

Figure 32.3 With a cannula, a total of 1.5 mL are injected per side (diluted 1:1) at the dermal-subdermal junction using two entry points: (a) zygomatic arch entry point and (b) midface entry point.

3. For preparation of the CaHA dilution, we recommend the ratios 1:1 and 1:2 of CaHA to saline solution.
4. Before each set of injections, the diluted product must be thoroughly mixed (5–10 times) and transferred to the syringe for injection, as its particles may sediment and settle on the walls of the syringe.
5. The resulting diluted CaHA is administered subdermally with retrograde linear threads to the middle and lower third of the face (Figure 32.2). Injections are made along uniform lines from the periphery to the center, from top to bottom. The needle is inserted with the bevel up to the full length at the minimum angle to the skin surface subdermally. The steel of the needle or cannula is not visible, but the retraction is visualized.
6. At the midpoint of the zygomatic arch 1 cm in front of the hairline, the skin is punctured with a 22G, 70 mm cannula. Injections are carried out by the vector method (fanning technique), subdermally (Figure 32.3). The distance between the vectors should be 0.5–0.7 mm.

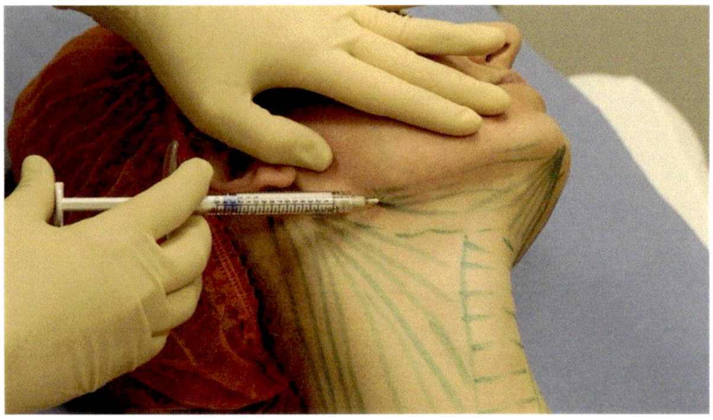

Figure 32.4 A total of 1.5 mL are injected per side from three entry points (diluted 1:2) at the dermal-subdermal junction.

7. An additional puncture for the introduction of the cannula is carried out from the lower point of the zygomatic bone, and 1.5 mL of diluted product are injected on each side of the face.
8. In the submental zone, a dilution ratio of 1:2 is advised (1.5 mL CaHA are mixed with 3 mL of saline solution). The puncture is made from the points of projection at the lateral angles of the submandibular triangle and the projection of the apex of the submental chord (Figure 32.4). Use a 22G, 70 mm cannula and inject 0.5 mL of the diluted product for each point of the cannula.
9. In the neck, a dilution of 1:2 CaHA with saline is used (1.5 mL CaHA are mixed with 3 mL saline). In the area of the scapular-tracheal triangle, the administration of the diluted product is carried out using a needle in a linear retrograde technique.
10. In the zone of the carotid triangle, the sternoclavicular-mastoid area, work with a 22G, 70 mm cannula is recommended. The insertion point for the cannula is placed in the upper corner of the carotid triangle and injection is done using a fanning technique.
11. In the large supraclavicular fossa, injections are made by means of a needle, from the center to the periphery, with retrograde linear threads.
12. In the area of the décolletage, it is possible to work both with a 22G, 50 mm cannula and a needle. The dilution and volume of the injected product is similar to that of used in the neck.

See also Figure 32.5 and Video 32.1 for end result and technique of MesoCaHA visualization, respectively.

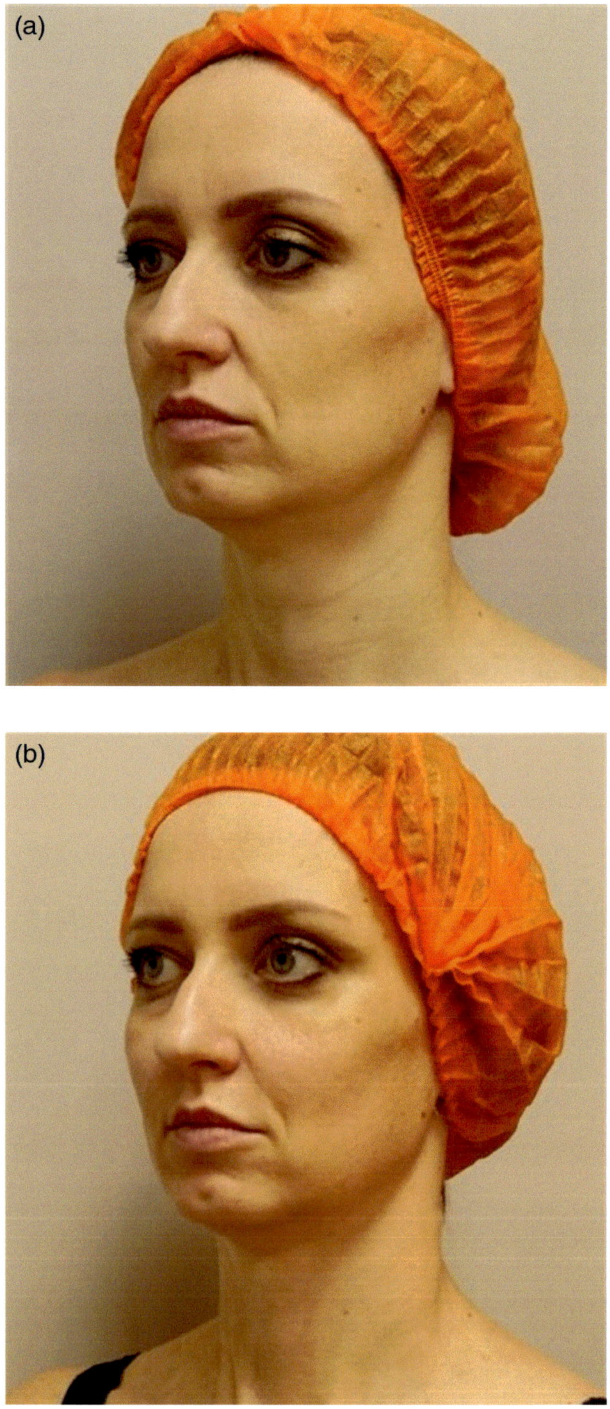

Figure 32.5 (a) Before and (b) results four months post-treatment.

32.3 AFTERCARE

After the procedure, an active massage using an anti-inflammatory (or arnica-enriched) ointment is recommended for a better distribution of the injected material. Irregularities after the procedure are acceptable; however, a hazy appearance is not (white deposits of material visible due to excessive superficial injection). For the fastest regeneration, it is advised to apply a pro-regenerative cream for sensitive skin, which has additional calming and healing effects.

Video 32.1 MesoCaHA technique.

REFERENCES

[1] B. Bode-Lesniewska et al., "Distribution of the large aggregating proteoglycan versican in adult human tissues," *J Histochem Cytochem*, vol. 44, no. 4, pp. 303–312, 1996.

[2] M. A. Ruiz Martínez et al., "Role of proteoglycans on skin ageing: A review," *Int J Cosmet Sci*, vol. 42, no. 6, pp. 529–535, 2020.

[3] K. S. Midwood et al., "Tissue repair and the dynamics of the extracellular matrix," *Int J Biochem Cell Biol*, vol. 36, no. 6, pp. 1031–1037, 2004.

[4] K. E. Kubow et al., "Mechanical forces regulate the interactions of fibronectin and collagen I in extracellular matrix," *Nat Commun*, vol. 6, no. 1, pp. 1–11, 2015.

[5] M. Bonta et al., "The process of ageing reflected by histological changes in the skin," *Romanian J Morphol Embryol*, vol. 54, no. Suppl 3, pp. 797–804, 2013.

[6] M. El-Domyati et al., "Intrinsic aging vs. photoaging: A comparative histopathological, immunohistochemical, and ultrastructural study of skin," *Exp Dermatol*, vol. 11, no. 5, pp. 398–405, 2002.

[7] S. H. Shin et al., "Skin aging from mechanisms to interventions: Focusing on dermal aging," *Front Physiol*, vol. 14, 2023.

[8] T. Pavicic, "Calcium hydroxylapatite filler: An overview of safety and tolerability," *J Drugs Dermatol*, vol. 12, no. 9, pp. 996–1002, 2013.

[9] K. M. Coleman et al., "Neocollagenesis after injection of calcium hydroxylapatite composition in a canine model," *Dermatol Surg*, vol. 34, no. Suppl 1, 2008.

[10] Y. Yutskovskaya et al., "A randomized, split-face, histomorphologic study comparing a volumetric calcium hydroxylapatite and a hyaluronic acid-based dermal filler," *J Drugs Dermatol*, vol. 13, no. 9, pp. 1047–1052, 2014.

[11] Y. A. Yutskovskaya, E. A. Kogan, "Improved neocollagenesis and skin mechanical properties after injection of diluted calcium hydroxylapatite in the neck and décolletage: A pilot study," *J Drugs Dermatol*, vol. 16, no. 1, pp. 68–74, 2017.

[12] M. H. Graivier et al., "Calcium hydroxylapatite (Radiesse) for correction of the mid- and lower face: Consensus recommendations," *Plast Reconstr Surg*, vol. 120, no. Suppl 6, 2007.

Extremities

Correction of Skin Laxity of the Upper Arms

33

WOUTER J. PEETERS AND JANI VAN LOGHEM

33.1 INTRODUCTION

CaHA stimulates dermal remodeling via neocollagenesis processes whereby collagen type I gradually replaces collagen type III [1]. Histological examination suggests a cycle in which the highest deposition of new collagen and elastin occurs around four months after injection, with stability achieved by nine months. In patients younger than 40 years old, neocollagenesis and neoelastogenesis are so strong that one single treatment results in a significant clinical improvement within four months. In those cases, reinjecting can be proposed after 24 to 36 months. In patients older than 40 years, where neocollagenesis is a slower process, retreatment is proposed after four months to enhance dermal remodeling. Sometimes a third treatment session is needed to achieve the optimal aesthetic effect, with maintenance injections every 12 to 18 months thereafter [2].

CaHA has been extensively used for facial rejuvenation and HIV-associated lipoatrophy, with few complications, similar to those of non-infected individuals [3]. When injected in retrograde fashion, using cannulas with the described dilutions, it is unlikely to cause adverse events.

33.2 THE MULTILAYER APPROACH

For injection placement, see Figure 33.1.

33.2.1 Step-by-Step Technique

1. Make markings with the patient in upright position. Mark the area of concern, as well as visible superficial veins that should be avoided during the procedure. In the neck, the superficial jugular vein is at risk. In the legs, varicose veins can be punctured easily, which causes long lasting bruises and, in some cases, permanent discoloration of the skin. Also, the injection points are marked. When a 50 mm or 70 mm cannula is used, two to four injection points suffice to treat the whole area (Figure 33.1).
2. The patient is installed and prepped with chlorhexidine or betadine solution. Thick and firm cannulas of 22–25G are preferred; hence, administer a local anesthetic at the injection points before entering the cannula.
3. CaHA is then diluted and mixed just before injection to avoid phase separation.
4. The homogenous mixture is injected using a 22–25G needle in a retrograde fashion. In arms, legs, abdomen, and gluteal areas, a multilayered approach is advised. First, the cannula is entered as superficially as possible in the superficial dermis. The cannula will gently scrape the underside of the dermis to encourage maximal biostimulation.
   - *First layer*: Stretch the skin with the non-dominant hand, enter the cannula parallel to the skin, and inject minimal amounts of the homogenous mixture retrograde, scraping the

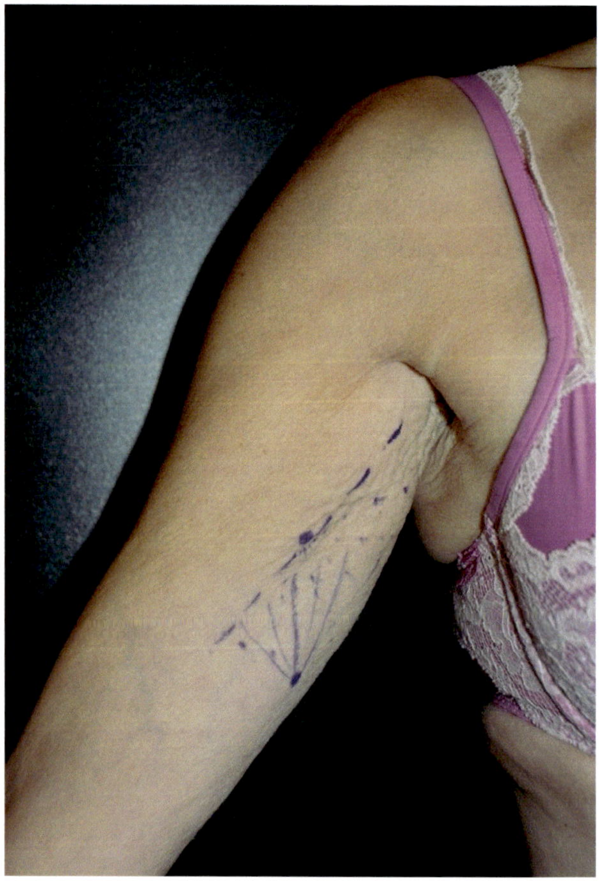

Figure 33.1 Marking the treated area and injection points in an upright position.

DOI: 10.1201/9781003617129-33

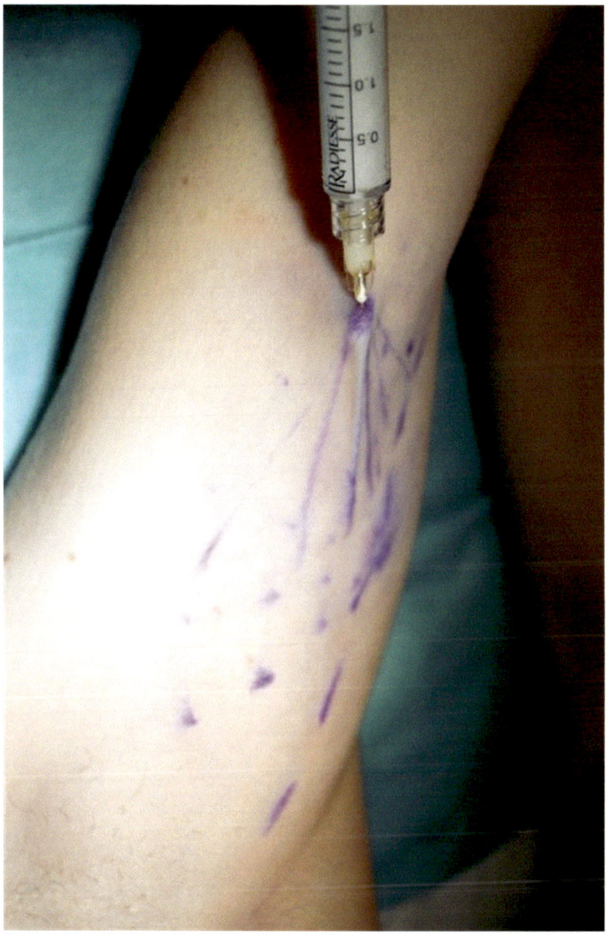

Figure 33.2 Injecting the first layer. Note that the cannula is inserted as superficially as possible in the superficial dermal layers.

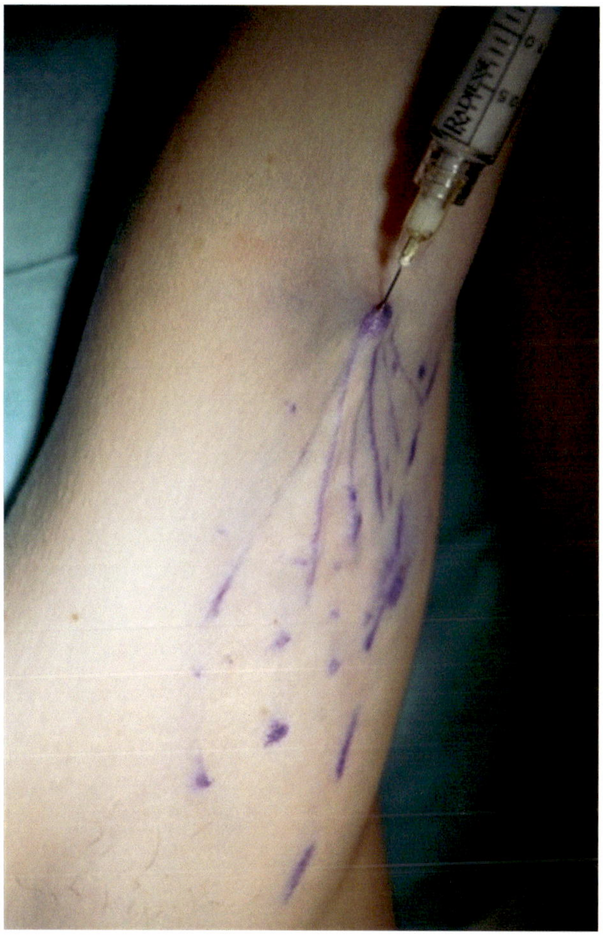

Figure 33.3 Injecting the second layer. Note that the cannula is inserted in a 45° angle. The cannula is pushed until resistance of the superficial fascia can be felt. Then product is injected in a retrograde fashion.

dermis (Figure 33.2). Use the full length of the cannula but avoid contacting the dermis with the cannula tip, especially when the cannula is inserted completely. Aggressive puncturing of the dermis from the inside can be unpleasant and painful for the patient.

This first thin layer of diluted CaHA will improve skin thickness, firmness, and elasticity.

- *Second layer*: Enter the cannula in a 45° angle gently until you feel the resistance of the superficial fascia; inject retrograde, connecting the superficial fascia with the dermal structures (Figure 33.3). This second layer of diluted CaHA will stimulate, reinforce, and thicken the already existing collagen fibers between these two skin layers, which results in a measurable lifting of the overlying tissues.

5. Due to superficial placement in very thin skin and hyperdilution of the product, temporary irregularities can occur (Figure 33.4).

See also Figure 33.5 for post-treatment results.

33.3 CANNULA TECHNIQUE IN THE UPPER ARM

For injection placement, see Figure 33.6.

33.3.1 Step-by-Step Technique

1. Disinfect the upper arm, including axilla.
2. Mark the area that needs to be treated; usually this is an oval area.
3. Use 1.5 mL CaHA per 100 cm^2 surface area; usually 3 mL are applied in this region.
4. Dilute CaHA between 1:1 and 1:3 (depending on severity of laxity) and use a 25G, 50 mm cannula or a 22G, 70 mm cannula.
5. Position the patient relatively horizontally for the comfort of the patient and ease of injection.
6. Consider bending the cannula for ease of handling the syringe.
7. Stretch the skin in the direction of injection to control the correct depth of the cannula. Make sure the cannula is at the dermal–subdermal junction (Figure 33.7).

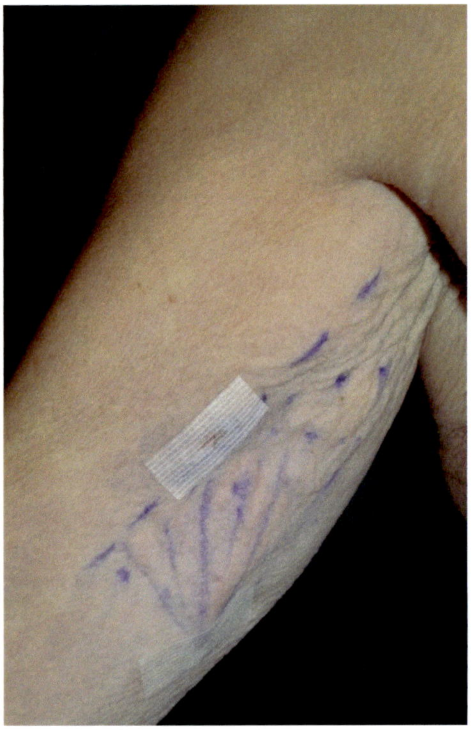

Figure 33.4 Temporary irregularities at the end of the procedure.

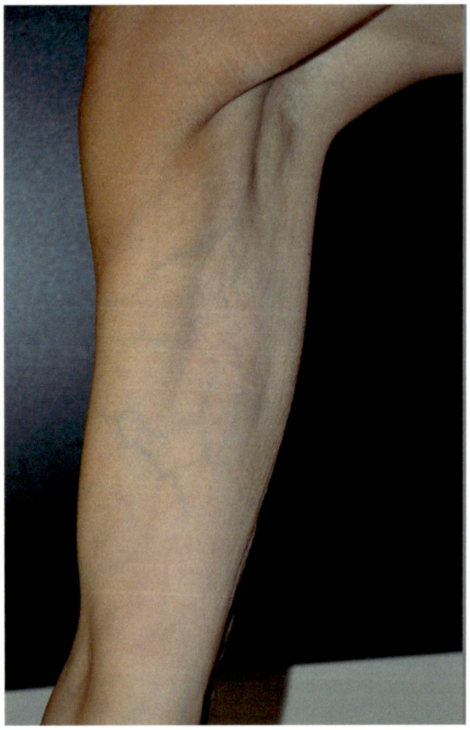

Figure 33.5 Result at four months, resulting in a firmer, healthier, and more hydrated appearance of the skin.

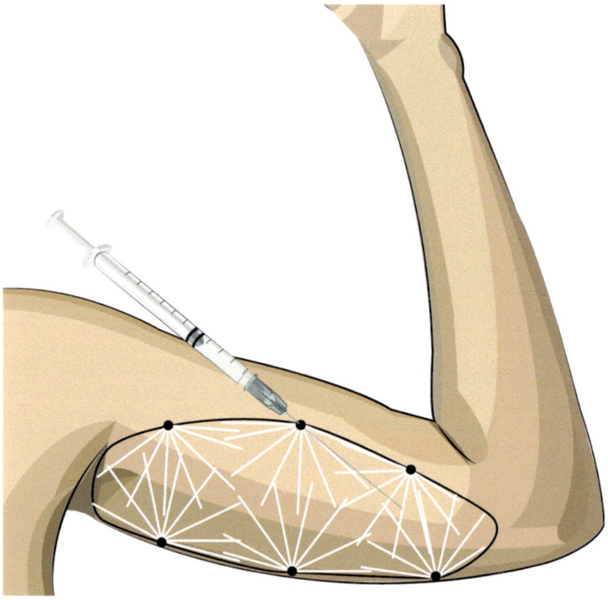

Figure 33.6 Diluted CaHA at the upper arm using the cannula technique. The white lines indicate retrograde linear threads of diluted CaHA at the dermal–subdermal junction.

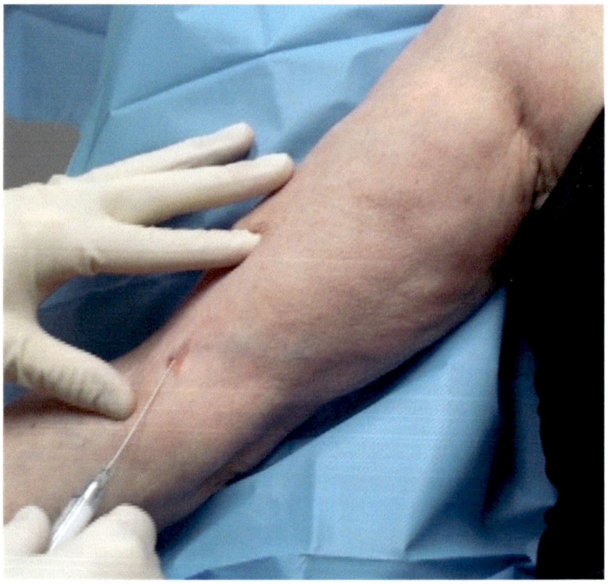

Figure 33.7 Stretch the skin in the direction of the cannula and inject in a retrograde fashion.

8. Slowly inject approximately 0.05–0.1 mL per retrograde injection in a fanning pattern.
9. Repeat until all the marked skin has a thin layer of diluted CaHA.

33.4 NEEDLE TECHNIQUE IN THE UPPER ARM

For injection placement, see Figure 33.8.

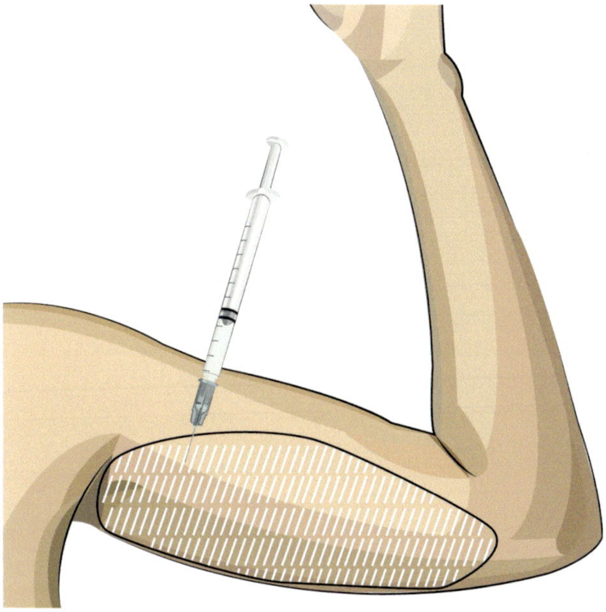

Figure 33.8 Diluted CaHA at the upper arm using the sharp needle technique. The white lines indicate retrograde linear threads of diluted CaHA at the dermal–subdermal junction.

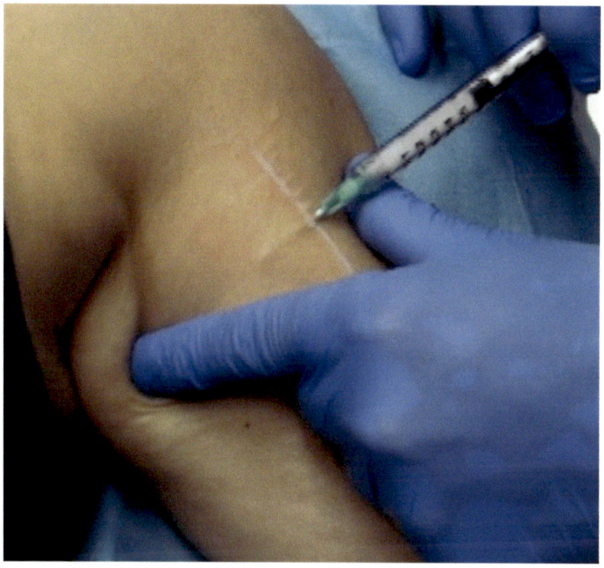

Figure 33.9 Sharp needle parallel to the retrograde linear threads.

33.4.1 Step-by-Step Technique

1. Disinfect the upper arm including the axilla; mark and position as described above.
2. Use 1.5 mL CaHA per 100 cm^2 surface area in this region.
3. Dilute CaHA 1:3 and use a 27–28G needle for injection.
4. Stretch the skin in the direction of injection to control the correct depth of the needle. Make sure the needle is in the superficial subdermal plane and avoid any product placement in the dermis. Superficial (dermal) placement of diluted CaHA may lead to product visibility immediately after the procedure and visible and palpable collagen strands a few weeks and months later. Especially in very thin skin, this causes very aesthetically disturbing results.
5. Slowly inject approximately 0.05 mL per retrograde injection in parallel to the retrograde linear threads (Figure 33.9).
6. Repeat until all the marked skin has a thin layer of diluted CaHA.

See also Figure 33.10 and Videos 33.1–33.3 for before and after results and application techniques, respectively.

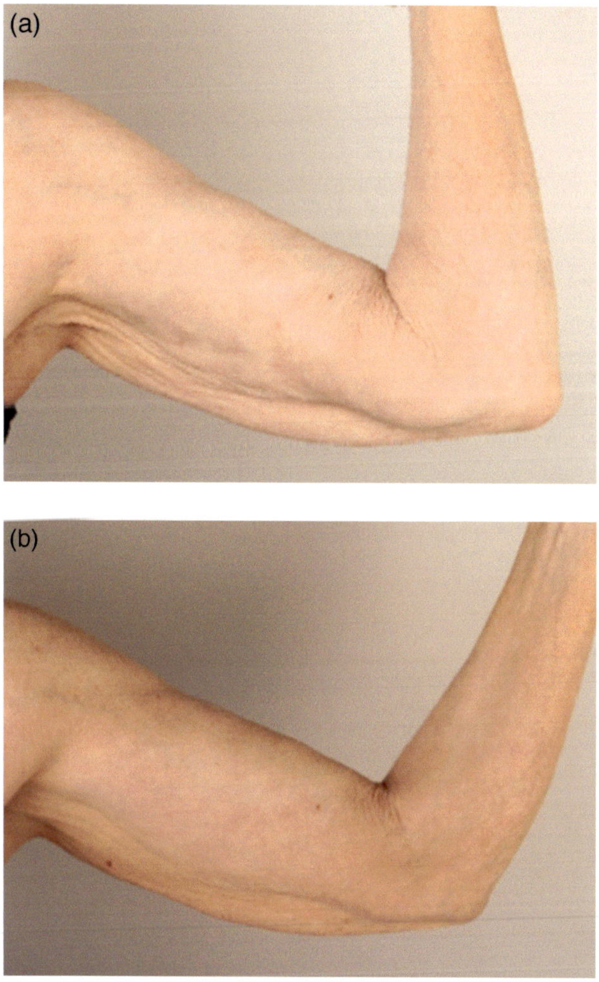

Figure 33.10 Before (a) and 15 months after (b) treatment with CaHA (3 mL per side; dilution 1:3).

33.5 AFTERCARE

When the saline is resorbed, irregularities disappear spontaneously within hours (Figure 33.11). We do not recommend massages or pressure garments after the

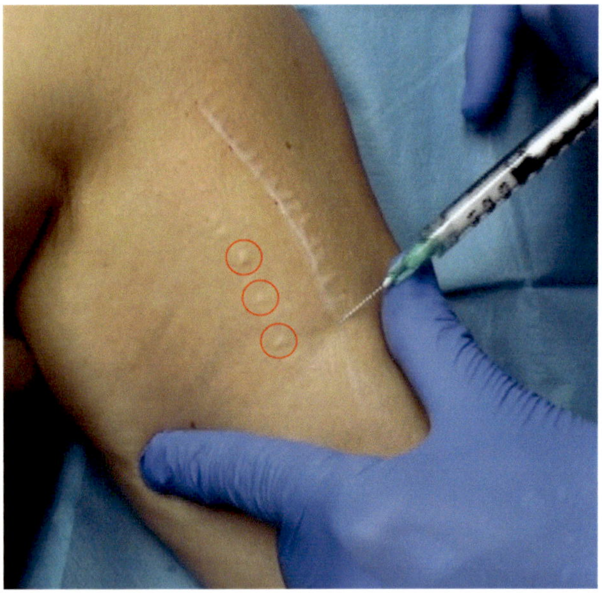

Figure 33.11 Irregularities due to the product placement usually recede within hours. Treatment with the needle technique has a higher chance of irregularities which may last longer but will recede spontaneously as well.

treatment. Vitamin K cream can be advised to speed up the resorption of a bruise. Clinical improvement can be expected no earlier than three months post-treatment. If necessary, additional treatment can be suggested then.

33.6 ADDITIONAL TREATMENTS FOR OPTIMAL RESULTS

Additional neocollagenesis stimulating techniques will improve the outcome (microfocused ultrasound, radiofrequency, lasers, peels, needling, etc.).

Video 33.1 Upper arm rejuvenation: cannula 1.

Video 33.2 Upper arm rejuvenation: cannula 2.

Video 33.3 Upper arm rejuvenation, hyperdiluted Radiesse: both cannula and sharp needle techniques.

REFERENCES

[1] Y. Yutskovskaya et al., "A randomized, split-face, histomorphologic study comparing a volumetric calcium hydroxylapatite and a hyaluronic acid-based dermal filler," *J Drugs Dermatol*, vol. 13, no. 9, pp. 1047–1052, 2014.

[2] K. Goldie et al., "Global consensus guidelines for the injection of diluted and hyperdiluted calcium gydroxylapatite for skin tightening," *Dermatol Surg*, vol. 44, no. Suppl 1, pp. S32–S41, 2018.

[3] F. Chirico et al., "Complications following non-surgical aesthetic treatments in HIV+ patients receiving antiretroviral therapy: A 12-years experience," *Appl Sci*, vol. 11, no. 9, p. 4059, 2021.

Extremities

34

Hand Rejuvenation

TATJANA PAVICIC, SEBASTIAN COTOFANA AND POLINA HOLOVINA

34.1 INTRODUCTION

Hands can reveal one's age as reliably as the face through a combination of fine lines, wrinkles, photo damage, and volume loss. In a questionnaire study conducted to determine factors that characterize the age of hands, people were asked to examine unaltered photographs of female hands and estimate women's age bracket (younger than 20 years, 20–30 years, 30–40 years, etc.) [1]. Young hands were found to be characterized by fullness, lack of veins, and lack of wrinkles, and in most cases, participants were able to accurately estimate the age of each woman in the unaltered photographs. Aged hands may therefore conflict with the appearance of a rejuvenated face.

Laser and other similar treatments can be used to decrease photo damage and to address fine lines and wrinkles. Fillers such as CaHA can be used to address volume loss, which also aid in wrinkle and fine line reduction. This chapter will briefly review hand anatomy, and the rationale for using CaHA for hand augmentation, before discussing a new technique for optimal hand rejuvenation.

34.2 RATIONALE FOR USING CAHA FOR HAND REJUVENATION

CaHA has several characteristics that make it an ideal agent for hand augmentation. In a two-step mechanism of action, the CaHA microspheres are first distributed at the injection site by their soluble carrier gel, which also provides immediate volume replacement. This is followed by a period of microsphere-induced activation of fibroblasts and neocollagenesis [2–4]. The aesthetic benefits from CaHA injection are therefore not just a result of the volume of product injected but also of the long-term stimulation of the patient's own collagen production, which ensures a long-lasting correction [5,6]. The components are all biodegradable and eventually reabsorbed naturally by the host's metabolic processes.

CaHA also has an optimal balance of viscoelasticity, allowing it to deform enough to be injected without excessive extrusion force and to be molded. Nevertheless, it is elastic enough to provide durable correction via its ability to resist external pressure once implanted [7]. These properties allow CaHA to integrate with the tissue, providing a natural appearance and feel. In addition to replacing lost volume, the opaque nature of CaHA can also help to conceal the color of veins and tendons, making them less visible.

CaHA is currently the only FDA-approved filler for hand augmentation based on the results of a randomized controlled trial in 101 patients who received a CaHA bolus in the dorsal hands or no treatment [8]. Controls were crossed over at three months, and all subjects were followed for six months [8]. CaHA-treated hands showed statistically and clinically significant improvements compared with control hands, along with high patient and physician satisfaction and no serious adverse events. Statistically significant improvements in the CaHA-treated hands were observed using validated hand grading scales, at 6 and 12 months, with only minor and short-lived adverse events [8,9] The results were supported by a separate randomized controlled trial in 114 patients who were randomized 3:1 to CaHA treatment and untreated control groups. Effectiveness was assessed by blinded investigators using a validated hand grading scale [10]. A total of 75% of CaHA-treated subjects achieved a ≥1-point improvement on the hand grading scale ($P < 0.0001$) at 3 months (primary endpoint), a response that was generally maintained at 12 months. The proportions of subjects reporting improvement ranged from 98% at 3 months to 86% at 12 months.

34.3 HAND ANATOMY

With the increasing demand for hand rejuvenation procedures, anatomical studies of the dorsum of the hand have been conducted to determine the optimal location for filler deposition and the safest injection technique [11–13]. Based on dissections of fresh cadaveric hands and duplex ultrasound investigation of healthy hands, the safest plane to apply volumizing material was found to be the undersurface of the dermis in a thin fatty layer known as the superficial dorsal lamina (Figure 34.1) [12]. The absence of major veins and sensory nerves explains why injections in this plane are significantly less likely to be related to adverse events (Figure 34.1).

In contrast, the fascial plane, located between the dermis and the tendons, with its numerous fibrous septa and blood vessels, was deemed unsuitable because of a greater risk of injuring the innervation, vasculature, and tendons [12,13].

DOI: 10.1201/9781003617129-34

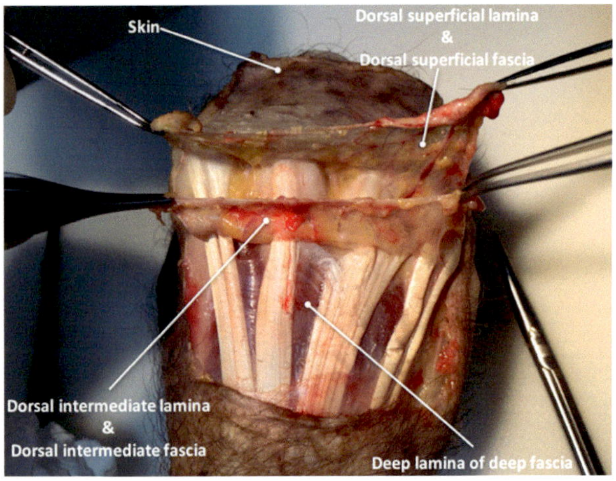

Figure 34.1 Cadaveric hand studies illustrate the plane of injection for CaHA–the superficial dorsal superficial lamina. This thin fatty layer is devoid of major veins and sensory nerves, making injections in this plane less likely to result in adverse events.

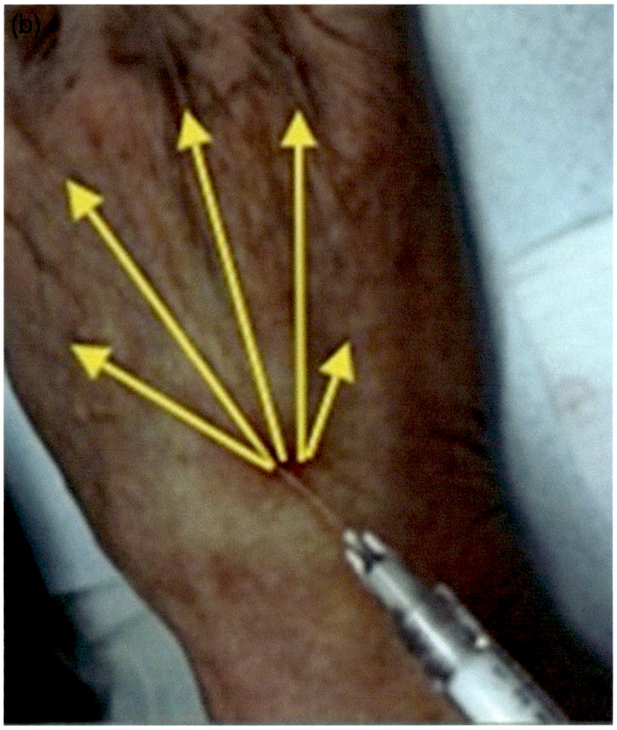

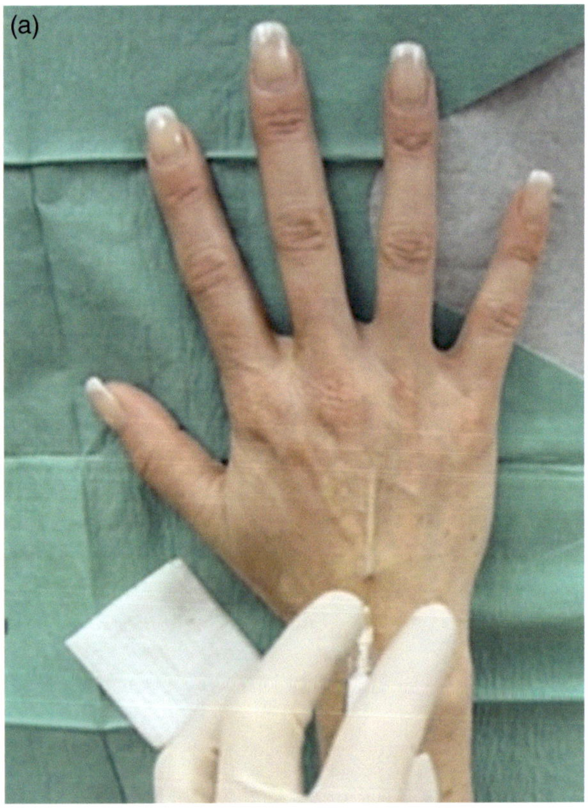

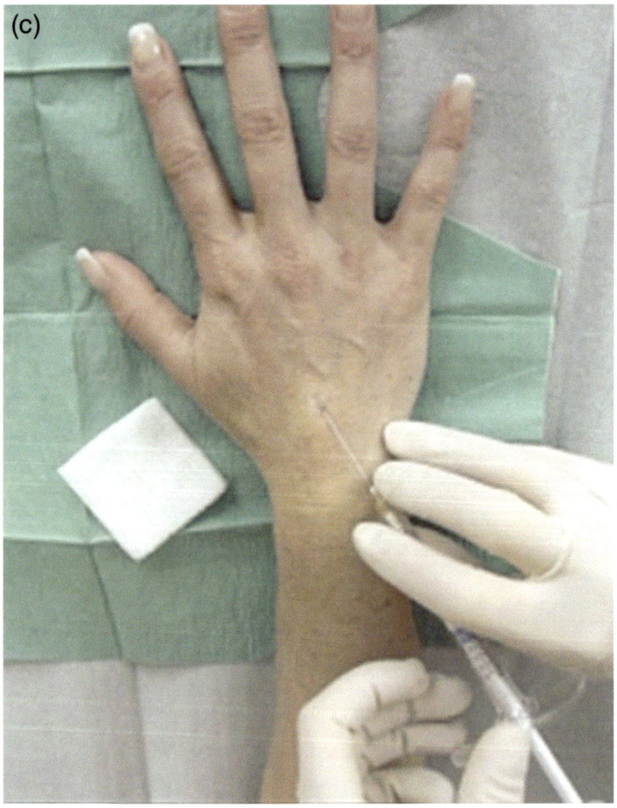

Figure 34.2 (a–c) CaHA is injected subdermally (0.2–0.9 mm) into the dorsum of the hand from a single entry point using a 22G, 70 mm cannula and a proximal-to-distal fanning technique. (Image courtesy of Sebastian Cotofana, MD).

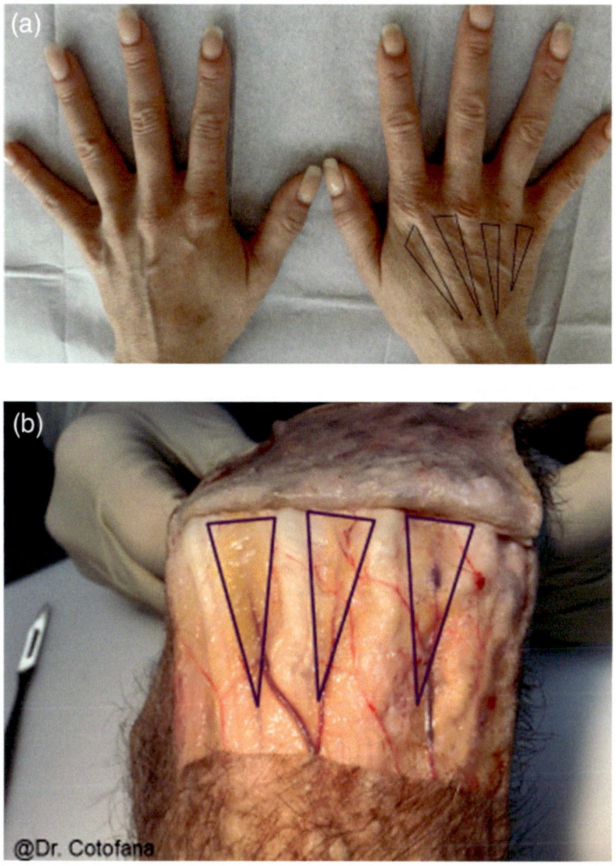

Figure 34.3 (a–b) CaHA is injected in a series of triangles between the tendinous bands with the triangle tip located proximally and the base distally; note the intrametacarpal fat distribution.

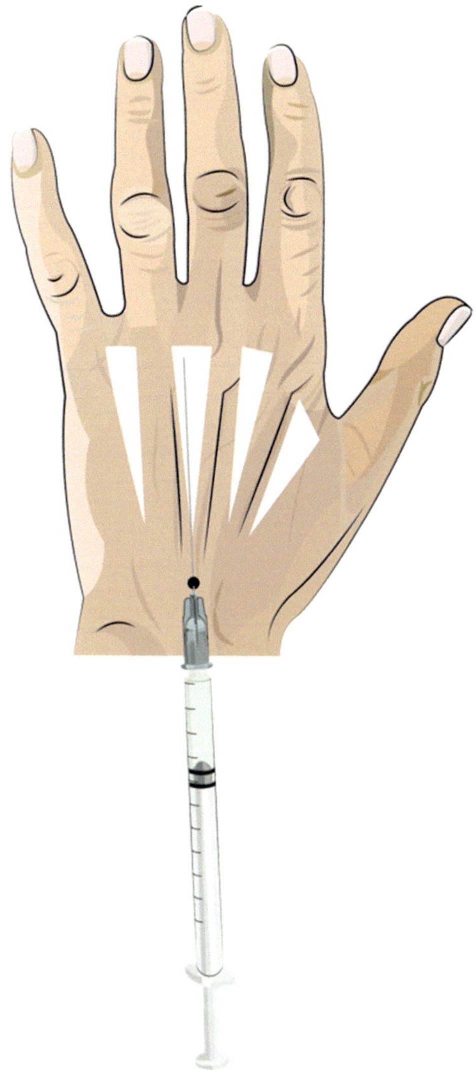

Figure 34.4 Rejuvenation of the dorsum of the hand using the cannula technique. The black dot illustrates the entry point of the cannula, and the white triangles refer to atrophic areas and, therefore, subdermal target sites for CaHA.

Further information on optimal approaches for hand augmentation with CaHA has been provided by a recent retrospective study on 220 individuals that examined safety and treatment outcomes with respect to the use of needle or cannula and chosen injection technique (bolus, tenting, proximal-to-distal fanning, distal-to-proximal single line) over 11 years of use [12]. Adverse events were reported in 32 individuals (7.3% of hands) in the first two weeks and were mostly related to swelling, pain, and erythema. Use of a needle was associated with a greater risk of adverse events than a cannula (OR 7.57, 95% CI 3.76–15.24; $P < 0.001$), and the proximal-to-distal fanning technique was found to have the lowest odds ratio for adverse events (Figures 34.2–34.3).

34.4 CAHA HAND INJECTION CANNULA TECHNIQUE

Based on the above findings, the authors propose the following technique for optimal hand rejuvenation with CaHA. The technique is based on the skin-scraping-threading technique described by Lefebvre-Vilardebo *et al.* [13] but with only a single entry point.

For injection placement, see Figure 34.4.

34.4.1 Step-by-Step Technique

1. The hand is cleaned and disinfected before being placed palm down on a procedure table with a sterile cloth beneath.
2. Using a 21G needle, an insertion point for the cannula is made. In sensitive patients, local anesthesia with lidocaine and adrenaline (1:200000) can be applied at the insertion point (Figure 34.5).
3. From this single entry point, CaHA diluted 1:1 with 0.9% NaCl and lidocaine mixture is injected using a 22G blunt, stiff 70 mm cannula and a proximal-to-distal (towards the fingers) fanning technique (Figure 34.2). A total of 1.5 mL is injected per hand (i.e. 1.5 mL volume, which represents 0.75 mL CaHA).

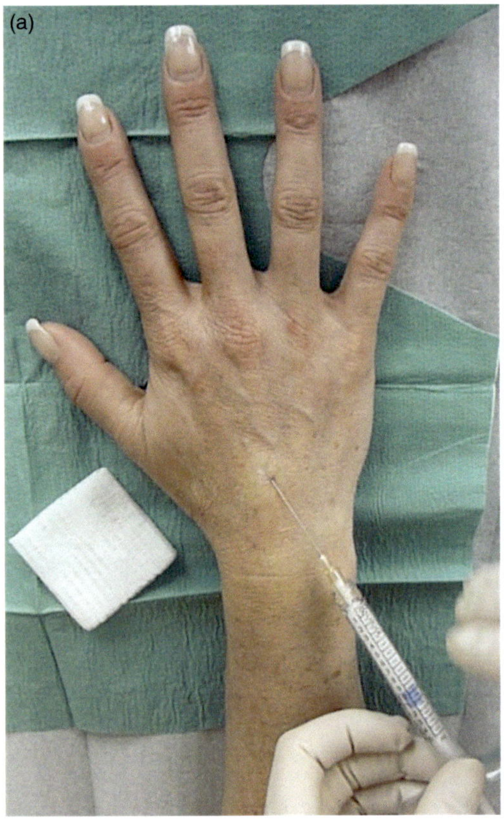

4. With the bevel pointing upwards, the cannula is advanced by scraping along the bottom of the dermis, twirling if any resistance is met. Tenting of the skin should be avoided, as this also lifts all the underlying structures.
5. Using the fanning technique, CaHA is injected in a retrograde and anterograde manner in a series of triangles between the tendinous bands, with the triangle tip located proximally and the base distally (see Figure 34.3).
6. The hand is then gently massaged to ensure even distribution.

34.5 CAHA HAND INJECTION SHARP NEEDLE TECHNIQUE

For injection placement, see Figure 34.6.

34.5.1 Step-by-Step Technique

1. Clean and disinfect the hand before placing it palm down on a procedure table with a clean cloth underneath.
2. Use a 30G needle and lidocaine with adrenaline (1:200000) to hydrodissect the skin from the fascia. Start injecting from the distal part of the dorsum

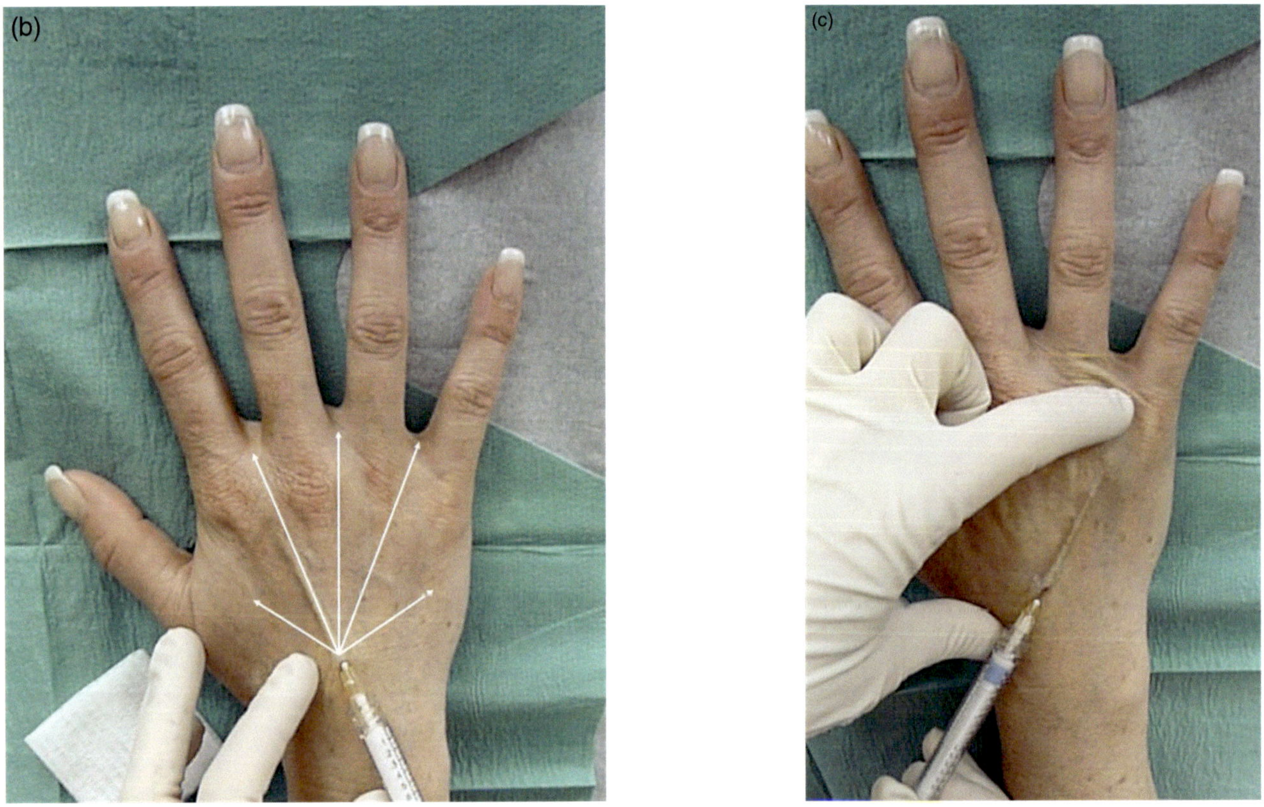

Figure 34.5 A single entry point suffices for treatment of the hand dorsum when using a 22G, 70 mm cannula. (a) The cannula is introduced at the immediate subdermal level, (b) the arrows indicate the direction of the retrograde linear threads, and (c) the skin is stretched with the non-dominant hand to facilitate remaining in the correct anatomical layer.

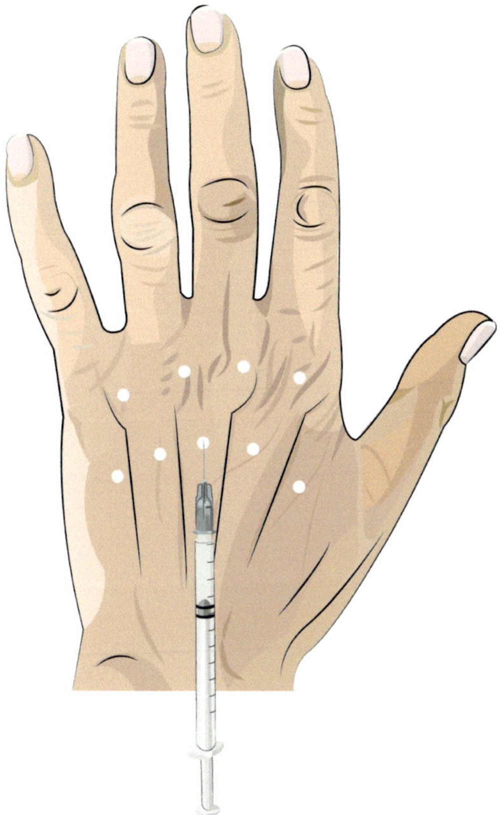

Figure 34.6 Hand rejuvenation treatment using the sharp needle technique. The white dots illustrate the injection sites to deposit CaHA.

(Figure 34.7a) of the hand and move proximally (Figure 34.7b).

3. After hydrodissection, a mixture 1:1 of diluted CaHA with 0.9% NaCl and lidocaine is injected using a 27G, 19 mm needle in the newly created space (Figure 34.8).
4. Place small boluses of CaHA in a retrograde, fanning fashion. A total of 1.5 mL is injected per hand (i.e. 1.5 mL volume, which represents 0.75 mL CaHA).
5. To ensure even distribution of the product, gently massage the hand following a proximal direction (Figure 34.9a). Consider adding an antibiotic cream.

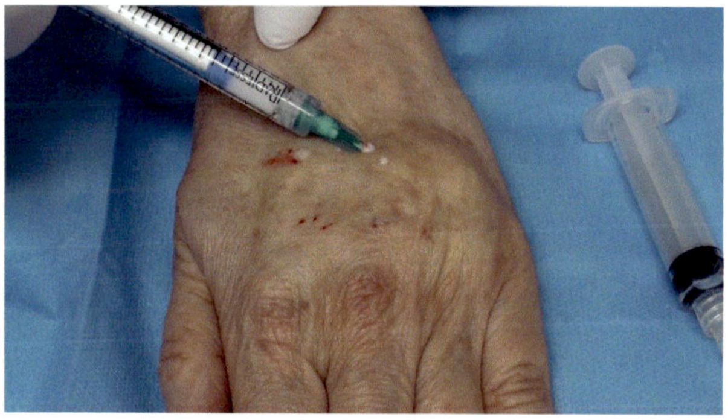

Figure 34.8 Sharp needle technique consists of CaHA deposition in retrograde, linear threads using multiple injection sites.

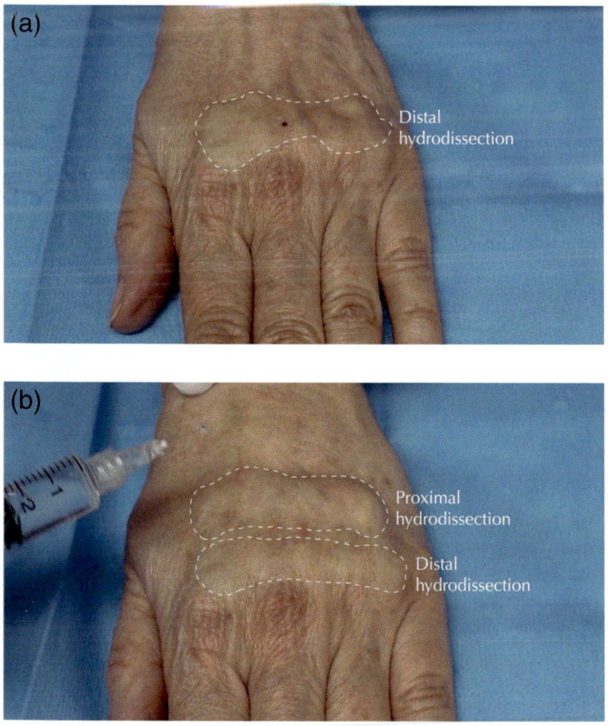

Figure 34.7 (a) Distal to (b) proximal hydrodissection of the hand dorsum to separate the skin from the fascia using diluted lidocaine with adrenaline.

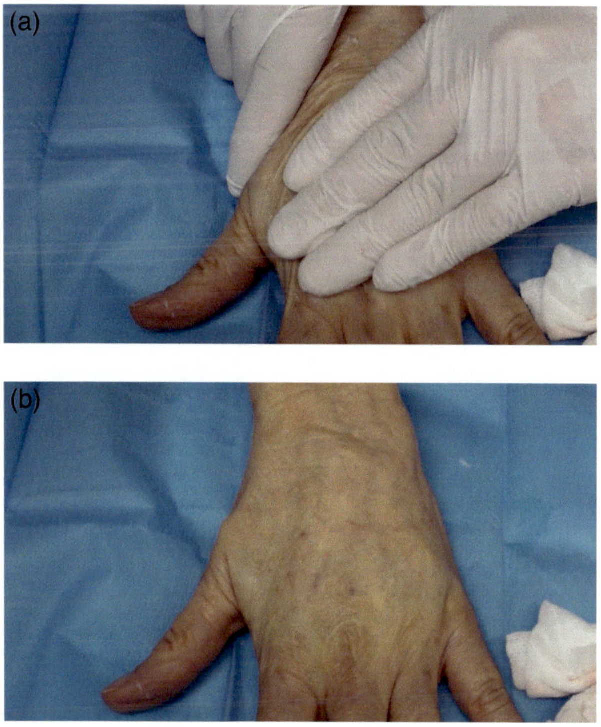

Figure 34.9 After treatment, (a) a massage from dorsal to proximal is warranted to even out the product and (b) achieve a smooth result.

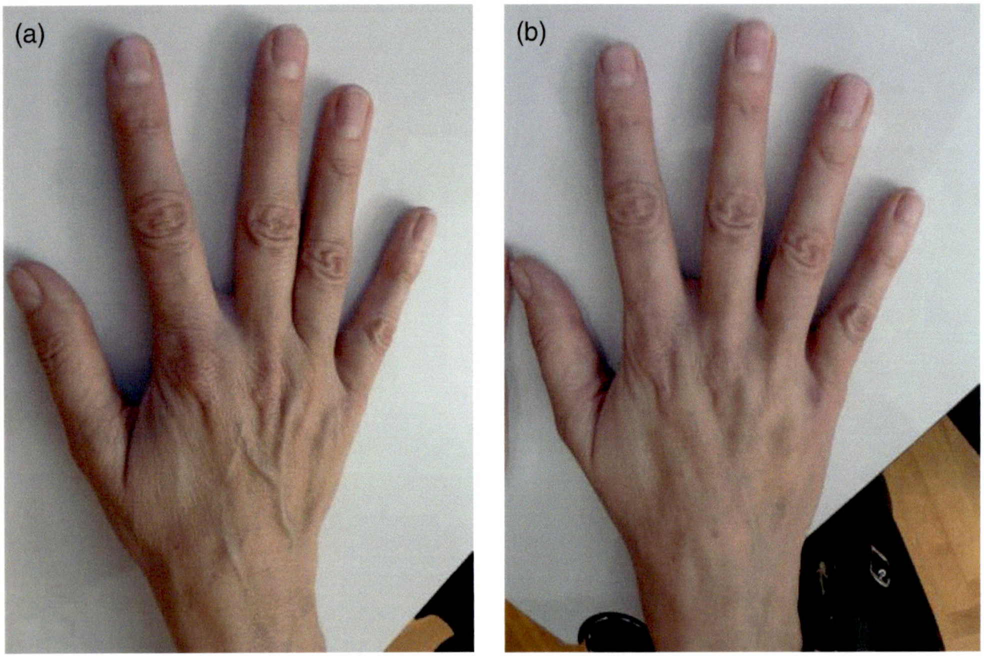

Figure 34.10 Before and after treatment of the dorsum of the hands with 1.5 mL of CaHA (Courtesy Dr. Tatjana Pavicic).

See further Figure 34.9b and Videos 34.1–34.2 for results and application techniques, respectively.

34.6 AFTERCARE

Injection of CaHA into the fingers is not recommended, as repeated movement can cause the product to accumulate over the knuckles and form nodules. A follow-up at eight weeks is recommended to determine if a second treatment is required. Beneficial effects can be expected to last up to 12 months in most patients based on results from published studies [9,14]. Patients should be advised to avoid activities such as gardening or dish washing for one week after treatment to prevent any infection entering at the cannula insertion point.

Adverse events in published studies have been few and of short duration and consisted mostly of bruising, erythema, and edema [8,9,12,14,15]. With the use of the proximal-to-distal fanning technique, these events are likely to be reduced even further.

Video 34.1 Hand rejuvenation: cannula technique.

Video 34.2 Hand rejuvenation: sharp needle technique.

REFERENCES

[1] R. D. Bains et al., "Hand aging: Patients' opinions," *Plast Reconstr Surg*, vol. 117, no. 7, pp. 2212–2218, 2006.

[2] A. L. Berlin et al., "Calcium hydroxylapatite filler for facial rejuvenation: A histologic and immunohistochemical analysis," *Dermatol Surg*, vol. 34, no. Suppl 1, pp. S64–S67, 2008.

[3] K. M. Coleman et al., "Neocollagenesis after injection of calcium hydroxylapatite composition in a canine model," *Dermatol Surg*, vol. 34, no. Suppl 1, Jun. 2008, https://doi.org/10.1111/J.1524-4725.2008.34243.X.

[4] E. S. Marmur et al., "Clinical, histologic and electron microscopic findings after injection of a calcium hydroxylapatite filler," *J Cosmet Laser Ther*, vol. 6, no. 4, pp. 223–226, Dec. 2004, https://doi.org/10.1080/147641704100003048.

[5] Y. Yutskovskaya et al., "A randomized, split-face, histomorphologic study comparing a volumetric calcium hydroxylapatite and a hyaluronic acid-based dermal filler," *J Drugs Dermatol*, vol. 13, no. 9, pp. 1047–1052, Sep. 2014 [Online], http://www.ncbi.nlm.nih.gov/pubmed/25226004 (accessed Nov. 7, 2024).

[6] Y. A. Yutskovskaya, E. A. Kogan, "Improved neocollagenesis and skin mechanical properties after injection of diluted calcium hydroxylapatite in the neck and décolletage: A pilot study," *J Drugs Dermatol*, vol. 16, no. 1, pp. 68–74, Jan. 2017 [Online], http://www.ncbi.nlm.nih.gov/pubmed/28095536 (accessed Nov. 7, 2024).

[7] H. Sundaram et al., "Comparison of the rheological properties of viscosity and elasticity in two categories of soft tissue fillers: Calcium hydroxylapatite and hyaluronic acid," *Dermatol Surg*,

vol. 36, no. Suppl 3, pp. 1859–1865, Nov. 2010, https://doi.org/10.1111/J.1524-4725.2010.01743.X.

[8] M. Busso, R. Voigts, "An investigation of changes in physical properties of injectable calcium hydroxylapatite in a carrier gel when mixed with lidocaine and with lidocaine/epinephrine," *Dermatol Surg*, vol. 34, no. Suppl 1, Jun. 2008, https://doi.org/10.1111/J.1524-4725.2008.34238.X.

[9] M. P. Goldman et al., "Calcium hydroxylapatite dermal filler for treatment of dorsal hand volume loss: Results from a 12-month, multicenter, randomized, blinded trial," *Dermatol Surg*, vol. 44, no. 1, pp. 75–83, Jan. 2018, https://doi.org/10.1097/DSS.0000000000001203.

[10] J. L. Cohen et al., "A randomized, blinded study to validate the merz hand grading scale for use in live assessments," *Dermatol Surg*, vol. 41, pp. S384–S388, Dec. 2015, https://doi.org/10.1097/DSS.0000000000000553.

[11] S. M. Bidic et al., "Dorsal hand anatomy relevant to volumetric rejuvenation," *Plast Reconstr Surg*, vol. 126, no. 1, pp. 163–168, Jul. 2010, https://doi.org/10.1097/PRS.0B013E3181DA86EE.

[12] K. Frank et al., "The anatomy behind adverse events in hand volumizing procedures: Retrospective evaluations of 11 years of experience," *Plast Reconstr Surg*, vol. 141, no. 5, pp. 650e–662e, May 2018, https://doi.org/10.1097/PRS.0000000000004211.

[13] M. Lefebvre-Vilardebo et al., "Hand: Clinical anatomy and regional approaches with injectable fillers," *Plast Reconstr Surg*, vol. 136, no. 5, pp. 258S–275S, 2015, https://doi.org/10.1097/PRS.0000000000001828.

[14] N. S. Sadick, "A 52-week study of safety and efficacy of calcium hydroxylapatite for rejuvenation of the aging hand," *J Drugs Dermatol*, vol. 10, no. 1, pp. 47–51, Jan. 2011.

[15] G. F. Muti et al., "Calcium hydroxylapatite for augmentation of face and hands: A retrospective analysis in Italian subjects," *J Drugs Dermatol*, vol. 14, no. 9, pp. 948–954, Sep. 2015 [Online], https://pubmed.ncbi.nlm.nih.gov/26355612/ (accessed Jan. 22, 2025).

Extremities

Elbow Skin Quality Improvement

35

JANI VAN LOGHEM

35.1 INTRODUCTION

During the aging process, the skin loses collagen and elastin fibers, and both intrinsic and extrinsic factors influence aging of the elbow skin. As this specific skin is accustomed to being continuously stretched (by bending the arm), the skin is significantly thicker than that of the upper arm, with significant wrinkling as a result of collagen fibers breaking.

Even though liposuction is used for the removal of unwanted adipose tissue of the upper arms and brachioplasty aims to remove excess loose skin after substantial weight loss [1–3], these treatment modalities do not target the changes in skin quality. Diluted CaHA is an effective nonsurgical option that gives a significant increase of strength and elasticity to the skin and therefore causes reduction in skin laxity and improves the appearance of the elbow area [4].

35.2 ANATOMICAL DANGERS

Injection should be done as close to the dermis as possible, preferably at the immediate subdermal level. This location ensures avoiding branches of the brachial artery.

35.3 ELBOW CANNULA TECHNIQUE

For injection placement, see Figure 35.1.

35.4.1 Step-by-Step Technique

1. Disinfect the treatment area.
2. Mark the treatment area (a round or square) and the direction of the skin folds.
3. Mark the injection points, ideally three to four points from different sides of the drawn shape.
4. Dilute CaHA between 1:0.5 and 1:3 (depending on severity of laxity) by mixing CaHA with lidocaine and saline.
5. Use a long 22G cannula (50 or 70 mm) and accessory 21G needle.
6. If needed, anesthetize the entry points by injecting a small amount of adrenalized lidocaine.
7. Puncture the skin at the injection points with a 21G needle.
8. Insert the 22G cannula.
9. Stretch the skin in the direction of the cannula to control the correct depth of the cannula. Make sure the cannula stays at the immediate subdermal level.
10. If needed, the cannula can be bent with the bevel pointing upward to facilitate superficial placement.
11. Inject CaHA in a retrograde linear fanning fashion from each injection point (Figure 35.2).
12. Slowly inject approximately 0.05–0.1 mL per retrograde injection (Figures 35.3–35.4).
13. Repeat until the entire treatment area contains a thin layer of diluted CaHA.
14. If clear irregularities are observed, massage the entire area to warrant proper distribution of the product.

See also Figure 35.5 and Video 35.1 for before and after results and application technique, respectively.

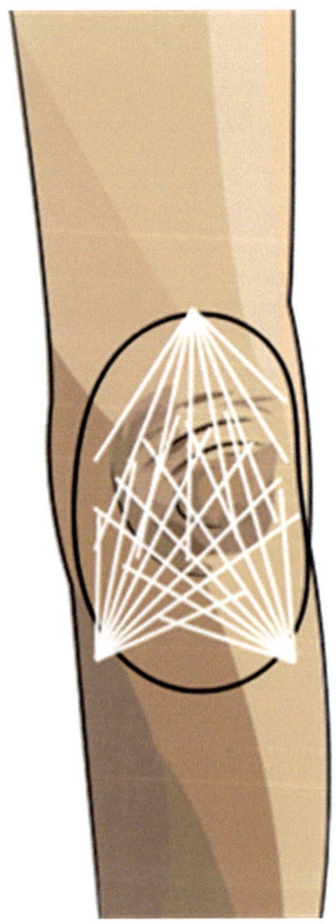

Figure 35.1 Diluted CaHA injection at the elbows using the cannula technique. The white lines indicate retrograde linear threads of diluted CaHA at the subdermal level.

DOI: 10.1201/9781003617129-35

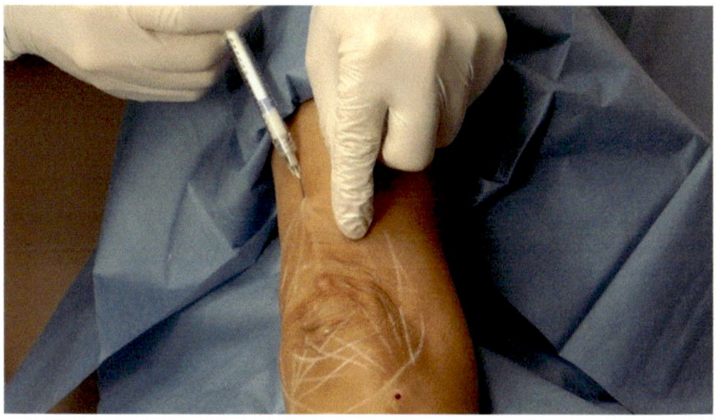

Figure 35.2 A 22G, 50 mm cannula is inserted in the first entry point and advanced at the immediate subdermal level. Several retrograde linear threads are injected using a fanning technique.

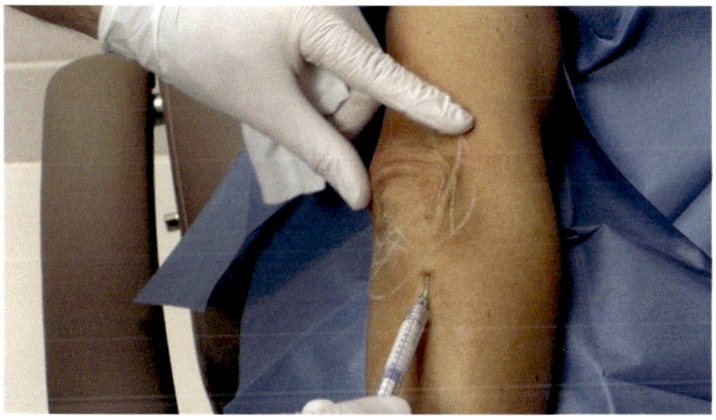

Figure 35.3 Injection from the second entry point.

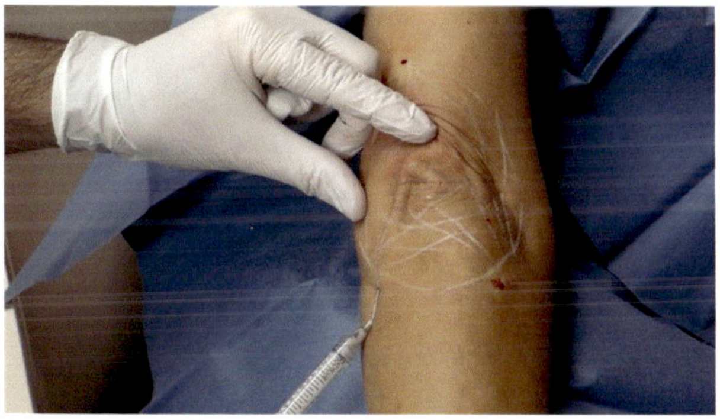

Figure 35.4 Injection from the third entry point.

35.5 AFTERCARE

Some swelling may be observed, although self-limiting. No specific after care is necessary other than to keep the entry points clean to prevent infection.

35.6 ADDITIONAL TREATMENTS FOR OPTIMAL RESULTS

Patients with more severe laxity or thicker skin may require combination therapy using other skin-tightening techniques (e.g. radiofrequency, microfocused ultrasound with visualization, microneedling, etc.) to achieve optimal results.

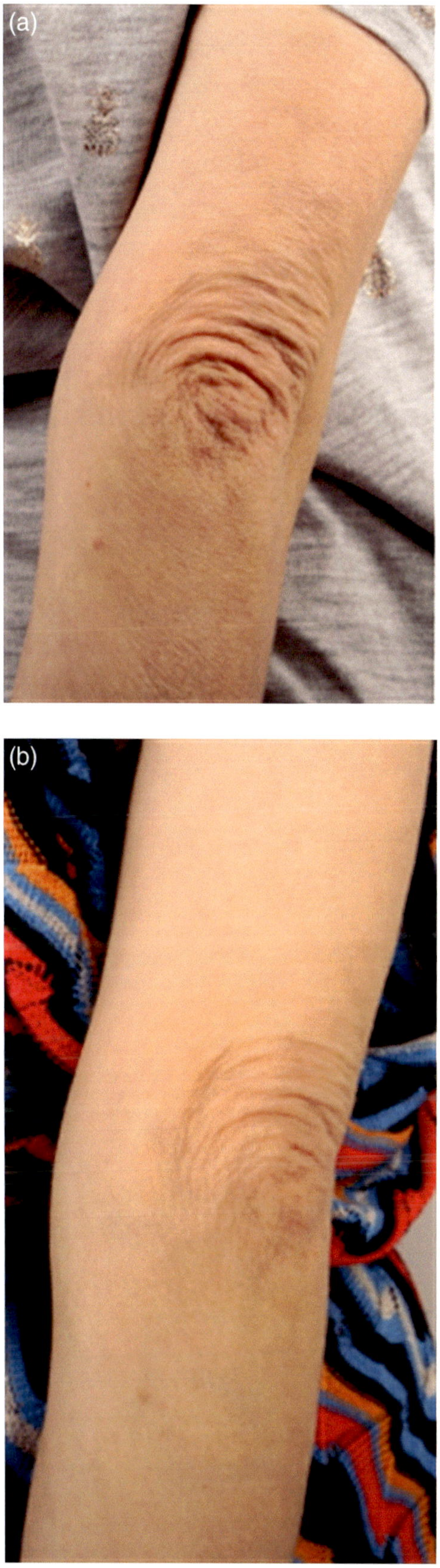

Figure 35.5 (a) Before and (b) three months post-treatment results using 1.5 mL CaHA per side, diluted with 0.5 mL 1% lidocaine and 1 mL saline.

Video 35.1 Elbow: cannula technique.

REFERENCES

[1] D. J. Hurwitz, S. W. Holland, "The L-brachioplasty: An innovative approach to correct excess tissue of the upper arm, axilla, and lateral chest," *Plast Reconstr Surg*, vol. 117, no. 2, pp. 403–411, 2006.

[2] D. J. Hurwitz, T. Neavin, "L-brachioplasty correction of excess tissue of the upper arm, axilla, and lateral chest," *Clin Plast Surg*, vol. 35, no. 1, pp. 131–140, 2008.

[3] D. J. Hurwitz, K. Jerrod, "L-brachioplasty: An adaptable technique for moderate to severe excess skin and fat of the arms," *Aesthet Surg J*, vol. 30, no. 4, pp. 620–629, 2010.

[4] K. Goldie et al., "Global consensus guidelines for the injection of diluted and hyperdiluted calcium hydroxylapatite for skin tightening," *Dermatol Surg*, vol. 44, no. Suppl 1, pp. S32–S41, 2018.

Extremities

36

Upper Leg Skin Quality Improvement

JANI VAN LOGHEM AND PIETER SIEBENGA

36.1 INTRODUCTION

With aging, the skin of the upper legs loses its tightness due to changes in the fibrous structure of the skin. This loss of collagen and elastin fibers, and changes in fat distribution, may then result in undesirable wrinkles and skin sagging. The phenomenon of skin flaccidity includes the development of *striae distensae* (also known as stretch marks) and/or cellulite [1–4], commonly affecting women more than men [5] and being more predominant in dark-skinned subjects [6]. Most often, these changes of the skin can be attributed to adolescence, a sudden change in weight, and/or pregnancy and can have a negative impact on the quality of life [7]. Hyperdiluted CaHA for the treatment of the anterior and posterior upper legs focuses on improving skin laxity and the appearance of cellulite and *striae*, increasing the strength and elasticity of the skin [7–9].

36.1.1 *Striae Distensae*

Striae distensae are a type of dermal scarring resulting from epidermal atrophy and loss of rete ridges [6]. This phenomenon has a higher incidence in puberty (6–86%), pregnancy (43–88%), and obesity (43%) [10], and its exact etiology remains unknown, but changes in the structure of collagen, mediated by hormonal changes, are thought to be the causative factors [8]. In these skin defects, CaHA can improve the appearance of *striae* by filling the stretch mark, thus enhancing its aesthetic look. Casabona *et al.* already proved the efficacy of CaHA, microneedling, and topical ascorbic acid combined for the treatment of *striae* [11], and in this chapter, we will also discuss the step-by-step procedure to treat this skin condition.

36.2 ANATOMICAL DANGERS

Injection should be done as close to the dermis as possible, at the dermal-subdermal junction. Varicose veins should be avoided to prevent extensive and possibly long-lasting ecchymoses.

36.3 UPPER LEG SHARP NEEDLE TECHNIQUE

For injection placement, see Figure 36.1.

36.3.1 Step-by-Step Technique

1. Disinfect the upper legs.
2. Mark the direction of the skin lines/wrinkles (Figure 36.2).
3. Dilute CaHA between 1:1 and 1:3 (depending on severity of laxity).
4. Use a long 27G, 38 mm cannula.
5. Stretch the skin in the direction of injection to control the correct depth of the needle. Make sure the needle is at the dermal-subdermal junction (Figure 36.3).
6. Inject CaHA in the direction of the skin line/wrinkle and crosshatch with multiple injections perpendicular to the wrinkle (Figure 36.4).

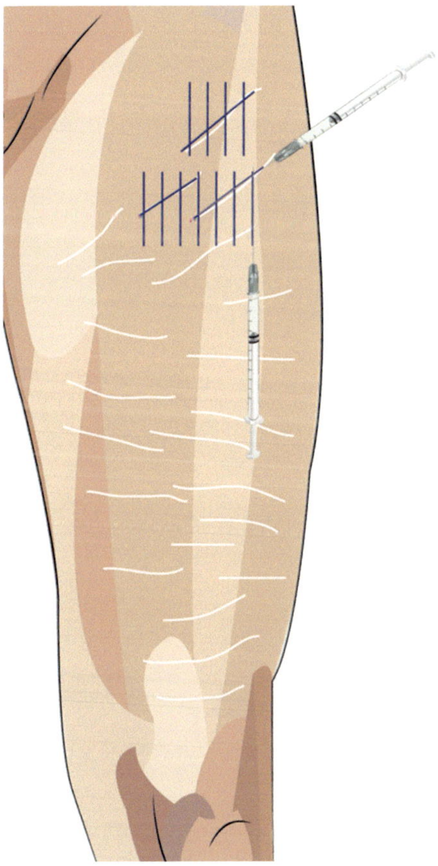

Figure 36.1 Diluted CaHA at the upper legs using the sharp needle technique. The white lines indicate direction of the wrinkles, and the blue lines indicate retrograde linear threads of diluted CaHA at the dermal–subdermal junction.

DOI: 10.1201/9781003617129-36

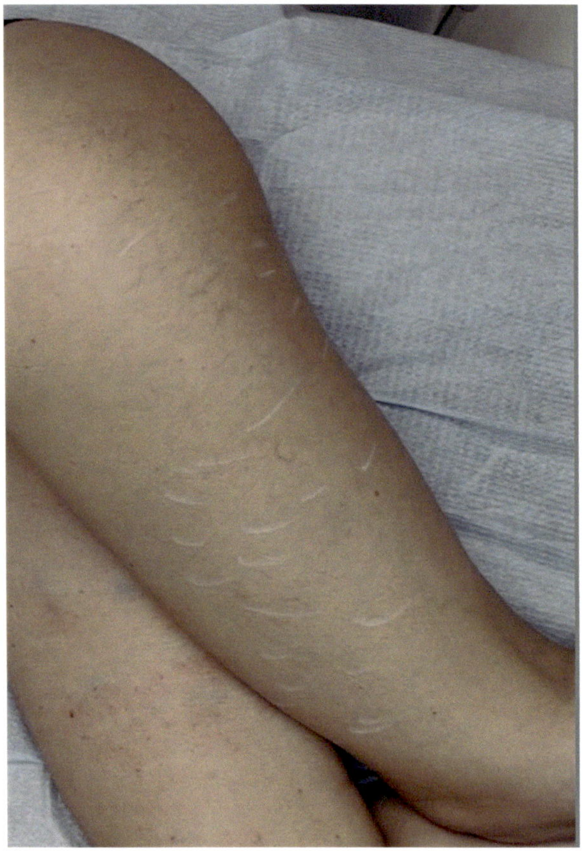

Figure 36.2 Marking the area to be treated.

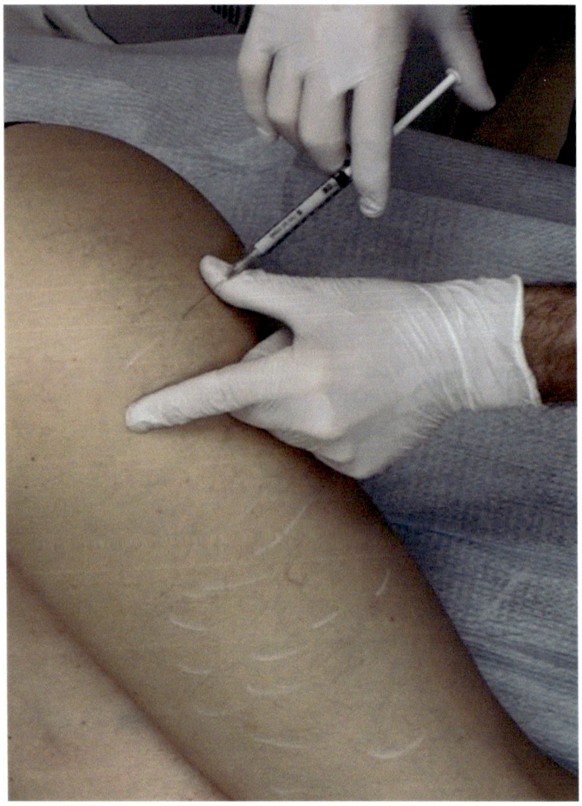

Figure 36.3 Stretch the skin in the direction of the needle and inject retrograde.

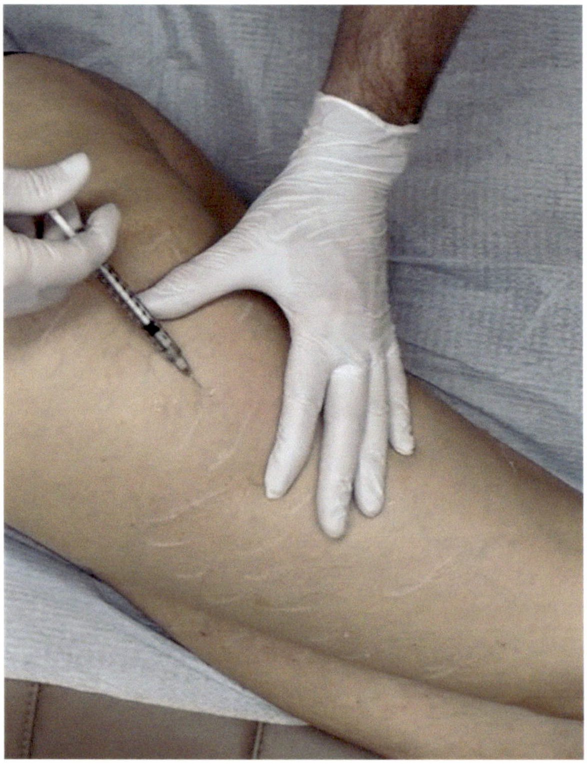

Figure 36.4 Perpendicular retrograde threads for extra skin tightening.

7. Slowly inject approximately 0.05–0.1 mL per retrograde injection.
8. Repeat until all of the marked skin has a thin layer of diluted CaHA.

See also Video 36.1 for application technique.

36.4 AFTERCARE

A post-injection vigorous massage is advised to ensure proper distribution of the product. Extensive bruising is possible in the presence of varicose veins.

36.5 ADDITIONAL TREATMENTS FOR OPTIMAL RESULTS

Patients with more severe laxity may require combination therapy using other skin-tightening techniques (e.g. radiofrequency, microfocused ultrasound with visualization, microneedling, etc.) to achieve optimal results.

Video 36.1 Upper legs: needle technique.

REFERENCES

[1] B. Barankin et al., "The skin in pregnancy," *J Cutan Med Surg*, vol. 6, no. 3, pp. 236–240, 2002.

[2] M. L. Elsaie et al., "Striae distensae (stretch marks) and different modalities of therapy: An update," *Dermatol Surg*, vol. 35, no. 4, pp. 563–573, 2009.

[3] S. Luebberding et al., "Cellulite: An evidence-based review," *Am J Clin Dermatol*, vol. 16, no. 4, pp. 243–256, 2015.
[4] K. Goldie et al., "Global consensus guidelines for the injection of diluted and hyperdiluted calcium hydroxylapatite for skin tightening," *Dermatol Surg*, vol. 44, no. Suppl 1, pp. S32–S41, 2018.
[5] N. Mendes et al., "A narrative review of current striae treatments," *Healthcare*, vol. 10, no. 12, p. 2565, 2022.
[6] A. M. Oakley, B. C. Patel, "Stretch Marks," *StatPearls* [internet], 2023: https://www.ncbi.nlm.nih.gov/books/NBK436005/.
[7] V. Cogorno Wasylkowski, "Body vectoring technique with Radiesse(®) for tightening of the abdomen, thighs, and brachial zone," *Clin Cosmet Investig Dermatol*, vol. 8, pp. 267–273, 2015.
[8] G. Singh, L. P. Kumar, "Striae distensae," *Indian J Dermatol Venereol Leprol*, vol. 71, no. 5, pp. 370–372, 2005.
[9] G. Casabona, G. Pereira, "Microfocused ultrasound with visualization and calcium hydroxylapatite for improving skin laxity and cellulite appearance," *Plast Reconstr Surg Glob Open*, vol. 5, no. 7, 2017.
[10] N. Mendes et al., "A narrative review of current striae treatments," *Healthcare*, vol. 10, no. 12, p. 2565, 2022.
[11] G. Casabona, P. Marchese, "Calcium hydroxylapatite combined with microneedling and ascorbic acid is effective for treating stretch marks," *Plast Reconstr Surg Glob Open*, vol. 5, no. 9, 2017.

Extremities

37 Calf Augmentation

JANI VAN LOGHEM AND PIETER SIEBENGA

37.1 INTRODUCTION

Benslimane described that both the symmetry of the curve distribution and progression from knee to ankle, as well as the vertical straightness, seem to be the most important features that define attractive legs [1]. The shape of the calf is determined by the development of the soleus and gastrocnemius muscles, the length and orientation of the crural bones, and the distribution of subcutaneous fat. Deformities, asymmetries, and/or atrophy due to disease (e.g. polio or trauma) or congenital disabilities, such as tibial torsion, *pes planus*, or *genu valgus*, can give reason for cosmetic calf augmentation [2–4]. With a rising demand for minimal invasive treatments, calf augmentation using CaHA has increased in popularity. Injection with CaHA can add volume to the calves and reshape the lower legs. Alternative treatments to dermal fillers include silicone implants, autologous fat transplantation, and injection with hyaluronic acid [2,5–9].

37.2 DANGER ZONES

Intramuscular injection may result in compartment syndrome. However, when staying in the correct subcutaneous plane, the risk is negligible.

37.3 CALF AUGMENTATION CANNULA TECHNIQUE

37.3.1 Step-by-Step Technique

1. Mark the treatment area with the patient in standing position whilst standing on their toes for better assessment. Consult with the patient about which area(s) they find important to augment.
2. Thoroughly disinfect the treatment area. Keep disinfecting throughout the treatment. Also disinfect the feet to avoid possible contamination of the cannula during treatment.
3. Mark the points of maximum projection of the muscles (Figure 37.1).
4. Anesthetize and make pre-holes at predetermined places (Figure 37.2).
5. Infiltration with lidocaine before injection of CaHA injection may be considered.
6. Use standard diluted CaHA (0.3 mL of lidocaine per 1.5 mL of CaHA).

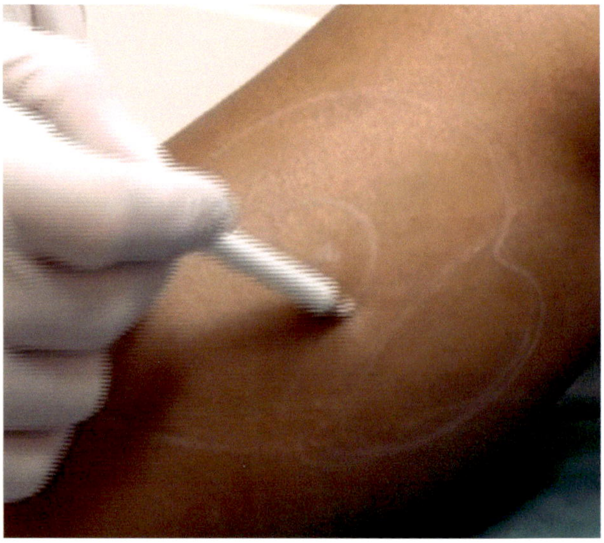

Figure 37.1 Markings of the area to be treated for more projection or reduction of the flattening. The apex of the muscle is marked for extra projection.

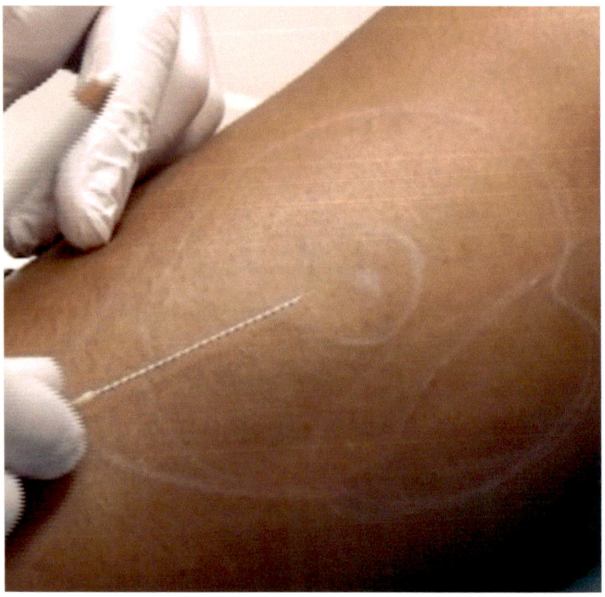

Figure 37.2 Determine the places for the pre-hole. Bear in mind the length of the cannula. The tip of the cannula must be able to reach the center of the apex.

DOI: 10.1201/9781003617129-37

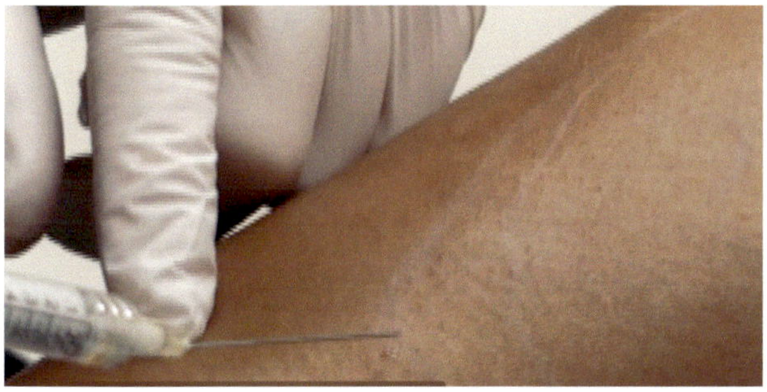

Figure 37.3 Bend the cannula to gain easier access to the correct anatomical plane.

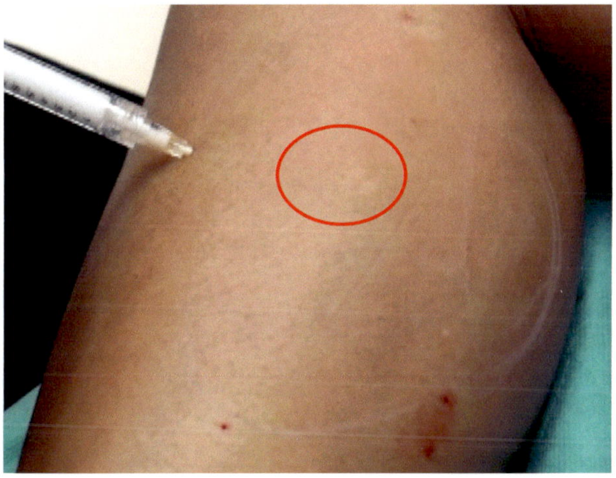

Figure 37.4 Inject extra product in the apex for maximum projection in this area. The red circle indicates the apex.

7. Inject the CaHA in a fanning technique with 0.05–0.1 mL per retrograde linear thread. The use of a 25G, 50 mm cannula is advised.
8. Bend the cannula slightly to make it easier to keep the cannula tip pointing superficial (Figure 37.3). Stay in the subcutaneous plane while avoiding an intramuscular administration possibly resulting in compartment syndrome.
9. Keep the apex in mind. This point of maximum projection needs more product to be injected (during fanning technique or extra bolus if needed) (Figure 37.4).
10. Even out the CaHA at the end of the treatment with a gentle massage.

See further Video 37.1 for application technique.

Video 37.1 Calf augmentation: cannula technique.

REFERENCES

[1] F. Benslimane, "The Benslimane's artistic model for leg beauty," *Aesthetic Plast Surg*, vol. 36, no. 4, pp. 803–812, 2012.

[2] L. H. Pereira et al., "Bilateral calf augmentation for aesthetic purposes," *Aesthetic Plast Surg*, vol. 36, no. 2, pp. 295–302, 2012.

[3] L. N. Carlsen, "Calf augmentation—a preliminary report," *Ann Plast Surg*, vol. 2, no. 6, pp. 508–510, 1979.

[4] R. A. Gutstein, "Augmentation of the lower leg: A new combined calf-tibial implant," *Plast Reconstr Surg*, vol. 117, no. 3, pp. 817–826, 2006.

[5] D. Melita, A. Innocenti, "Surgical calf augmentation techniques: Personal experience, literature review and analysis of complications," *Aesthetic Plast Surg*, vol. 43, no. 4, pp. 973–979, 2019.

[6] P. Hedén et al., "Body shaping and volume restoration: The role of hyaluronic acid," *Aesthetic Plast Surg*, vol. 33, no. 3, pp. 274–282, 2009.

[7] I. Niechajev, C. Krag, "Calf augmentation and restoration: Long-term results and the review of the reported complications," *Aesthetic Plast Surg*, vol. 41, no. 5, pp. 1115–1131, 2017.

[8] G. S. Mundinger, J. E. Vogel, "Calf augmentation and reshaping with autologous fat grafting," *Aesthet Surg J*, vol. 36, no. 2, pp. 211–220, 2016.

[9] K. Andjelkov et al., "Safety and efficacy of subfascial calf augmentation," *Plast Reconstr Surg*, vol. 139, no. 3, pp. 657e–669e, 2017.

Extremities

38

Foot Rejuvenation

JANI VAN LOGHEM AND PIETER SIEBENGA

38.1 INTRODUCTION

The human foot is perhaps one of the most complex parts of the body. It contains 26 bones; 33 joints; and over 100 tendons, muscles, and ligaments. The foot is responsible for locomotion and to ensure the balance of the body's weight on two legs. The skin protects the internal structures from injury and infection. Atrophy of the structures due to aging leads to a reduction of volume, mainly of the muscles and fat, in turn leading to skin laxity and more prominent veins, tendons, and bones. This "skeleton-like" appearance is regarded as aesthetically unpleasant, and treatment with CaHA gives a smooth, supple, and renewed appearance by increasing skin thickness and reducing the visibility of blood vessels (Figure 38.1).

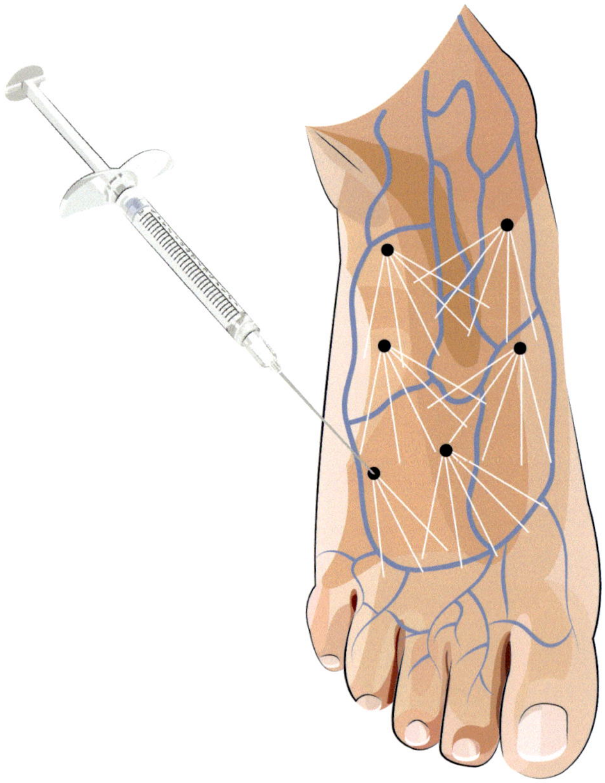

Figure 38.1 Diluted CaHA at the dorsum of the foot legs using blunt cannula. The black dots indicate the entry sites, whereas the white lines indicate retrograde linear threads of diluted CaHA at the dermal–subdermal junction. Care should be taken to avoid hitting the venous system (blue vascularization).

38.2 ANATOMICAL DANGERS

When injected at the right anatomical level, between the dermis and superficial fascia, risks of complications are very low. However, the veins are attached to the superficial fascia, so in order to avoid extensive bruising, care should be taken to avoid them.

38.3 FOOT REJUVENATION CANNULA TECHNIQUE

For injection placement, see Figure 38.1.

38.3.1 Step-by-Step Technique

1. Disinfect the feet.
2. Mark the treatment area (Figure 38.2).
3. Anesthetize the entry points and make a pre-hole with the correct needle (23G needle for a 25G cannula, 50 mm or 21G needle for a 22G cannula, 50 mm).
4. Dilute CaHA 1:3; a total of 1–1.5 syringe is needed per foot.
5. Injection should be done subcutaneously. Stay above the superficial fascia and the blood vessels. Injecting CaHa in this location will reduce the visibility of the veins (Figure 38.3).
6. Inject retrograde threads of 0.05–0.1 mL per thread with the bevel up, employing the fanning technique.
7. Repeat until the marked treatment area has been treated completely. Approach the cannula from the lateral part of the dorsum of the foot and advance it to the middle of the dorsum for easier access and more optimal control of the cannula in the correct anatomical plane. Hydrodissection can separate the dermis and the fascia to avoid inadvertent injection and injury of the blood vessels (Figure 38.4).

DOI: 10.1201/9781003617129-38

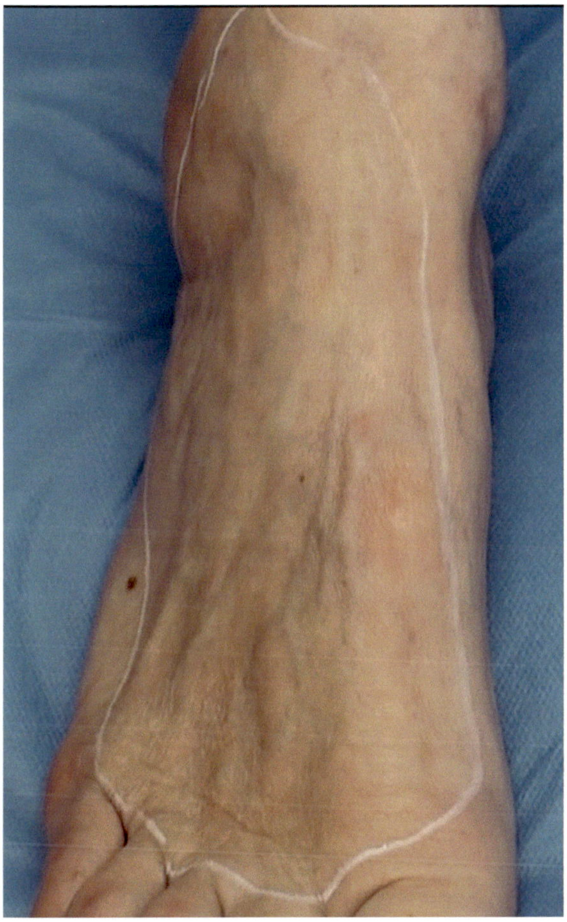

Figure 38.2 Marking the area to be treated on the dorsum of the foot.

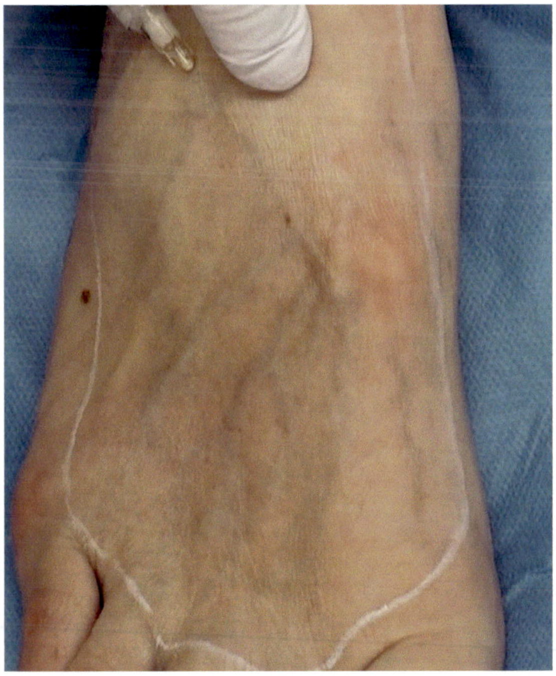

Figure 38.3 It is important to stay above the superficial fascia to avoid trauma of the blood vessels and the underlying structures (bones, joints, ligaments, etc.). Moreover, it will cover the veins to give a more aesthetic result.

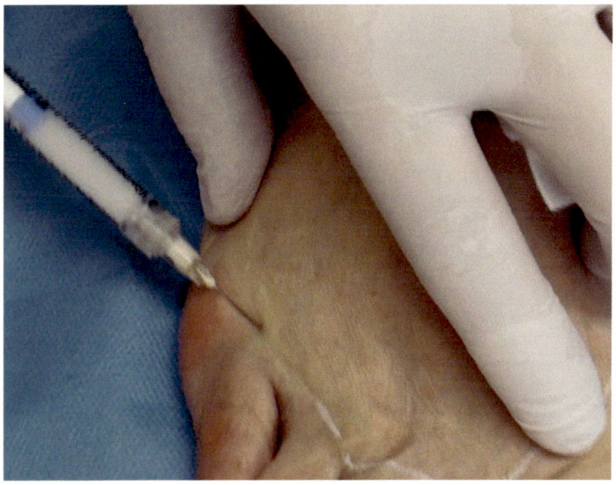

Figure 38.4 A lateral approach leads to a better control of the cannula to stay in the correct anatomical layer.

See further Video 38.1 to visualize the application technique.

38.4 AFTERCARE

Cover the entry point to prevent infections when the patient is wearing socks.

Video 38.1 Dorsal foot rejuvenation: cannula technique.

Intimate Areas

39

Rejuvenation of Labia Majora and Mons Pubis

JANI VAN LOGHEM, JOB THUIS, AND PIETER SIEBENGA

39.1 INTRODUCTION

Cosmetic procedures of the female genital area are becoming increasingly popular nowadays. In fact, the International Society for Aesthetic Plastic Surgery, recognized as the world's leading professional organization for board-certified aesthetic plastic surgeons, reported rises in vaginal aesthetic procedures, peaking with an increase of 45% in 2016 [1]. Just like other parts of the body, genitalia are subjected to age-related changes. A loss of subcutaneous fat as well as dermal loss of collagen and elastin in the mons pubis and labia majora is commonly thought to increase laxity and rhytids of the skin, giving it an aged appearance [2,3]. The thickness of the skin and vascularization are affected by the hormonal changes during menopause [4], as estrogen levels are reduced with age. Moreover, the labia minora-to-labia majora ratio shifts to a more prominent labia minora compared with the labia majora [5]. These changes not only affect the aesthetic appearance of the genital area but may also influence women's self-esteem [6].

There is no standardized approach for female genital augmentation, but authors have reported the use of CaHA to rejuvenate the external appearance of the vulva by tightening the skin on the mons pubis and labia majora [7,8], especially in advanced cases of atrophy [9].

39.2 ANATOMICAL DANGERS

Possible anatomical dangers during the rejuvenation procedure of the pubis and the labia include the posterior labial artery, the transverse perineal artery, and the inferior rectal artery, all shown in Figure 39.1.

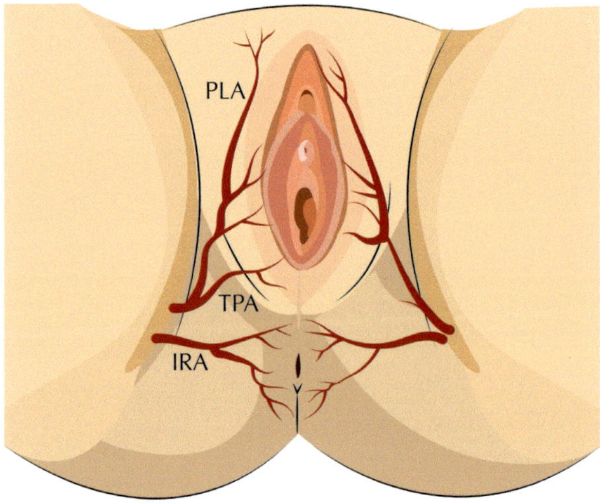

Figure 39.1 Arterial danger zones for the rejuvenation of the mons pubis and labia majora are: posterior labial artery (PLA), transverse perineal artery (TPA), and inferior rectal artery (IRA).

39.3 CANNULA TECHNIQUE FOR LABIA MAJORA AND MONS PUBIS REJUVENATION

For injection placement, see Figure 39.2.

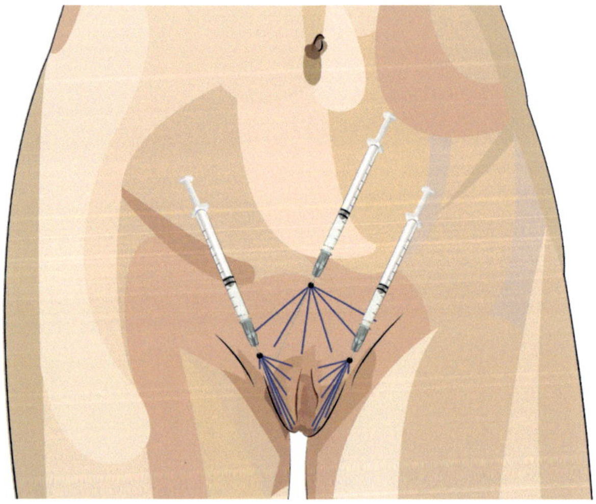

Figure 39.2 Rejuvenation of the vulva using diluted CaHA. Blue lines indicate retrograde linear threads of diluted CaHA.

39.3.1 Step-by-Step Technique

1. Disinfect and mark the treatment area.
2. Dilute 1.5 mL CaHA with up to 0.6 mL of lidocaine with adrenaline so the product easily spreads to the tissue but retains volumizing capacity.
3. Anesthetize and make three entry points with a 21G needle: one entry point per labia majora (Figure 39.3) and one in the midline of the mons pubis (Figure 39.4).
4. Use a 22G, 70 mm cannula and inject the CaHA in linear retrograde threads in the dermal-subdermal junction. Use half a syringe per side for the labia.
5. Only treat the anterior part of the labia majora. The risk of product migration to the lowest point

DOI: 10.1201/9781003617129-39

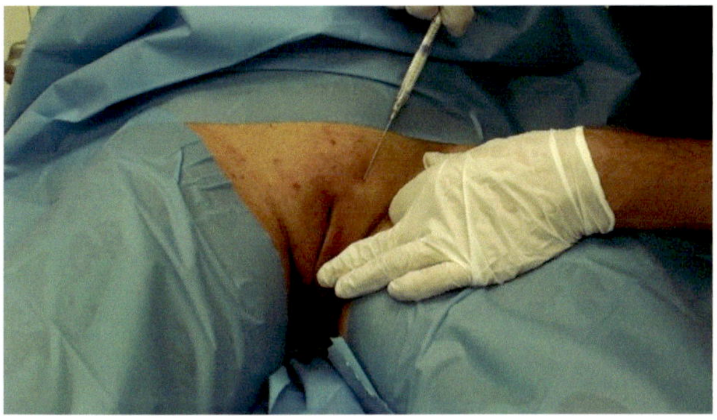

Figure 39.3 Labia majora treated with half a syringe per side.

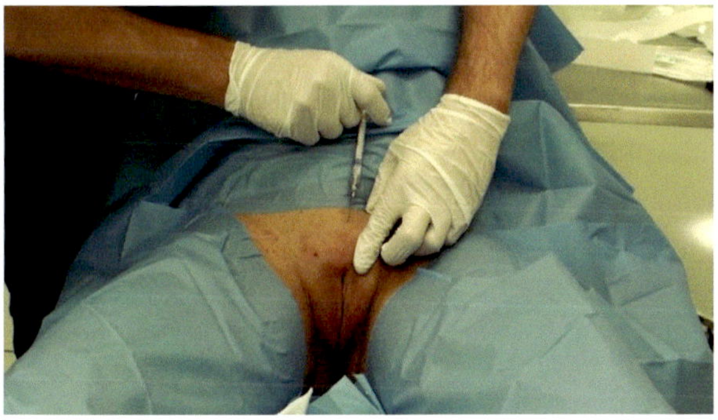

Figure 39.4 Mons pubis treated with half a syringe per side.

increases when the posterior part of the labia majora is also treated. This will result in a dissatisfactory aesthetic result.

See also Figure 39.5 and Video 39.1 for before and after results and application technique, respectively.

39.4 ADDITIONAL TREATMENTS FOR OPTIMAL RESULTS

Rejuvenation of the vulva may be combined with a hyaluronic acid filler or autologous fat injection for augmentation of the female genital area. Other plastic/cosmetic surgical procedures that can be considered in combination with the rejuvenation of the female genitalia include labiaplasty, clitoral hood reduction, vaginoplasty, and perineoplasty. Pigmented areas react well to TCA peels or lasers, and the skin quality improvement observed with CaHA may be further enhanced after applying such techniques.

REFERENCES

[1] L. Triana et al., "Trends in surgical and nonsurgical aesthetic procedures: A 14-year analysis of the international society of aesthetic plastic surgery—ISAPS," *Aesthetic Plast Surg*, vol. 48, no. 20, pp. 4217–4227, 2024.

[2] C. A. Hamori, "Aesthetic surgery of the female Genitalia: Labiaplasty and beyond," *Plast Reconstr Surg*, vol. 134, no. 4, pp. 661–673, 2014.

[3] S. H. Kim et al., "Rejuvenation using platelet-rich plasma and lipofilling for vaginal atrophy and lichen sclerosus," *J Menopausal Med*, vol. 23, no. 1, pp. 63–68, 2017.

[4] R. L. Binder et al., "Histological and gene expression analysis of the effects of menopause status and hormone therapy on the vaginal introitus and labia majora," *J Clin Med Res*, vol. 11, no. 11, pp. 745–759, 2019.

[5] B. Hersant et al., "Labia majora augmentation combined with minimal labia minora resection: A safe and global approach to the external female genitalia," *Ann Plast Surg*, vol. 80, no. 4, pp. 323–327, 2018.

[6] G. J. Alter, "Aesthetic labia minora and clitoral hood reduction using extended central wedge resection," *Plast Reconstr Surg*, vol. 122, no. 6, pp. 1780–1789, 2008.

[7] J. A. van Loghem, "Use of calcium hydroxylapatite for augmentation of the labia majora and mons pubis," vol. 2, no. 1, pp. 010–013, 2017 [online], www.sciresliterature.org/Dermatology/DCR-ID15.pdf.

[8] V. de Carvalho Amaral, "Fios de PDO, hidroxiapatita de cálcio e ácido l-polilático para flacidez vulvar—indicações, técnica e resultados," *Surg Cosmet Dermatol*, vol. 15, no. 0, pp. 1–5, 2023.

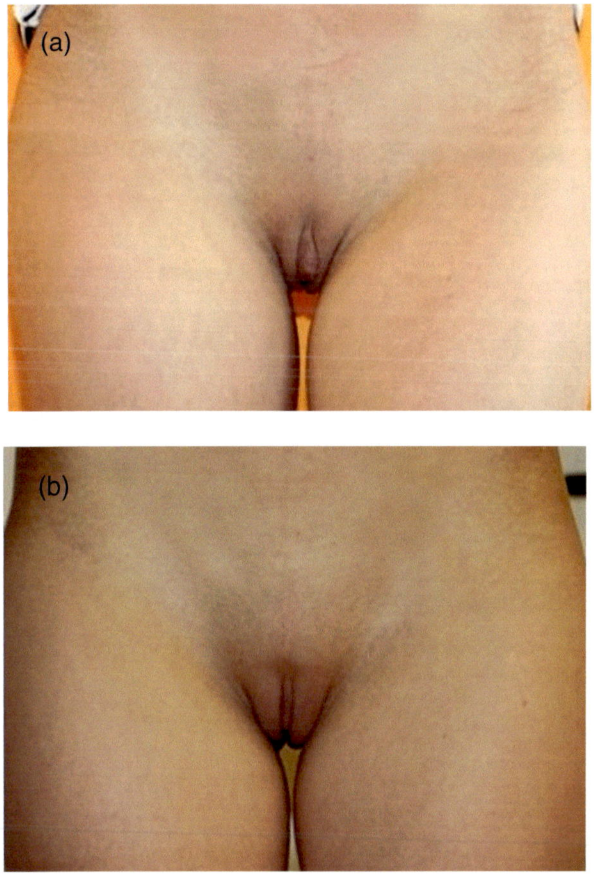

Figure 39.5 (a) Before and (b) three months after treatment with 6 mL CaHA in the labia majora (reproduced with permission from ref 7).

[9] C. L. Vilela et al., "Treatment of atrophy of the labia majora: Calcium hydroxyapatite or hyaluronic acid?," *Aesthetic Plast Surg*, vol. 48, no. 3, pp. 472–477, 2024.

Video 39.1 Labia major rejuvenation: cannula technique.

Intimate Areas

40

G-Spot Augmentation

JANI VAN LOGHEM

40.1 INTRODUCTION

Mentions of the existence of an erogenous zone inside the anterior wall of the vagina date back to ancient texts, such as a 7th-century poem in the Kama Sutra, which later in 1950s was referred to the Gräfenberg spot (or G-spot). Evidence supporting the existence of the G-spot remains controversial [1,2], but research has shown a direct correlation between the thickness of the urovaginal space (space between vagina and urethra) and the capacity to achieve orgasms by vaginal stimulation, most likely of the internal clitoris [3]. In fact, its volume represents a favorable factor for the above-mentioned orgasms where women capable of achieving internal clitoris orgasms presented higher lengths and volumes of this area [4]. Battaglia *et al.* have also suggested the influence of serum androgens and time since last intercourse in the volume of such an anatomical structure [4]. Additionally, other reports have also shown the efficacy of HA injections in this area to increase sexual sensation [5].

In the current chapter, we show a technique to increase the volume of the G-spot region using CaHA. As this is a procedure that has not received regulatory approval, we advise the physician to include some additional paperwork—not just the informed consents and medical questionnaires—such as the validated female sexual function index (FSFI) questionnaire [6]. We also recommend that an assistant always be present before, during, and after the procedure. Contraindications to the procedure are pregnancy, gynecological or psychiatric disease, sexual dysfunctions (problems with the female sexual response cycle: arousal, plateau, orgasm, resolution), emotional/psychological problems, or sexually transmitted diseases.

40.2 ANATOMICAL DANGERS

Anatomical danger zones include the vaginal artery, the uterine artery, and the vaginal venous plexus.

Care must be taken not to inject large boluses, as injection in the venous vasculature has been reported to cause lung embolism [7]. Maximum amounts of 0.1 mL in retrograde linear threads are recommended.

40.3 NEEDLE TECHNIQUE FOR G-SPOT AUGMENTATION

For injection placement, see Figure 40.1.

40.3.1 Step-by-Step Technique

1. The patient should have an empty bladder.
2. Place the patient in the gynecological chair.
3. Ask the patient to locate the G-spot with a finger (it should be approximately 5 cm from introitus).
4. Mark on their finger the point at the introitus and measure the distance to the fingertip. This is the distance to the G-spot from the introitus (Figure 40.2).
5. When the patient does not know the location of her G-spot, introduce one gloved finger into the vagina and move the index finger down over the anterior vaginal wall.
6. Ask the patient to indicate "yes" when the feeling of having to urinate is felt. Mark with a marker on the glove the point at which the finger is at the introitus and measure the distance to the fingertip. This is the distance to the G-spot from the introitus. For the remaining patients who do not feel the urge to urinate on digital stimulation, a 5 cm distance can be assumed.

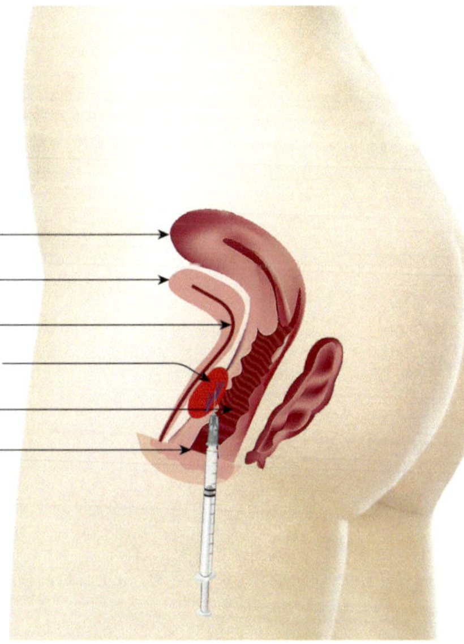

Figure 40.1 CaHA for G-spot augmentation. The red area indicates the target area (approximately 5 cm from the introitus with a length of ~18 mm). Blue lines indicate retrograde linear threads of CaHA.

DOI: 10.1201/9781003617129-40

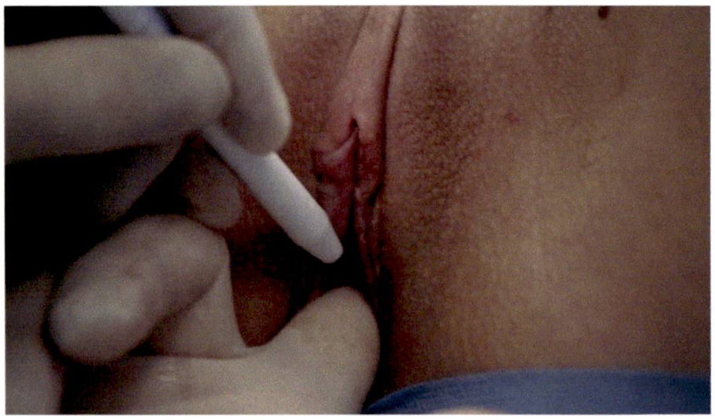

Figure 40.2 Marking of distance from introitus to G-spot.

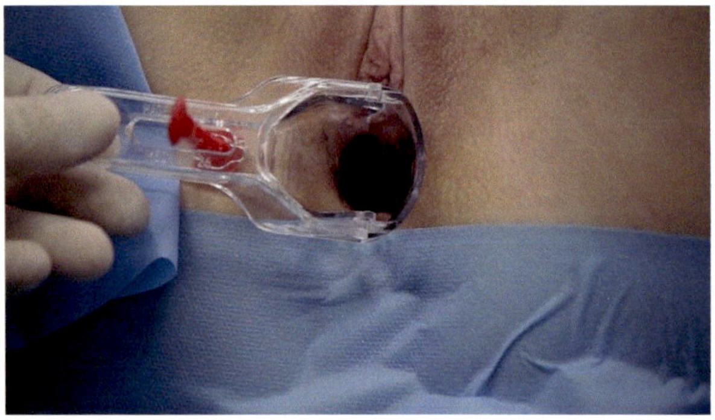

Figure 40.3 Speculum insertion without rotation.

7. If available, an intravaginal ultrasound measurement can be made of the urethrovaginal space (the distance between the anterior vaginal wall and the urethra) at the location of the G-spot (so the measured distance from the introitus). This can be compared with a measurement after the treatment.
8. Place the (lubricated) speculum into the vagina. Do not rotate, as the anterior wall should remain accessible for injection, and fix the speculum open (Figure 40.3).
9. Introduce the marked gloved finger with the marking at the introitus. Press against the anterior vaginal wall and ask the patient if this is indeed the right location. Mark the location of the G-spot with a marker on the mucosa.
10. Disinfect with chlorhexidine without alcohol to prevent stinging.
11. Optionally, apply sterile local lidocaine gel for topical anesthesia for 5 minutes.
12. Inject 1 mL 1% lidocaine with adrenaline 1:200000 neutralized with bicarbonate into the G-spot. Inject very slowly to prevent pain (Figure 40.4).
13. Use a 25–27G needle, 20 mm cannula and bend it slightly for ease of injection.
14. Inject 0.5–1 mL of standard diluted CaHA (0.3 mL lidocaine per 1.5 mL syringe of CaHA) into the submucosal space using a fanning technique with 0.05–0.1 mL linear threads with slow injection

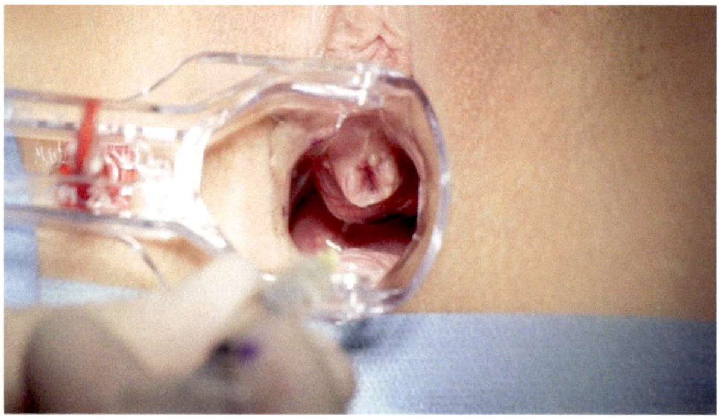

Figure 40.4 The marking on the anterior wall is the target to inject lidocaine.

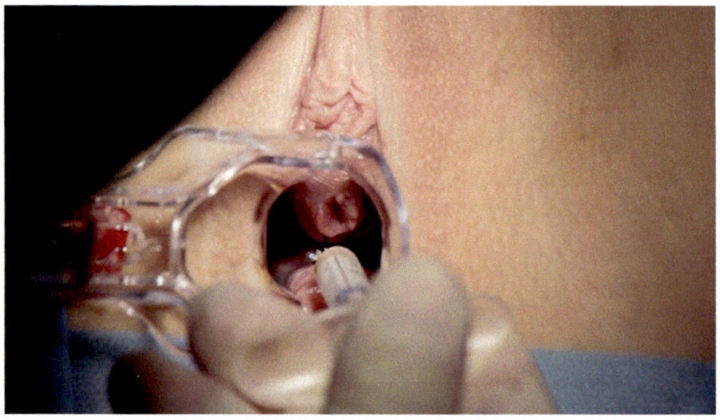

Figure 40.5 CaHA injection of small retrograde linear threads.

and slow retrograde movement of the needle in the mid-line over the length of the marked area (Figure 40.5).

15. Make sure to strictly stay submucosal to avoid injury of the urethra and bladder.
16. After the injection, a second intravaginal ultrasound measurement can be made to check the increase in urethrovaginal thickness.
17. Insert a tampon into the vagina and instruct patient to leave it there and refrain from sexual activity for at least four hours.

See also Video 40.1 to visualize the application technique.

40.4 AFTERCARE

Request the patient return in one month for a follow-up appointment and fill out the FSFI questionnaire again. The results of the procedure can be objectified with the key included in the FSFI questionnaire. Patients who showed no improvement in sexual sensation can be given a retouch treatment.

Video 40.1 G-spot augmentation: needle technique.

REFERENCES

[1] T. M. Hines, "The G-spot: A modern gynecologic myth," *Am J Obstet Gynecol*, vol. 185, no. 2, pp. 359–362, 2001.

[2] V. Puppo, G. Puppo, "Anatomy of sex: Revision of the new anatomical terms used for the clitoris and the female orgasm by sexologists," *Clin Anat*, vol. 28, no. 3, pp. 293–304, 2015.

[3] G. L. Gravina et al., "Measurement of the thickness of the urethrovaginal space in women with or without vaginal orgasm," *J Sex Med*, vol. 5, no. 3, pp. 610–618, 2008.

[4] C. Battaglia et al., "3-D volumetric and vascular analysis of the urethrovaginal space in young women with or without vaginal orgasm," *J Sex Med*, vol. 7, no. 4, pp. 1445–1453, 2010.

[5] A. Moore et al., "Proceedings of the world meeting on sexual medicine, Chicago, USA, August 26–30 2012," *J Sex Med*, vol. 9, no. Suppl 4, pp. 183–298, 2012.

[6] R. Rosen et al., "The Female Sexual Function Index (FSFI): A multidimensional self-report instrument for the assessment of female sexual function," *J Sex Marital Ther*, vol. 26, no. 2, pp. 191–205, 2000.

[7] H. J. Park et al., "Hyaluronic acid pulmonary embolism: A critical consequence of an illegal cosmetic vaginal procedure," *Thorax*, vol. 65, no. 4, pp. 360–361, 2010.

Intimate Areas

41

Rejuvenation of the Buttocks and Hip Dip Contouring

JANI VAN LOGHEM, POLINA HOLOVINA, AND PIETER SIEBENGA

41.1 INTRODUCTION

The shape of the buttocks is an important aesthetic feature in many cultures. As with most other areas of the body, the buttocks are subjected to age-related changes. Gluteal ptosis, as a result of volume loss and skin laxity, and alterations in the skin morphology, such as *striae distensae* and cellulite, have led to an increased patient demand to rejuvenate and/or reshape the buttocks. Trochanteric depressions, known as "hip dips", can be constitutional from a pronounced muscle definition or as a result of the aging process [1].

A wide variety of techniques have been introduced to rejuvenate and reshape the buttocks. Proper evaluation of the patient's wishes is essential in the decision of which treatment will lead to the most optimal results. CaHA can be used as a monotherapy or as part of a multidimensional approach in the treatment of skin laxity and cellulite. Lifting the buttocks (reshaping) may also be achieved with CaHA, although these results are less pronounced than, for example, a surgical buttock lift.

41.2 CELLULITE

Cellulite is a term used to characterize the altered topography of the skin (e.g. dimpled or *"peau d'orange"*-like appearance) located most frequently on the buttocks and the posterior outer thighs [2]. In females, it has a high prevalence of about 80–90%, although cellulite remains rare in males [3]. Cellulite is thought to be a multifactorial condition influenced by dimorphism of subcutaneous connective tissue, abnormalities of the circulatory system, inflammatory and hormonal processes, and localized differences in tissue tension [4,5]. When treating cellulite, it is imperative to increase the strength and elasticity of both the dermis and superficial fascia. This can be accomplished via remodeling and neocollagenesis. In a recent study in women with moderate-to-severe cellulite, it was found that CaHA, in combination with microfocused ultrasound with visualization, was able to significantly improve the cellulite after only one treatment [6]. Both treatments are known for their skin-tightening ability, as they remodel the dermis and collagenous structures in the superficial fascia with neocollagenesis and elastogenesis [7].

41.3 ANATOMICAL DANGERS

Injecting in the dermal-subdermal junction for buttock augmentation is a safe approach. Anatomical dangers in the gluteal region, such as branches from the sacral plexus, the sciatic nerve, and branches of the internal iliac artery, are to be considered (Figure 41.1).

41.4 CANNULA TECHNIQUE FOR BUTTOCK REJUVENATION

For injection placement, see Figure 41.2.

41.4.1 Step-by-Step Technique

1. Disinfect the buttocks.
2. Mark the treatment area and divide the buttocks in four equal quadrants. If needed, the banana roll may be included.
3. Dilute CaHA between 1:2 and 1:6 (depending on severity of laxity). On average, a 1:3 dilution should be sufficient.
4. Anesthetize and make entry points with a 21G needle (Figure 41.3).
5. Use a 22G, 70 mm cannula and inject the CaHA in linear retrograde threads in the dermal–subdermal junction. Use one to two syringes per side. For

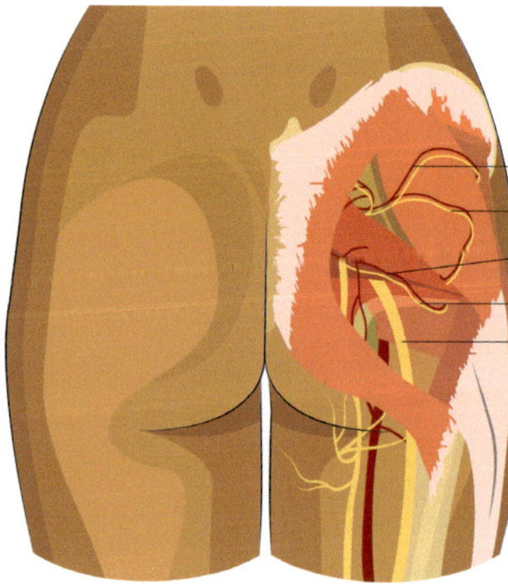

Figure 41.1 Arterial danger zones of the gluteal region are the superior and inferior gluteal arteries and nerves and the sciatic nerve.

DOI: 10.1201/9781003617129-41

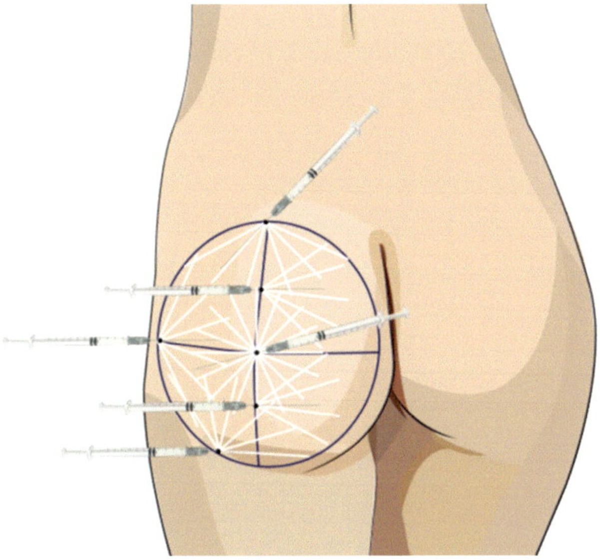

Figure 41.2 Diluted CaHA used to treat the cellulite of the buttocks using the cannula technique. The blue lines indicate the treatment area where the buttocks are divided in four quadrants, and the white lines indicate retrograde linear threads of diluted CaHA at the dermal–subdermal junction.

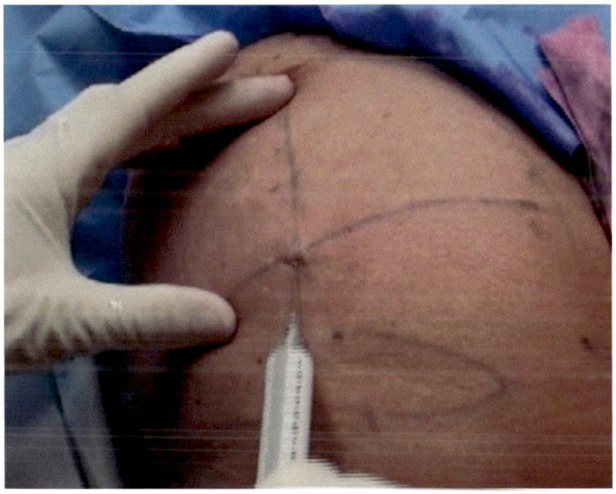

Figure 41.3 Markings of the area to be treated. When injecting larger quantities of CaHA, a 10 mL syringe can be used.

optimal results, repeat the treatment for a total of three sessions with an interval of three to four months between each session.

41.5 SHARP NEEDLE TECHNIQUE FOR BUTTOCK REJUVENATION

For injection placement, see Figure 41.4.

41.5.1 Step-by-Step Technique

1. Prepare the buttocks in the same manner as with the cannula technique (disinfect, mark, and anesthetize).
2. Dilute CaHA between 1:2 and 1:6 (depending on severity of laxity). On average, a 1:3 dilution will be sufficient.
3. Use a long (38 mm) 27G needle.
4. For skin laxity, linear threads will be sufficient; for the treatment of cellulite, it is necessary to cross-hatch (Figure 41.5). Inject CaHA at the dermal–subdermal junction for optimal results.
5. Repeat the treatment after three to four months if needed.

See further Figure 41.6 and Video 41.1 for before and after results and application of sharp needle technique, respectively.

41.6 SHARP NEEDLE TECHNIQUE FOR HIP DIP CONTOURING

For injection placement, see Figure 41.7.

41.6.1 Step-by-Step Technique

1. Assess and mark the area with two concentric circles: the outer circle marks the whole area of depression, and the smaller circle marks the area most depressed (Figure 41.8).
2. Disinfect the area to treat.
3. Use a 27G, 20 mm needle and start injecting from the epicenter of the biggest depression while lifting the tissue with the non-dominant hand.
   NOTE: Inject at the deep subdermal layer a maximum of 0.2 mL per bolus.

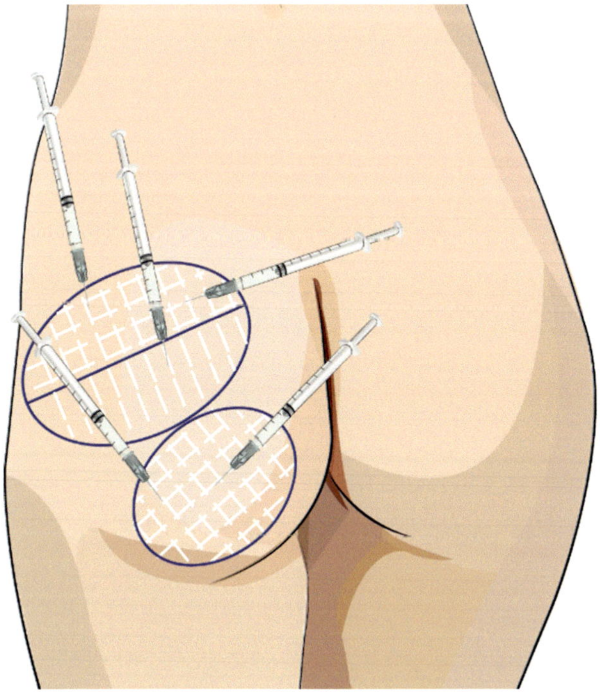

Figure 41.4 Diluted CaHA injection at the buttocks using the sharp needle technique. The white lines indicate retrograde linear threads of diluted CaHA at the dermal–subdermal junction.

4. Retract, reorient, and readvance the needle with its full length after each injection.
5. Start injecting from the center of the depression towards the periphery. While moving to the periphery, gradually decrease the overall volume of the product, creating a "gradient effect" (Figure 41.9).
6. Assess the result; add more product, if needed.

41.7 CANNULA TECHNIQUE FOR HIP DIP CONTOURING

For injection placement, see Figure 41.10.

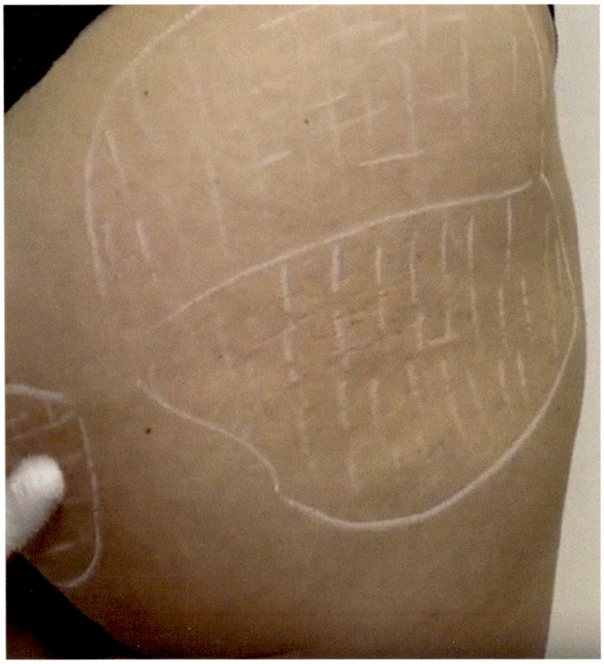

Figure 41.5 Markings of the treatment area. The upper area will be cross-hatched in order to treat the stretch marks in the most optimal manner. The lower area contains some creases but no stretch marks, and retrograde linear threads will suffice.

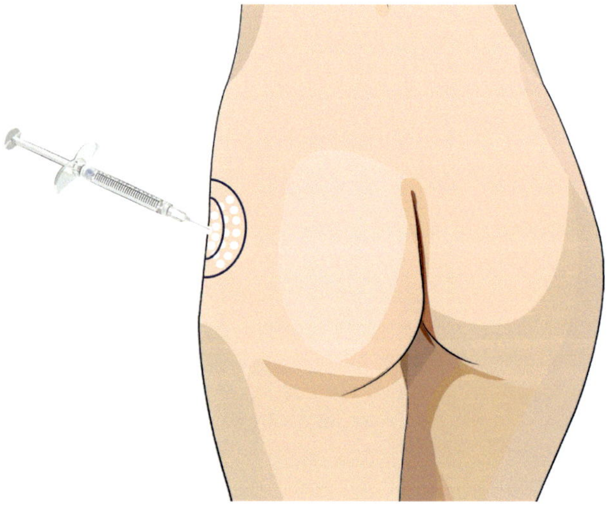

Figure 41.7 Schematic drawing of CaHA injection with a sharp needle for hip dip contouring using two concentric circles as reference points. The outer circle shows the entire depression of the hip, whereas the inner circle indicates the most depressed area.

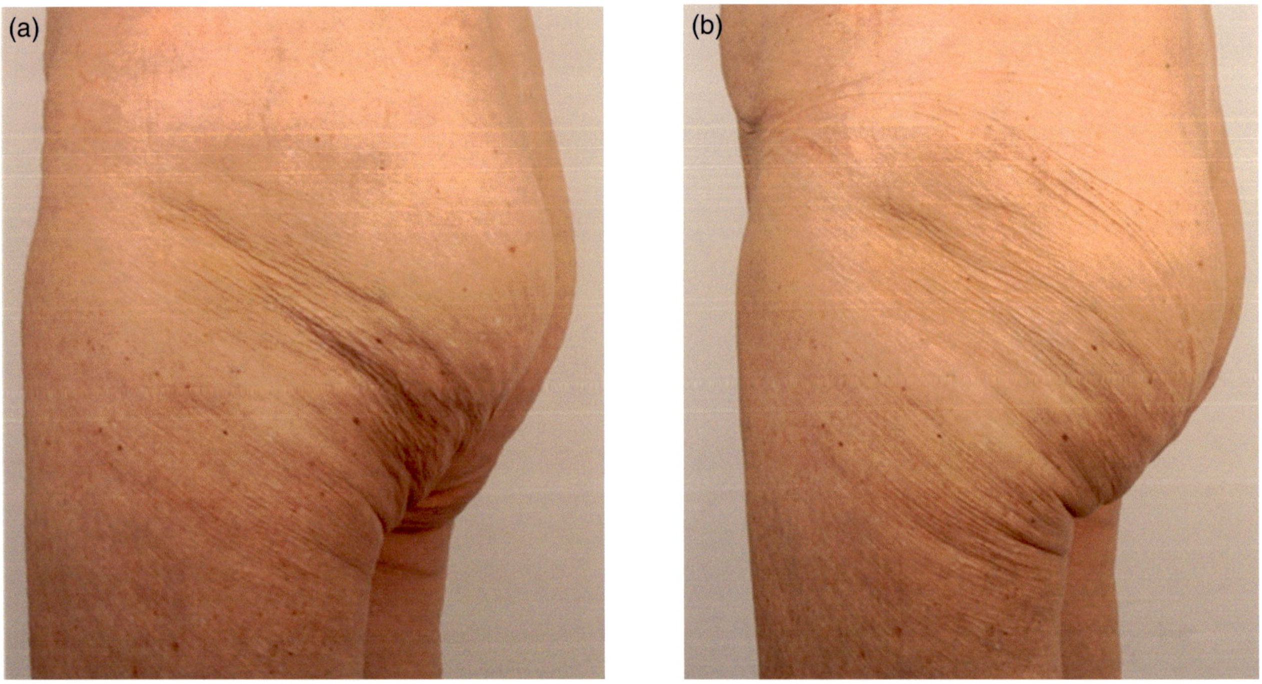

Figure 41.6 Before (a) and three months after (b) 12 mL CaHA per side.

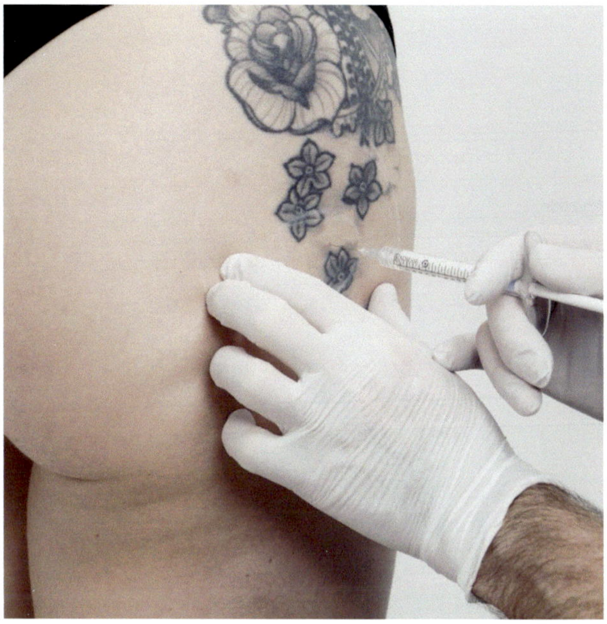

Figure 41.8 Markings of the treatment area to correct the hip dip.

41.7.1 Step-by-Step Technique

1. Just like in the needle technique, assess and mark the area to treat with two concentric circles (Figure 41.11).
2. Disinfect the injection area.
3. Choose your entry points for the cannula in the area of the most depression and use local anesthesia to numb the region; create the openings for the cannula (Figure 41.12).
4. Advance a 22G, 50 cm cannula to the deep subcutaneous plane. With the tip of the cannula facing the muscle, start injecting boluses of 0.2 mL on top of the muscle (Figure 41.13).
5. After each bolus, reposition the cannula for additional safety.
6. Moving to the periphery, continue with a fanning technique in the subcutaneous, creating a "gradient effect" an ensuring even distribution of the volume. Inject 0.1–0.2 mL in a retrograde fanning fashion.
7. Assess the result; add more product, if needed.

See further Figure 41.14 and Videos 41.2–41.3 for before and after results and application techniques, respectively.

41.8 AFTERCARE

A vigorous massage post-injection is advised to ensure proper distribution of the product. Extensive bruising is possible due to the presence of superficial veins.

41.9 ADDITIONAL TREATMENTS FOR OPTIMAL RESULTS

In most cases, monotherapy will not create the desired results for the patient. CaHA is used for skin quality

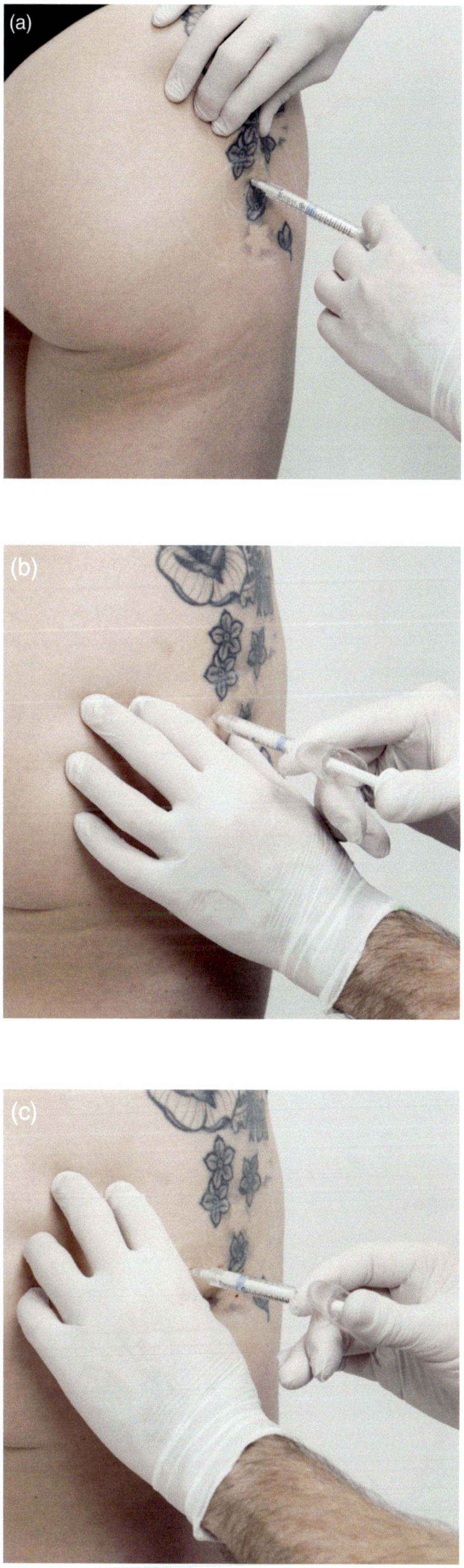

Figure 41.9 Treatment sequence of the hip dip moving from the epicenter of the depression (a) and toward the periphery (b and c) using a sharp needle.

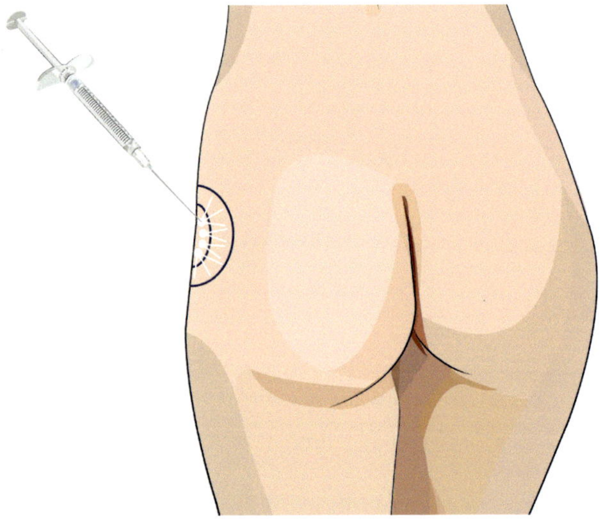

Figure 41.10 Schematic drawing of CaHA injection with cannula for hip dip contouring using two concentric circles as reference points. The cannula entry points are drawn into the innermost concentric circle, where the most pronounced depression is, and the product is distributed in a retrograde fanning fashion.

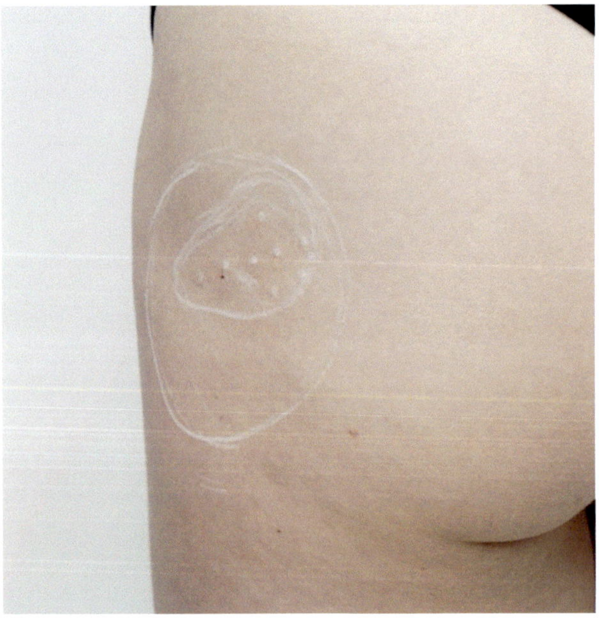

Figure 41.11 Markings of the treatment area to correct the hip dip using a cannula.

improvement, tightening, and lifting of the buttocks but has very limited volume-enhancing capacity with small amounts of product, and it does not reduce the subcutaneous cellulite *septae*. A multi-modal approach is therefore often necessary. Depending on the indication, CaHA can be combined with additional therapies listed in Table 41.1.

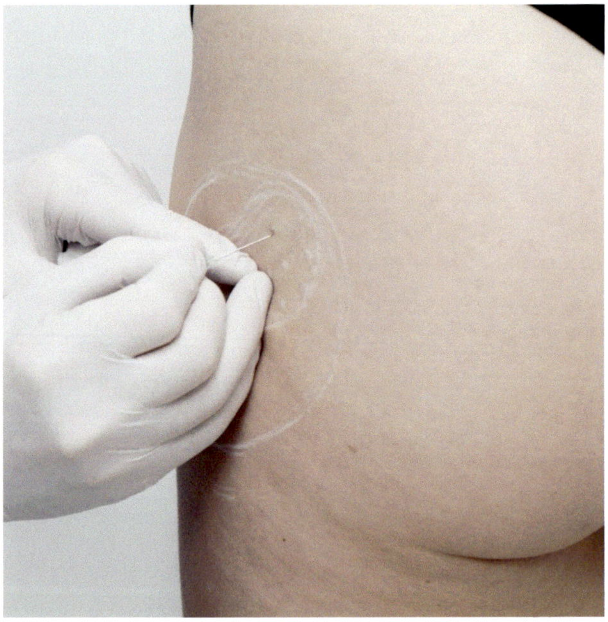

Figure 41.12 Cannula entry points made with a needle within the most depressed area of the hip.

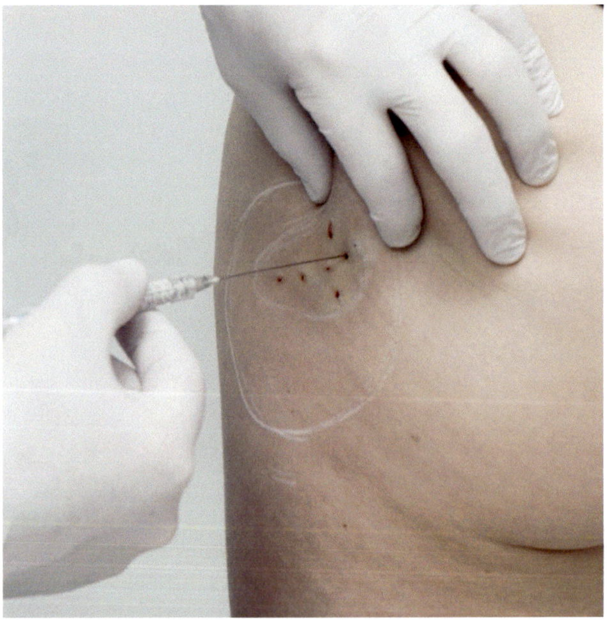

Figure 41.13 Cannula advanced through the entry holes to treat the hip dip.

Video 41.1 Buttock rejuvenation: needle technique.

Video 41.2 Hip dips: sharp needle technique.

Video 41.3 Hip dips: cannula technique.

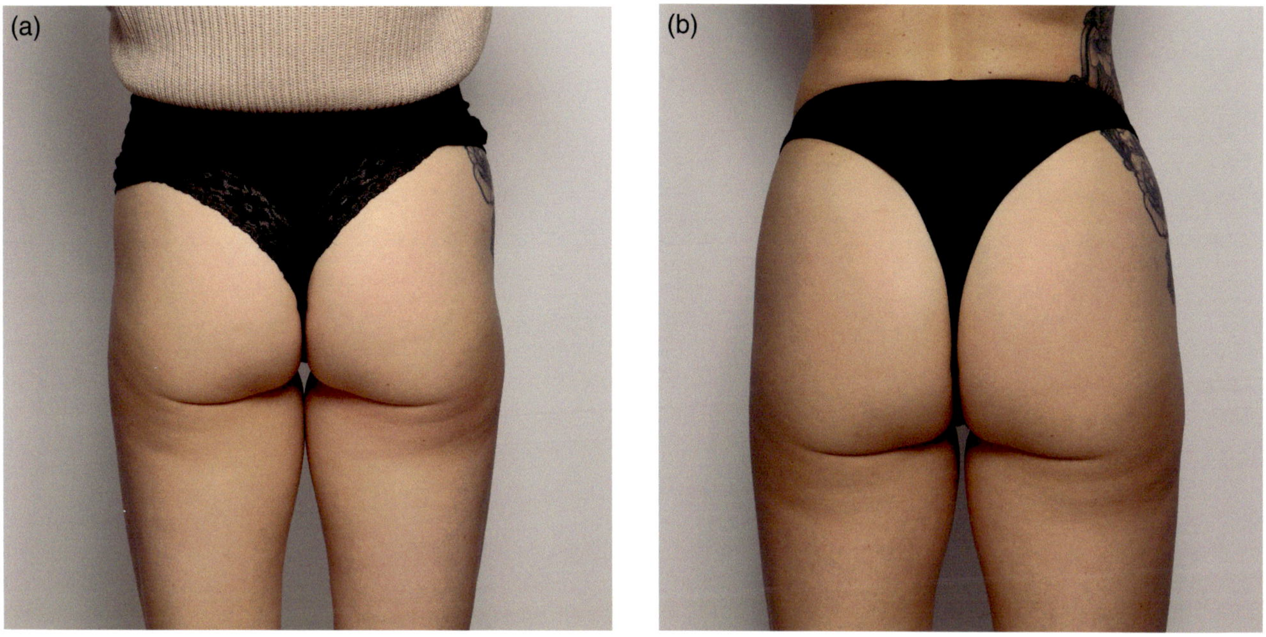

Figure 41.14 Before (a) and one month after (b) results after 6 mL per side of CaHA to treat hip depressions.

Table 41.1 Combination Therapies with CaHA for the Treatment of the Buttocks

Indication	Treatment Options
Skin laxity	• Microfocused ultrasound with visualization • Radiofrequency • Subcutaneous laser • Diluted CaHA
Volume loss	• Volumizing hyaluronic acid filler • CaHA in large amounts • Autologous fat transfer (lipofilling) • Surgical buttock lift • (Silicone) implant
Volume excess	• Liposuction • Radiofrequency • Cryolipolysis • Injection lipolysis
Cellulite	• Subdermal release of subcutaneous fibrous septae • Aggressive liposuction

Source: Adapted from ref 7.

REFERENCES

[1] L. Lourenco et al., "Hip dips technique: Filling lateral depressions with hyaluronic acid of large particles," *Skin Health Dis*, vol. 4, no. 6, 2024.

[2] D. P. Friedmann et al., "Cellulite: A review with a focus on subcision," *Clin Cosmet Investig Dermatol*, vol. 10, p. 17, 2017.

[3] E. Emanuele, "Cellulite: Advances in treatment: Facts and controversies," *Clin Dermatol*, vol. 31, no. 6, pp. 725–730, 2013.

[4] M. M. Avram, "Cellulite: A review of its physiology and treatment," *J Cosmet Laser Ther*, vol. 6, no. 4, pp. 181–185, 2004.

[5] B. Publishing, G. E. Piérard, "Commentary on cellulite: Skin mechanobiology and the waist-to-hip ratio," *J Cosmet Dermatol*, vol. 4, no. 3, pp. 151–152, 2005.

[6] G. Casabona, G. Pereira, "Microfocused ultrasound with visualization and calcium hydroxylapatite for improving skin laxity and cellulite appearance," *Plast Reconstr Surg Glob Open*, vol. 5, no. 7, 2017.

[7] K. M. Coleman, J. Pozner, "Combination therapy for rejuvenation of the outer thigh and buttock: A review and our experience," *Dermatologic Surg*, vol. 42, pp. S124–S130, 2016.

Intimate Areas

42

Penile Augmentation

JOHN LEONARDO

42.1 INTRODUCTION

Patients often express a desire to increase the size of their penis. Some are insecure about how they are perceived by other men (locker room syndrome) or by their partner [1,2]. Until recently, the treatment options were limited to traction devices [3,4] and surgery [5–9]. Nowadays, there are effective nonsurgical options to enhance the male genitalia, including dermal filler injections [10–12]. In this chapter, special mention of penile augmentation with CaHA will be made.

To the best of our knowledge, there is no published evidence of CaHA used for penile augmentation, although similar materials have been proposed [13]. The scientific community argues in favor of such nonsurgical approaches due to their inexpensiveness, low invasiveness, and fewer adverse effects than surgical cosmetic procedures. However, some authors imply that careful consideration must be taken when using such materials so that hypersensitivity type I reactions are not triggered, and re-applications might be necessary due to the resorbable nature of these fillers [14,15]. Therefore, CaHA represents an ideal choice due to its low incidence of granuloma formation, its ability to stimulate fibroblasts for collagen synthesis producing long-lasting effects, and its smooth texture when blended with normal saline.

The main concern during CaHA application in the penis is causing vascular occlusion, especially to the dorsal arteries, which supply circulation to the *corpora cavernosa* (see danger zones). Thus, administration of CaHA is advised with blunt-tip cannulas in anatomical layer 4 (subfascial). A vein visualization system is also recommended to visualize the venous system during the procedure [16,17]. Additionally, hair causes visual artifact when using such devices, and therefore it is recommended that the patient shave the shaft of the penis two to three days prior to procedure to allow any nicks or cuts to heal. An initial scan with the vein visualizer will aid in selecting the correct entry point with the introducer needle.

Just like in G-spot augmentation (Chapter 40), the use of CaHA for penile augmentation is deemed off label by the FDA; therefore, careful consideration must be made when patients and physicians decide to embark on this journey. Per the author's suggestion and endorsed by the European Association of Urology [18], besides consent forms, a psychological assessment through medical questionnaires (such as the male genital self-image scale) should be filled out to evaluate the satisfaction level of the patient [19,20] and potential penile dysmorphic disorders [21].

42.2 DANGER ZONES

During penile augmentation, neurovascular danger zones to be aware of consist of the superficial dorsal vein (below Dartos fascia), the dorsal artery, the deep dorsal vein, and the dorsal nerve (below the Buck's fascia) (Figure 42.1).

42.3 CANNULA TECHNIQUE FOR PENILE AUGMENTATION

For injection placement, see Figure 42.2.

42.3.1 Step-by-Step Technique

1. Disinfect the area to perform dorsal penile nerve block or simply apply topical local anesthesia such as 30% lidocaine or 20% benzocaine/10% lidocaine/10% tetracaine.
2. If topical local anesthesia is applied, cleanse the remnants off the penis and disinfect.
3. Apply a constriction ring around the testicles and penis to allow the penis to become semi-engorged.
4. The penis must be erect during the procedure to minimize contour irregularity; therefore injection of Trimix (papaverine, phentolamine, and prostaglandin E1) is used. With a 31G needle, inject 0.3 mL Trimix 0.3 mL to the base of the penis at either the 2 or 10 o'clock position of the penis in cross-section. Remove constriction ring once an erection has been achieved.

   NOTE: The patient must be screened for recent use of PDE5 inhibitors, as Trimix in conjunction with these medications may lead to priapism. Patients must be instructed to avoid use as the procedure date approaches.
5. Disinfect area once more.
6. Introduce a 21G trochar needle mid-shaft at either the 2 or 10 o'clock position of the penis in cross-section. Utilize AccuVein to determine the ideal location to avoid puncturing a blood vessel.
7. Prepare a 1:1 dilution of CaHA or even a standard dilution (0.3 mL lidocaine mixed with 1.5 mL CaHA) and a 22G, 70 mm injection cannula.

DOI: 10.1201/9781003617129-42

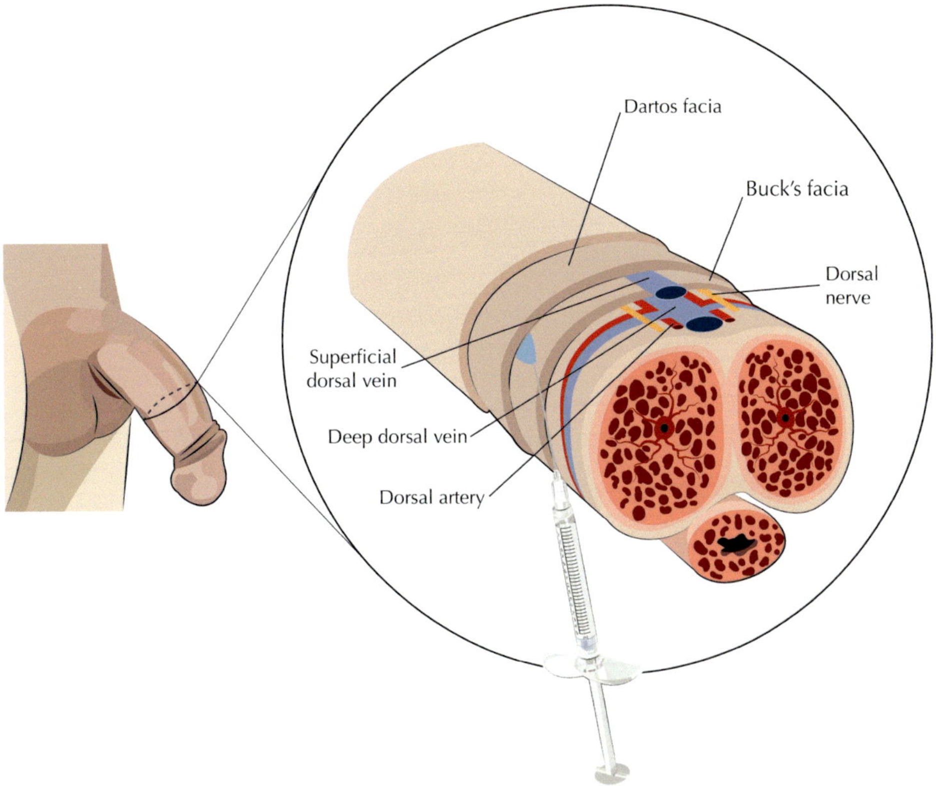

Figure 42.1 Neurovascular danger zones in the penis include the superficial dorsal vein below the Dartos fascia and the deep dorsal vein, together with the deep artery and nerve, right below the Buck's fascia. The augmentation procedure should be performed in between the Dartos and Buck's fascias.

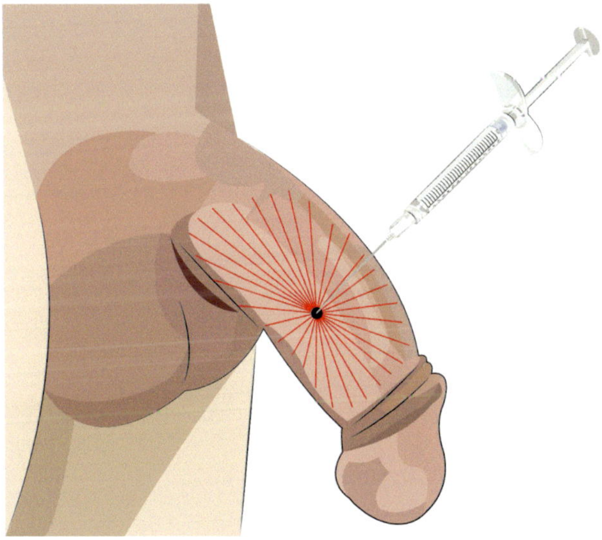

Figure 42.2 Schematic illustration of penile augmentation with CaHA.

8. Introduce the 22G cannula through Buck's fascia and inject the CaHA in linear retrograde threads in the subfascial plane, preferably under the guidance of a vein visualization system. Do not go too superficially to avoid nodule formation and not too distally (i.e. beneath the glans), as the skin in this area is too thin for the CaHA (Figure 42.3).

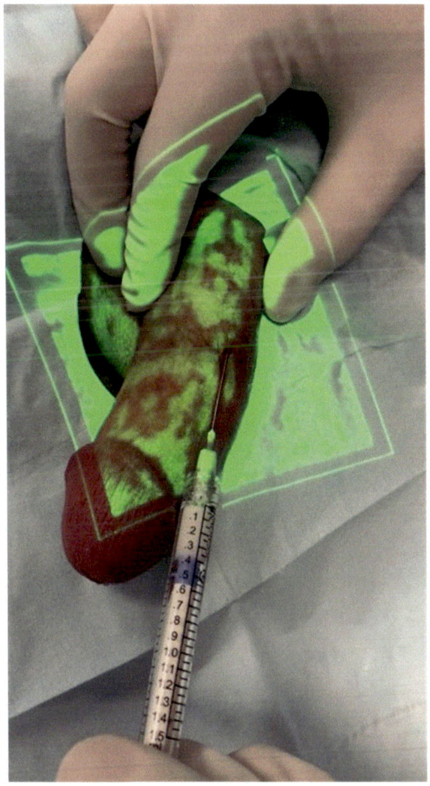

Figure 42.3 Injection of diluted CaHA under AccuVein guidance from a mid-shaft lateral entry point.

9. Apply 1/4 of the product to each quadrant of the penis delineated by the 8 o'clock to 2 o'clock position and the 4 o'clock to 10 o'clock position on the dorsum of the penis below midshaft and above. It is acceptable to cross midline to even out the distribution of the product.
10. Massage the product to minimize contour irregularity. It is best to perform this while the patient is erect. Previous warning to the patient of this part of the procedure is advised.

See Figure 42.4 for six-month assessment and Video 42.1 for application technique.

42.4 AFTERCARE

Further massage of the penis a few days after the procedure is advised to smooth out any potential lumps or uneven deposition of the product. There is risk of transmission of HIV or hepatitis via bodily fluids from the injection sites; therefore, sex can be practiced using physical barriers the first three days post-procedure (this is more pertinent if the patient is not aware of the health status of their partner). Repetition of the treatment should be considered depending on the three-month assessment, although most of the time it is required to add girth or to smooth out any contour irregularities due to uneven distribution or migration of the product. After the second session, contour irregularities are typically unnoticeable.

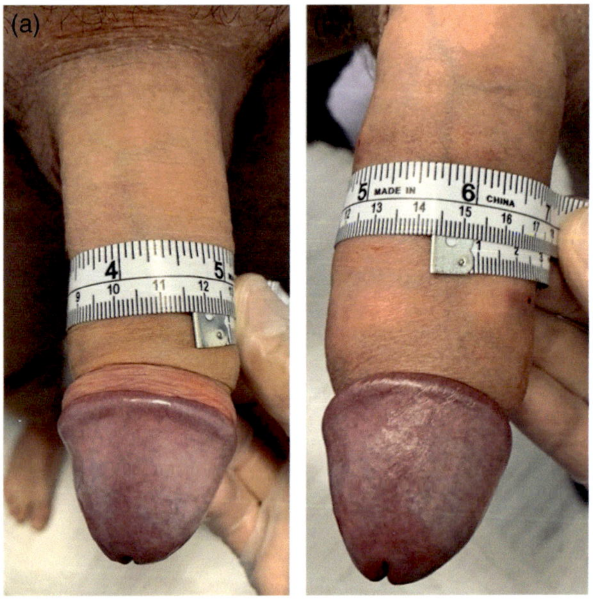

Figure 42.4 Before (a) and six months after (b) 9 mL of CaHA diluted with 9 mL saline in two sessions, six weeks apart (patient also received 1 mL hyaluronic acid [CPM-I] proximal to the glans within the distal shaft). In this case, penile circumference improved from 11.6 cm to 14.3 cm.

42.5 ADDITIONAL TREATMENT OPTIONS

A HA product with high elasticity is recommended to add volume below the glans on the shaft. Use caution with uncircumcised patients, as too much volume in this area may lead to phimosis. HA, however, will allow the product to be dissolved by hyaluronidase.

Special attention should be paid to patients presenting a high degree of penile dissatisfaction, and nonmedical and self-inflicted alternatives should be discouraged. There is a vast body of evidence reporting self-penile augmentation using foreign material [22,23]. These articles mostly report granulomatous inflammatory foreign-body reaction resulting in penile pain, swelling, induration, purulent secretion, and ulceration, which can lead to fatal outcomes such as circumcision and surgical excision of the skin [24].

> **Video 42.1** Penile augmentation: cannula technique.

REFERENCES

[1] J. Oates, G. Sharp, "Nonsurgical medical penile girth augmentation: Experience-based recommendations," *Aesthet Surg J*, vol. 37, no. 9, pp. 1032–1038, 2017.

[2] M. C. Hehemann et al., "Penile girth enlargement strategies: What's the evidence?," *Sex Med Rev*, vol. 7, no. 3, pp. 535–547, 2019.

[3] P. Gontero et al., "A pilot phase-II prospective study to test the 'efficacy' and tolerability of a penile-extender device in the treatment of 'short penis'," *BJU Int*, vol. 103, no. 6, pp. 793–797, 2009.

[4] M. Nikoobakht et al., "Effect of penile-extender device in increasing penile size in men with shortened penis: Preliminary results," *J Sex Med*, vol. 8, no. 11, pp. 3188–3192, 2011.

[5] Z. Jin et al., "Tissue engineering penoplasty with biodegradable scaffold maxpol-T cografted autologous fibroblasts for small penis syndrome," *J Androl*, vol. 32, no. 5, pp. 491–495, 2011.

[6] D. H. Kang et al., "Efficacy and safety of penile girth enhancement by autologous fat injection for patients with thin penises," *Aesthetic Plast Surg*, vol. 36, no. 4, pp. 813–818, 2012.

[7] N. Mertziotis et al., "Is V-Y plasty necessary for penile lengthening? Girth enhancement and increased length solely through circumcision: Description of a novel technique," *Asian J Androl*, vol. 15, no. 6, pp. 819–823, 2013.

[8] O. Shaeer, "Girth augmentation of the penis using flaps 'Shaeer's augmentation phalloplasty': The superficial circumflex iliac flap," *J Sex Med*, vol. 11, no. 7, pp. 1856–1862, 2014.

[9] L. Xu et al., "Augmentation phalloplasty with autologous dermal fat graft in the treatment of 'small penis'," *Ann Plast Surg*, vol. 77, no. Suppl 1, pp. S60–S65, 2016.

[10] T. Il Kwak et al., "The effects of penile girth enhancement using injectable hyaluronic acid gel, a filler," *J Sex Med*, vol. 8, no. 12, pp. 3407–3413, 2011.
[11] D. Y. Yang et al., "Tolerability and efficacy of newly developed penile injection of cross-linked dextran and polymethylmethacrylate mixture on penile enhancement: 6 months follow-up," *Int J Impotence Res*, vol. 25, no. 3, pp. 99–103, 2012.
[12] L. Casavantes et al., "Penile girth enhancement with polymethylmethacrylate-based soft tissue fillers," *J Sex Med*, vol. 13, no. 9, pp. 1414–1422, 2016.
[13] C. Manfredi et al., "Penile girth enhancement procedures for aesthetic purposes," *Int J Impot Res*, vol. 34, no. 4, pp. 337–342, 2021.
[14] L. Baumann, "Collagen-containing fillers: Alone and in combination," *Clin Plast Surg*, vol. 33, no. 4, pp. 587–596, 2006.
[15] M. T. Kim et al., "Long-term safety and longevity of a mixture of polymethyl methacrylate and cross-linked dextran (Lipen-10®) after penile augmentation: Extension study from six to 18 months of follow-up," *World J Mens Health*, vol. 33, no. 3, p. 202, 2015.
[16] G. S. K. Lee, "Use of AccuVeinTM for preventing complications from accidental venipuncture when administering dermal filler injections," *J Cosmet Laser Ther*, vol. 17, no. 1, pp. 55–56, 2015.
[17] K. W. Law et al., "Use of the AccuVein AV400 during RARP: An infrared augmented reality device to help reduce abdominal wall hematoma," *Can J Urol*, vol. 25, no. 4, pp. 9384–9388, 2018.
[18] M. Falcone et al., "European association of urology guidelines on penile size abnormalities and dysmorphophobia: Summary of the 2023 guidelines," *Eur Urol Focus*, vol. 10, no. 3, pp. 432–441, 2024.
[19] D. Herbenick et al., "The development and validation of the male genital self-image scale: Results from a nationally representative probability sample of men in the United States," *J Sex Med*, vol. 10, no. 6, pp. 1516–1525, 2013.
[20] S. N. P. Davis et al., "The index of male genital image: A new scale to assess male genital satisfaction," *J Urol*, vol. 190, no. 4, pp. 1335–1339, 2013.
[21] D. Veale et al., "Penile dysmorphic disorder: Development of a screening scale," *Arch Sex Behav*, vol. 44, no. 8, pp. 2311–2321, 2015.
[22] A. E. Dellis et al., "Paraffinoma, siliconoma and co: Disastrous consequences of failed penile augmentation—a single-centre successful surgical management of a challenging entity," *Andrologia*, vol. 50, no. 10, p. e13109, 2018.
[23] J. N. Svensøy et al., "Complications of penile self-injections: Investigation of 680 patients with complications following penile self-injections with mineral oil," *World J Urol*, vol. 36, no. 1, pp. 135–143, 2018.
[24] K. H. Pang et al., "Complications and outcomes following injection of foreign material into the male external genitalia for augmentation: A single-centre experience and systematic review," *Int J Impotence Res*, vol. 36, no. 5, pp. 498–508, 2023.

Hair Loss

A Novel Approach Using CaHA in Hair Loss Treatment: A Preliminary Study

43

FADI HAMADANI, AINA CERVERA-BAREA, AND JANI VAN LOGHEM

43.1 INTRODUCTION

Hair loss is a widespread concern in aesthetic medicine, with androgenetic alopecia being the most common cause. Traditional treatments include topical and oral medications such as minoxidil and finasteride, along with procedural interventions like platelet-rich plasma (PRP) and hair transplantation. However, regenerative therapies are emerging as promising alternatives [1,2]. CaHA, widely used in facial volumization and skin biostimulation, may offer a novel approach to hair restoration. This chapter presents a preliminary clinical exploration of hyperdiluted CaHA as a treatment for mild to moderate hair loss.

Although CaHA is primarily used for collagen stimulation and volume restoration, its potential in hair restoration may be attributed to:

- *Dermal remodeling and improved scalp microenvironment.* CaHA injections may enhance extracellular matrix support (ECM), thereby optimizing follicular function [3].
- *Keratinocyte activation.* CaHA's contribution to ECM remodeling is considered to have a supportive role for keratinocyte function, known to be the main hair-producing cell type [4].
- *Angiogenesis stimulation.* Increased vascularization may improve follicle nourishment and promote hair growth [5].
- *Collagen and elastin production.* CaHA-induced fibroblast activation could enhance scalp elasticity and health, indirectly benefiting hair follicles [6,7].

43.2 CLINICAL OUTCOMES OF CAHA TREATMENT FOR HAIR LOSS

43.2.1 Patient Selection and Inclusion

The current protocol is suggested in patients with mild to moderate androgenetic alopecia. In case of men, they are eligible up to stage 2 of the Norwood–Hamilton classification. As for women, Ludwig classification stage 1 applies (early progression). History of autoimmune hair loss disorders or contraindications for injectables should be considered when treating these patients.

The protocol described here has been applied in patients from Dr. Hamadani's practice. Four of these patients received only CaHA (no adjunctive therapies), whereas the rest had been previously stabilized on minoxidil. A total of four patients completed the follow-up (six months) and demonstrated hair improvement. From these, two patients treated with CaHA alone showed increased hair density and improved scalp quality. The other two treated with CaHA and minoxidil demonstrated enhanced results beyond their baseline minoxidil response [8].

43.3 RISK AND COMPLICATION MANAGEMENT

Although no complications were observed in this preliminary study [8], potential risks derived from CaHA treatment (non-inflammatory nodules, vascular occlusion causing filler-induced alopecia or delayed inflammatory reactions) or the region to be treated, causing shock hair loss, should be disclosed during consultations [9–11].

Shock hair loss (also known as *telogen effluvium*) was not detected in any of the patients treated in this study, yet it is still a known risk in hair restoration procedures [12,13]. The exact mechanism remains unclear, but contributing factors are likely to include procedural trauma to the scalp, stress on hair follicles and injection-related disruption of the natural hair cycle [14]. Hair shedding *en masse* starts about two to three months after the precipitating event, but regrowth is possible since it is considered a temporary condition [15].

43.4 CANNULA TECHNIQUE FOR HAIR LOSS TREATMENT WITH CAHA

For injection placement, see Figure 43.1.

43.4.1 Step-by-Step Technique

1. Dilute CaHA in a 1:1 ratio (1.5 mL CaHA: 1.0 mL saline: 0.5 mL lidocaine); final volume of 3.0 mL per session.
2. Anesthetize the region where the cannula will be inserted with adrenalized lidocaine.

DOI: 10.1201/9781003617129-43

3. Using a 25G, 50 mm blunt-tip cannula, create two entry points at the subdermal plane: one at the frontal area of the scalp and one at the mid-scalp (Figure 43.2).
4. Use a fanning approach with small, retrograde injections of 0.05 mL per linear thread (Figure 43.3).
5. A multi-bolus technique ensures an even distribution across the treatment area.
6. Pay special attention to being gentle while advancing the cannula to minimize the risk of *telogen effluvium* [12,13,16].

See Video 43.1 for application technique.

Video 43.1 Hair loss treatment: cannula technique.

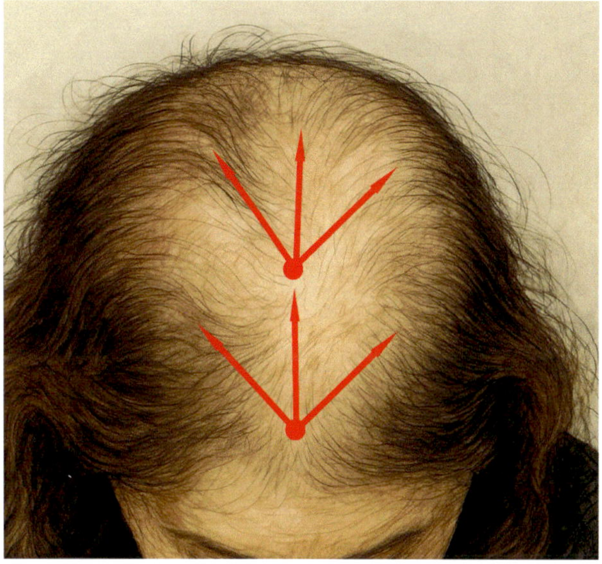

Figure 43.1 Schematic drawing of the injection technique of hyperdiluted CaHA in the scalp for the treatment of hair loss.

43.5 AFTERCARE

After CaHA injections in the scalp, minor side effects such as redness, swelling, or tenderness at the injection site can occur. These should subside within a few days, but the patient should refrain from touching, rubbing, or applying pressure to the treated area. Keeping the injected area clean and dry is of the utmost importance to prevent infections or other complications. However, hot water or steam on the treated area should be avoided for 24 hours, and hair products (gels or hairsprays) or styling, together with direct sunlight, tannings beds, saunas, and hot tubs, should be avoided for at least 48 hours post-treatment.

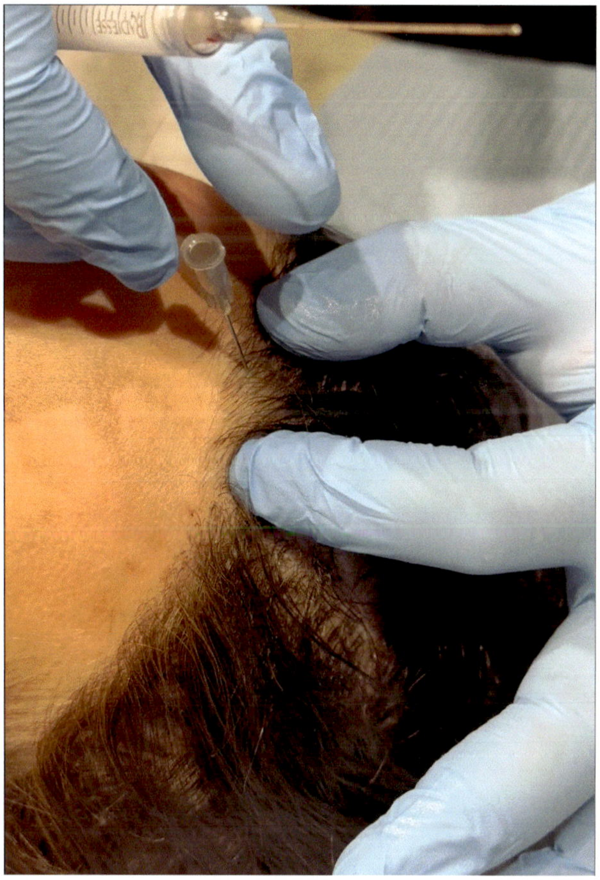

Figure 43.2 Entry point created at the frontal area of the scalp.

43.6 ADDITIONAL TREATMENTS FOR OPTIMAL RESULTS

To reduce the risk of *telogen effluvium* and support recovery, consider the following strategies. First, preventive hair loss medication is advised (namely minoxidil, finasteride, or dutasteride), initiated one month before treatment and continued for at least one year to reduce shedding and support regrowth [17].

Regenerative solutions should also be considered as complementary therapies to manage hair loss. Low-level laser therapy (LLLT) may support healing and regrowth [18]; PRP under stromal vascular fraction can strengthen follicles and reduce shock loss risk [19]; and exosomes, microneedling with nanofat, and fractional radiofrequency also show promise in stimulating growth and improving outcomes [2]. More importantly, hair regrowth is gradual, and patients should understand that improvement will occur slowly and steadily over several months [20].

43.7 FUTURE DIRECTIONS AND CONCLUSIONS

This study serves as proof-of-concept of the potential implementation of CaHA in hair restoration. Further

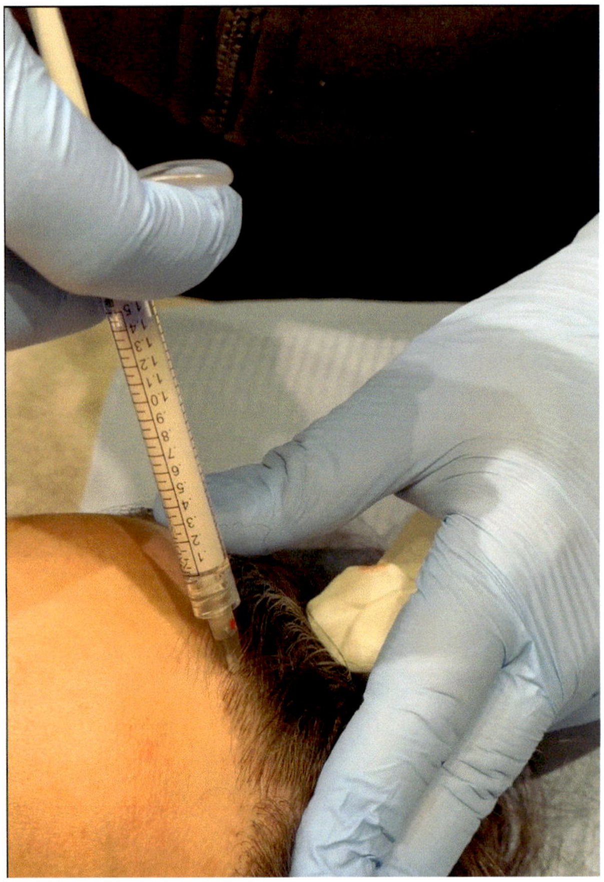

Figure 43.3 Insertion of the cannula (25G, 50 mm) at the frontal area of the scalp for the treatment of hair loss with CaHA using a retrograde fanning technique.

research, including larger-scale studies and histological evaluations, is needed to validate efficacy, refine dosing, and assess combination therapies. Repeated treatments at three-month intervals may also be explored [21].

The use of hyperdiluted CaHA in treating hair loss represents an innovative direction in aesthetic medicine. While early results are promising, further research is essential to fully understand its mechanism and optimize protocols. With careful patient selection, gentle technique, and appropriate adjunctive therapies, CaHA could become a valuable addition to the hair restoration toolkit.

REFERENCES

[1] P. Gentile, S. Garcovich, "Advances in regenerative stem cell therapy in androgenic alopecia and hair loss: Wnt pathway, growth-factor, and mesenchymal stem cell signaling impact analysis on cell growth and hair follicle development," *Cells*, vol. 8, no. 5, p. 466, 2019.

[2] Y. Shimizu et al., "Regenerative medicine strategies for hair growth and regeneration: A narrative review of literature," *Regen Ther*, vol. 21, pp. 527–539, 2022.

[3] J. van Loghem, "Calcium hydroxylapatite in regenerative aesthetics: Mechanistic insights and mode of action," *Aesthet Surg J*, vol. 45, no. 4, pp. 393–403, 2025.

[4] N. Corduff, "Introducing aesthetic regenerative scaffolds: An immunological perspective," *J Cosmet Dermatol*, vol. 22, no. S1, pp. 8–14, 2023.

[5] N. G. Lapatina, T. Pavlenko, "Diluted calcium hydroxylapatite for skin tightening of the upper arms and abdomen," *J Drugs Dermatol*, vol. 16, no. 9, pp. 900–906, 2017.

[6] B. Nowag et al., "Calcium hydroxylapatite microspheres activate fibroblasts through direct contact to stimulate neocollagenesis," *J Cosmet Dermatol*, vol. 22, no. 2, pp. 426–432, 2023.

[7] Y. A. Yutskovskaya, E. A. Kogan, "Improved neocollagenesis and skin mechanical properties after injection of diluted calcium hydroxylapatite in the neck and décolletage: A pilot study," *J Drugs Dermatol*, vol. 16, no. 1, pp. 68–74, 2017.

[8] F. Hamadani, "Unpublished data," 2025.

[9] R. F. Liu et al., "Alopecia with foreign body granulomas induced by Radiesse injection: A case report," *J Cosmet Laser Ther*, vol. 20, no. 7–8, pp. 462–464, 2018.

[10] A. Pulumati et al., "Fillers impacting follicles: The emerging complication of filler-induced alopecia," *Int J Dermatol*, vol. 63, no. 9, pp. 1131–1139, Sep. 2024.

[11] S. Albargawi et al., "Dermal filler-induced alopecia: A case report and literature review," *J Cosmet Dermatol*, vol. 24, no. 2, p. e16684, 2024.

[12] S. H. Loh et al., "Localized telogen effluvium following hair transplantation," *Ann Dermatol*, vol. 30, no. 2, p. 214, 2018.

[13] A. Gómez-Zubiaur et al., "Localized telogen effluvium of the donor area after hair transplant surgery in 12 patients," *Dermatol Surg*, vol. 47, no. 7, pp. 1023–1024, 2021.

[14] S. Harrison, R. Sinclair, "Telogen effluvium," *Clin Exp Dermatol*, vol. 27, no. 5, pp. 389–395, 2002.

[15] G. O. Chien Yin et al., "Telogen effluvium—a review of the science and current obstacles," *J Dermatol Sci*, vol. 101, no. 3, pp. 156–163, 2021.

[16] M. Küçüktaş, "Complications of hair transplantation," in: Kutlubay, Z., Serdaroglu, S., eds., *Hair and Scalp Disorders*. InTechOpen, 2017.

[17] A. Rossi et al., "Efficacy of the association of topical minoxidil and topical finasteride compared to their use in monotherapy in men with androgenetic alopecia: A prospective,

randomized, controlled, assessor blinded, 3-arm, pilot trial," *J Cosmet Dermatol*, vol. 23, no. 2, pp. 502–509, 2024.

[18] R. J. Lanzafame et al., "The growth of human scalp hair mediated by visible red light laser and LED sources in males," *Lasers Surg Med*, vol. 45, no. 8, pp. 487–495, 2013.

[19] P. Gentile et al., "The effect of platelet-rich plasma in hair regrowth: A randomized placebo-controlled trial," *Stem Cells Transl Med*, vol. 4, no. 11, pp. 1317–1323, 2015.

[20] M. Gupta, V. Mysore, "Classifications of patterned hair loss: A review," *J Cutan Aesthet Surg*, vol. 9, no. 1, p. 3, 2016.

[21] U. Wollina, A. Goldman, "Long lasting facial rejuvenation by repeated placement of calcium hydroxylapatite in elderly women," *Dermatol Ther*, vol. 33, no. 6, p. e14183, 2020.

Ultrasound Investigation of CaHA Treatment and Complications

44

AINA CERVERA-BAREA, TOM DECATES, LEONIE W. SCHELKE, PETER VELTHUIS, AND JANI VAN LOGHEM

44.1 INDICATIONS OF ULTRASOUND IMAGING IN CAHA FILLER TREATMENTS

In recent years, application of ultrasound techniques in the daily facial aesthetics practice has been found an invaluable tool to map underlying structures (vasculature, musculature, deep and superficial fat, periosteum, glands, etc.) and guide soft tissue filler injections [1]. The experienced clinical eye is of paramount importance to discern facial structures, but the choice of transducers and the settings that govern the process of image optimization are equally relevant [2].

Facial aesthetics can employ compact "hockey stick" probes, which allow better access to mobile and difficult-to-reach facial areas, enabling complete contact with the skin surface to reduce skin scattering artifacts, e.g., anisotropic effect [2,3]. The international working group DERMUS, with vast expertise in dermatologic ultrasound, together with the European Federation for Ultrasound in Medicine and Biology (EFSUMB) and a panel of 15 international experts that elaborated a modified Delphi consensus, strongly recommend the use of high-frequency transducers (e.g. 10–15 MHz) for dermatologic aesthetic applications [4–8]. Modern ultrasound transducers have broad bandwidth features built in to produce sharp, adjustable images at different depths and discern superficial vascular patterns and subtle features in sub-epidermal structures [2]. High variable-frequency ultrasound (HVFUS) transducers range from 6–18 MHz, with color Doppler frequencies ranging from 4 to 7 MHz [3]. This wide array of frequencies enables the visualization of skin layers at high ranges (14–15 MHz) or deeper tissues at lower ones (6–13 MHz) [3].

The use of real-time ultrasound techniques promotes a dual role for safety application and precise injection to ensure desirable results. As a calcium-based filler, CaHA reflects sound waves differently compared to HA, its non-synthetic counterpart (Table 44.1) [9]. In *pre-treatment stages*, ultrasound-mediated treatment planning gains importance when CaHA is injected in high-risk areas (Table 44.1) [10]. *During aesthetic interventions*, real-time ultrasound may aid physicians localize the needle/cannula and deposit CaHA at the desired anatomic layer (dermis, subcutaneous, interfascial, or periosteal). Spectral Doppler monitoring is particularly useful at this stage where vascular occlusions can occur, and on-the-spot adjustments can be made to ensure patient safety (Table 44.1) [2]. In *later phases of the treatment*, ultrasound is also advised to monitor changes and address overcorrections, dislocations, or vascular adverse events (Table 44.1) [11]. In some instances, filler dissolution may be necessary to prevent impending filler-induced skin necrosis (i.e. HA dissolution with hyaluronidase), and ultrasound guidance appears to significantly improve the chances of total recovery minimizing scarring [12]. A summary of advantages and indications of ultrasound guidance in the daily aesthetics practice can be found in Table 44.1.

Table 44.1 Ultrasound Indications before, during, and after CaHA Treatment

Before Treatment	During Treatment	After Treatment	References
• Record the width of the plane (superficial fatty layer for subcutaneous or fascia/SMAS for deep fatty layer/periosteum placement). • Assessment of vasculature in high-risk zones. • Educational tool for unexperienced injectors to "feel" the injection plane.	• Real-time guidance of injections. • Confirmation of filler deposit at a certain anatomical level. • Quantitative estimation of blood flow to avoid vascular occlusion.	• Deposited filler visualization. • Ultrasound-guided CaHA dilution with saline • Diagnose and monitor complications.	[3,12–17]

DOI: 10.1201/9781003617129-44

44.2 COMMON PITFALLS DURING DERMATOLOGIC ULTRASOUND

Based on current reports, we believe that common pitfalls during dermatologic ultrasound stem from (inexperienced) operators, the equipment used during ultrasound examinations, and the parameters or settings chosen to conduct the imaging. Deficient anatomical or clinical knowledge, inadequate training, and misinterpretation of findings account for *operator pitfalls* [18]. *Pitfalls derived from devices* usually relate to the use of low-frequency probes (<15 MHz), although nowadays the commonly used ultrasound devices in aesthetic clinics achieve frequencies of up to 20 MHz. Following recommendations from some authors, variable frequency transducers offer the best balance among spatial resolution and depth while generating sharp images of all skin layers and structures [19]. In the absence of the former probes, it has been suggested that possession of two devices, one that goes up to 24 MHz and another one for high-frequency ultrasound (up to 70 MHz), is helpful when visualizing superficial skin layers (epidermis and dermis) and posterior acoustic shadowing (PAS) artifacts from (diluted) CaHA [7,20]. Moreover, a copious amount of gel should also aid the recognition of skin structures in ultrasounds, in contrast to the little gel needed to image soft tissues [7,21]. The pitfalls derived from the method may result in artifact visualization (beyond the ones inherent to image processing) and can be caused by the wrong selection of the image mode or parameters or the absence of tailored presets that can enhance image quality and workflow efficiency [2,18]. An example of deficient imaging is the inadequate tilting of the probe (angle of ≃90° instead of ≤60°) that can lead to thrombosis misdiagnosis instead of normal flow detection [18]. Other parameter tweaks required for ultrasound optimization would include gain correction contributing to contrast enhancement and focus adjustment [2]. A comprehensive understanding and manipulation of ultrasound settings are indispensable for achieving optimal image quality.

44.3 SONOGRAPHIC CHARACTERIZATION OF CaHA

Soft tissue fillers present distinctive sonographic features. Authors have described CaHA deposits as hyperechoic bands that reflect most sound waves that do not change with time, producing PAS artifacts caused by the calcium particles (Figure 44.1 and Table 44.2) [22,23]. In contrast, HA appears as anechoic pseudocysts that decrease in size over time [9]. Importantly, different formulations of CaHA generate variable degrees of PAS. In a retrospective study, Wortsman *et al.* proved that undiluted versions of CaHA presented a strong PAS effect versus the mild PAS of diluted ones (1:1 to 1:6) [20]. In diluted formulations, these artifacts were more visible when switching to high-frequency probes (70 MHz), whereas in a mixed formulation with HA, PAS accounted for 0% [20].

44.4 SONOGRAPHIC EVALUATION OF SKIN LAYERS AND STRUCTURES ADJACENT TO THE SKIN

The skin is an easily accessible organ for ultrasound examination. However, its morphological and functional complexity makes it a challenging structure to image. The different cutaneous strata of the skin also share reciprocal layers when imaged with ultrasounds such as the outer layer (epidermis), the middle layer (dermis), and the deeper layer (subcutaneous or hypodermis). To understand the anatomical variability of the skin and adjacent organs, here we will discuss different sonography features of healthy facial

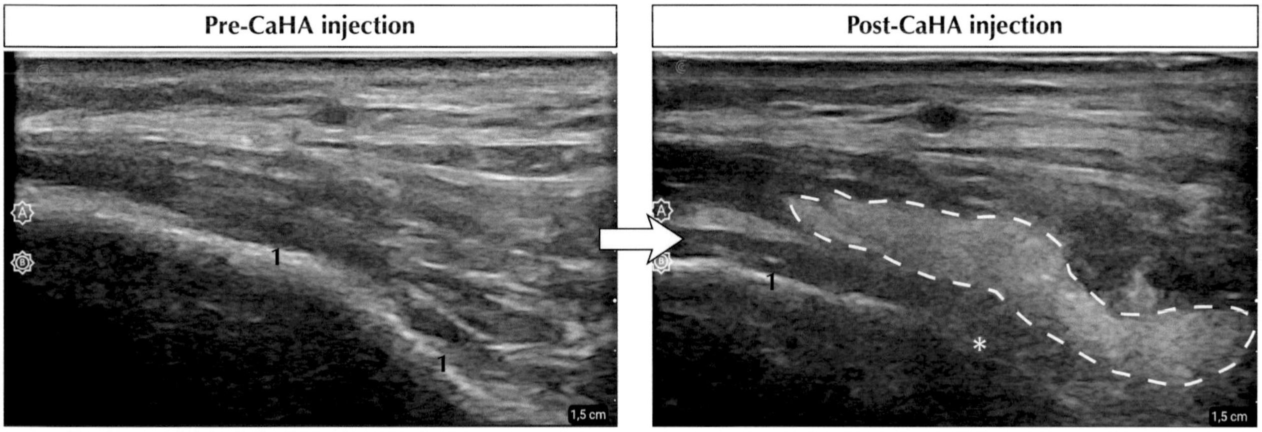

Figure 44.1 Ultrasound visualization of the temple before CaHA treatment (left) reveals a hyperechoic lining where the temporal bone (1) starts. After treatment (right) below the deep temporal fascia with non-diluted CaHA, the hyperechoic line from the bone fades below the CaHA depot (white, dashed line), creating a PAS effect (asterisk) typically characteristic of this tissue filler.

Table 44.2 Comparative Sonographic Characteristics of CaHA and HA

Tissue Filler	Echogenicity	Texture	Shape	Findings	Duration	References
CaHA	Hyperechoic	Coarse grain snowfall	Band-like	Posterior acoustic shadowing artifact due to calcium component	Constant product → no change over time	[11,22,24,25]
HA	Anechoic	Homogenous upon deposit → heterogeneous after tissue integration	Oval-shaped (pseudocyst)	No signs of internal echoes (mixed formulations with lidocaine show inner echoes)	Reduces over time	

structures and ultrasound protocols applied in CaHA filler treatments.

44.4.1 Epidermis

The *epidermis,* containing four epidermal layers (corneum, granulosum, spinosum, and basal), is the outer layer of the skin and typically ranges from 50–120 μm thickness depending on the area. The stratum corneum is an acellular structure that contains keratin and lipids and has high echogenic properties. In non-glabrous skin, and therefore less keratinized regions, the epidermis appears as a single, hyperechoic line (Figure 44.2) [19,26]. Instead, in heavily keratinized areas, such as thick, glabrous skin from palmar and plantar structures, a bilaminar hyperechoic structure is observed (Table 44.3) [19,26,27]. This outer layer is nourished through diffusional mechanisms [28], taking advantage of the epidermal–dermal junction; therefore, it does not show any vascular flow using color Doppler.

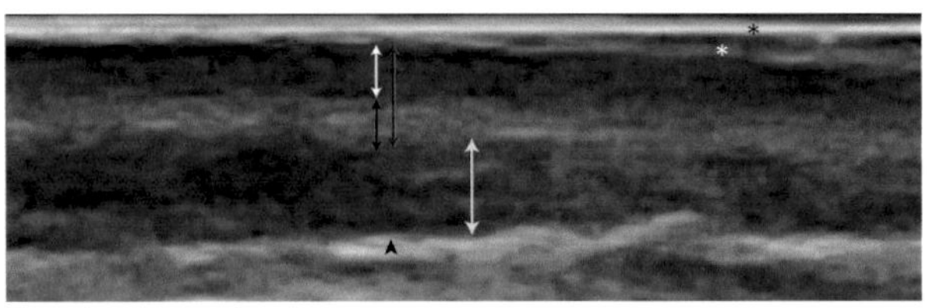

Figure 44.2 Ultrasound visualization of the most superficial cutaneous layers on the temple. Immediately after the transducer membrane (black asterisk) and the echo gel (hypoechoic band below the membrane), there is the epidermis (hyperechoic line; white asterisk), corresponding to the outermost layer of the skin. Following the epidermis, there is the dermis (red arrow), containing the superficial papillary dermis (white arrow) and the deep reticular dermis (black arrow). Below the dermis, we can find the subcutaneous/hypodermis layer (yellow arrow), followed by the superficial temporal fascia (black arrowhead).

44.4.2 Dermis

The middle layer of the skin is the *dermis,* where organized bundles of collagen provide mechanical functions and represent the extracellular matrix for the epidermis [26]. It is important to notice that the dermis is arranged in two layers: the *superficial papillary dermis* and the *deeper reticular dermis* (Figure 44.2). Contrary to the epidermis, the dermis—especially the reticular dermis—is also traversed by a complex vascular system (and other skin structures and appendages). The papillary dermis is nourished by superficial vascular capillaries that sprout from a candelabra-like plexus originated in the deep dermis. The latter also contains artery–vein anastomoses that help blood to bypass upper horizontal dermal vessels. In the process of percutaneous injection, in particular for dermal filler deposition, mild bleeding might occur. Color Doppler ultrasound examination gives an idea of real-time flow movement within the human body. In aesthetics, this is especially interesting to understand the vascular pattern and avoid inadvertent vessel injections. However, some authors have indicated that dermal vascularity is not commonly detectable on color Doppler, since at least 2 cm/s flow velocity is needed, and that only occurs if there is any dermal abnormality [29]. Others have even speculated the mechanism of detection, suggesting that the more hemoglobin molecules in superficial dermal layers might shield deeper hemoglobin ones, thus weakening the signal at greater penetration depths [26,30].

In terms of remodeling, the dermis is also an attractive region to administer CaHA, where mostly collagen is deposited, predominantly type I and type III. In here, the connective tissue is denser, but few elastic fibers are present, making it a pivotal player in sustaining mechanical forces and preventing the skin from sagging [26,31]. Ultrasound assessment of the healthy dermis appears by default as a hyperechoic band that is directly related to the collagen component (Table 44.3) [26,31], and typically no ultrasonographic differences between the papillary and reticular dermis are found (Table 44.3) [32]. However, trophic changes of the skin can impact the echogenic signs. In fact, De Rigal *et al.* described an additional sub-epidermal hypoechoic band (SLEB) in the papillary dermis of older individuals upon chronic sunlight exposure [33] (Table 44.3). This evidence allowed many authors to propose SLEB as a skin-aging parameter [34], where the thickness increases as a function of age [33,35]. Others still report that there is no direct correlation between SLEB thickness and age, and it has to do with dermal atrophy more than SLEB expansion [36]. In any case, SLEB remains an ultrasound sign of damaged skin and a target for CaHA treatment.

44.4.3 Subcutaneous or Hypodermis

The *subcutaneous* compartment is composed of fat tissue divided into lobules [26]. Each *fatty lobule* is divided by *fibro-vascular septa* containing a fibrous and a vascular element (Figure 44.2). The fibrous component of the septa consists of collagen and reticular fibers, whereas the vascular part contains arteries that supply blood and a venular–venous system that drains the hypodermis layer. The oxygenated blood is carried from the septa through a small muscular artery (250–500 μm diameter) that sprouts into centrilobular arterioles (100–300 μm diameter) and later capillaries, wrapping and nourishing each adipocyte individually [26]. The primary sonography sign of the subcutaneous layer is hypoechoic, with hyperechoic interspersed bands—corresponding to the septa—dividing the lobules (Table 44.3).

In the subcutaneous tissue, isolated vessels of <1 mm are readily visible as thin anechoic ducts, and their arrangement is clinically relevant, especially when occlusions take place (Figure 44.3 and Table 44.3) [3]. Arterial interferences have been linked to diffuse intralobular changes (mostly lobular panniculitis), whereas venous occlusions manifest with septal and paraseptal alterations (mostly septal panniculitis) [26,37].

44.4.4 SMAS and Deep Fascia

The *SMAS* is an organized continuous fibrous network in charge of connecting the muscles to the dermis, which belongs—together with the deep fascia—to the subcutaneous layer (Figure 44.4). The SMAS has been found to be in discontinuity at the midface, whereas in the temples, it is contiguous to the superficial temporal fascia [38]. Moving to the superior temporal line and up to the forehead, the temporal fascia becomes a continuum with the galea aponeurotica, which is the fibromuscular extension of SMAS [39]. Different SMAS have been described throughout time [40], but in this chapter we will use Zattar *et al.*'s description of the five types of SMAS considered during filler-based facial rejuvenation (Table 44.3) [41]. These five morphological SMAS also present regional diverse ultrasound responses, which will be subsequently defined. *Type I* belongs to the preparotideal region, rich in fat, which confers on it a hypoechoic effect with hyperechoic vertical septa, resembling *type V* SMAS and the hypodermis of other body regions. In *type II*, they describe a heterogenic hyperechoic subcutaneous, with a loss of definition in the dermal-hypodermal border. *Type III* can be found in the lower and upper eyelid, characterized for being a thin, fat-poor region, giving it hyperechoic features. The temporal and parotideal regions belong to *type IV* SMAS, showing hyperechoic horizontal lines, parallel to the skin. Zattar and others also described a *type 5* SMAS at the neck region. This one has a prominent hypoechoic subcutaneous, with parallel-to-skin fibrous septa in addition to vertical ones that connect the skin to the platysma muscle [41].

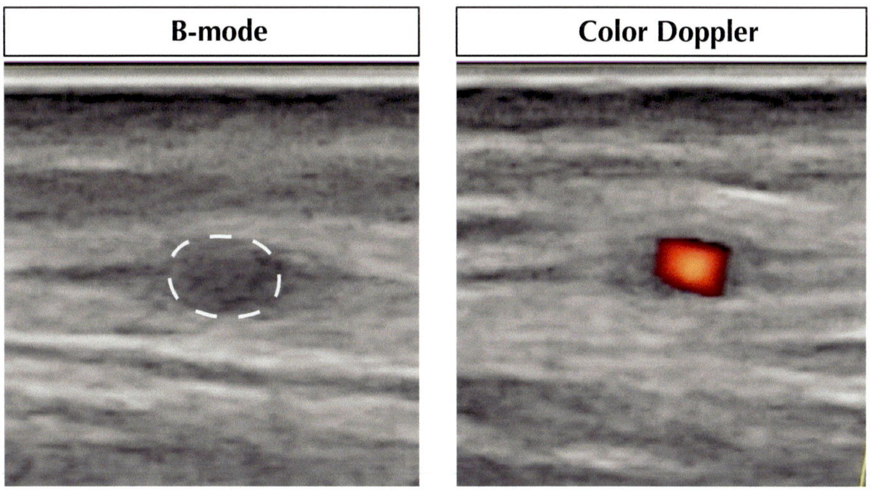

Figure 44.3 Ultrasound visualization of vessels is observed as echo-free ducts (white, dashed line) in B-mode grayscale (left). In the presence of color Doppler (right), vascular flow and pulsation – in the case of arteries – can be observed.

In the temples, we can also find the *interfascial plane* in between the superficial and deep temporal fascia layers (Figure 44.4 and Table 44.3) [42]. This region appears hypoechoic on grayscale ultrasound and is enclosed between the hyperechoic bands originating from the fascial layers [42]. The interfascial plane remains a target for temporal volumization (Figure 44.5), especially when strong, contracting muscles (i.e. temporalis muscle) traverse the region and a deeper placement could potentially cause migration or lumping of the product [39]. See further Video 44.1.

Video 44.1 Ultrasound-guided CaHA treatment for temporal volumization.

In addition to SMAS, in the deep hypodermis there is also the *deep fascia* (also known as intermediate fascia) [39] that connects the subcutaneous to the muscle (Figure 44.4 and Table 44.3). This dense connective tissue sheet appears as a hyperechoic band and is also known to be part of a thicker fibrofatty layer that fills the space between the superficial fascia and deeper structures [43]. The deep fascia adopts different thicknesses depending on the region it traverses, being thin and convergent in convex underlying structures and thick and divergent, forming deep fat entities, in concave ones [43].

44.4.5 Muscles

During ultrasound examination of the face, the *muscles* are visible when using high-frequency transducers (Figure 44.4) [44,45]. Skeletal muscle appears as a hypoechoic, fibrillary structure that presents dynamic maneuvers depending on its contractile state [29]. Muscles are arranged in spindles separated by hyperechoic adipose-fibrous septa known as perimysium, visible as hyperechoic linear bands in the longitudinal plane (Table 44.3) [26]. The muscle is contained in a loose connective sheath called

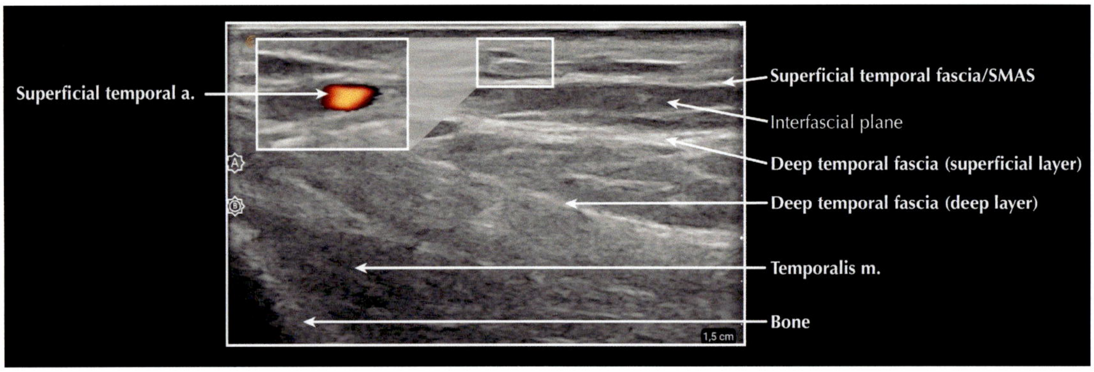

Figure 44.4 Visualization of skin structures using ultrasound.

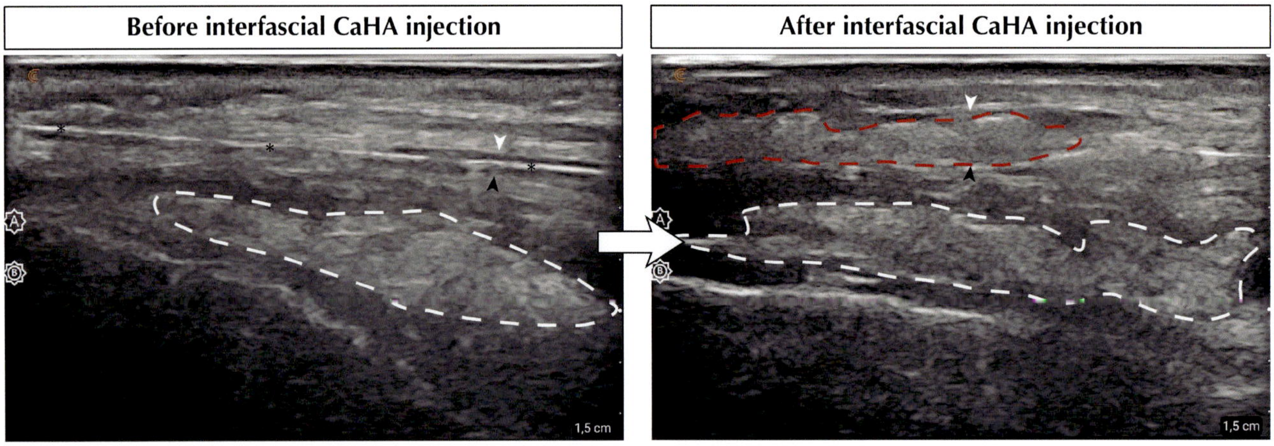

Figure 44.5 Ultrasound image before (left) and after (right) interfascial treatment with standard dilution of CaHA. The treatment was performed with a cannula (hyperechoic, white line; black asterisks) at the interfascial space between the superficial temporal fascia (white arrowhead) and the superficial lamina of the deep temporal fascia (black arrowhead). The same area was previously treated with CaHA (white, dashed line) at the level of the deep lamina of the deep temporal fascia. After treatment (right image), the new CaHA depot (red, dashed line) was visible at the interfascial space.

Table 44.3 Transducer Characteristics and Ultrasound Protocols to Visualize Cutaneous Layers and Structures Adjacent to the Skin

Skin Structure		Echogenicity	Frequency	Ultrasound Protocol	References
Epidermis	Non-glabrous skin	Hyperechoic layer	75–100 MHz	B-mode grayscale	[3–6,18,29,56]
	Glabrous skin (palmar and plantar region)	Bilaminar hyperechoic layer			
Dermis	Papillary or superficial dermis	• Healthy: hyperechoic • Elastosis: sub-epidermic low echogenic band (SLEB)	20–30 MHz	B-mode grayscale	[3–6,18,29,56]
	Reticular or deep dermis				
Subcutaneous/ hypodermis	Fatty lobules	Hypoechoic	• Superficial subcutaneous: 12–17 MHz • Deeper subcutaneous/ muscle: 7.5–12 MHz	B-mode grayscale + color Doppler	[18,19,26]
	Fibro-vascular septa	• Fibers: hyperechoic • Vasculature: anechoic tubular			
	Vessels ≥300 µm ø	Anechoic tubular	12 MHz	color Doppler	[57–60]
	~ 100 µm ø		18–22 MHz		
SMAS	Preparotideal (*type I*)	• Subcutaneous: hypoechoic • Vertical septa: hyperechoic	15–33 MHz	B-mode grayscale	[41,61]
	Chin and lip (*type II*)	• Subcutaneous: heterogeneous hyperechoic • Loss dermal-hypodermal border			
	Lower and upper eyelid (*type III*)	Hyperechoic thin line			
	Temporal and parotideal (*type IV*)	Hyperechoic horizontal lines (parallel to skin)			
	Cervical (*type V*)	• Subcutaneous: hypoechoic • Parallel and vertical septa: hyperechoic			
Fascias	Superficial and deep fascia layers	Hyperechoic bands	10–18 MHz	B-mode grayscale	[42,61,62]
	Interfascial plane	Hypoechoic			
Muscle	Muscles	Hypoechoic	10–15 MHz	B-mode grayscale	[3,44,45]
	Connective tissue (peri- and epimysium)	Hyperechoic bands (in longitudinal plane)			
Periosteum	Periosteum	• Healthy: not visible • Pathologic/periosteal reaction: hypoechoic thickening	10–15 MHz	B-mode greyscale + color Doppler	[44,49]
	Vasculature	• Healthy: negative color or power Doppler but detectable nutrient arteries • Pathologic/periosteal reaction: possible hyperemia on color Doppler			

Ø, diameter.

Table 44.4 Ultrasound Assessment of CaHA Complications

Complication	Facial Structures Involved	Echogenicity	Findings	Ultrasound Protocol	References
Early onset complications (within first 24-48 h post-injection)					
Vascular occlusion	Occlusion of facial arteries like facial, angular, dorsal and alar nasal, anterior and posterior ethmoidal, ophthalmic, or labial arteries	N/A	• Ischemia, blindness, mucosal or dermal necrosis* • Hypervascular turbulent artery or absence of visible flow with/without detectable filler blockage	B-mode grayscale + color Doppler	[14,63,64]
Edema	Inflammation of subcutaneous fat, lymphatic congestion	• Dermis: echogenicity • Hypodermis: echogenicity	Anechoic bands between the fatty lobules (severe stages)	B-mode grayscale	[65,66]
Late onset complications (after four months post-injection)					
Chronic inflammation	Dermis and hypodermis of injection region(s)	• Dermis: echogenicity • Hypodermis: echogenicity	Regional hypervascularity with slow-flow vessels	B-mode grayscale + color Doppler	[63]
Non-infectious nodule/lump†	Injection region	Focal accumulation can be visualized as hyperechoic deposition	• Remains unchanged upon compression • Variable degree of hypervascularity	B-mode grayscale + color Doppler	[22,67–69]
Panniculitis	Hypodermis of injection region(s)	• Lobular/"foggy" pattern: echogenicity + diffuse and bright pattern • Septal/"cobblestone" pattern: echogenicity lobules • Mixed pattern: echogenicity lobules + septa	• Lobular: hypo/hypervascularity • Septal: hypo/hypervascularity	B-mode grayscale + color Doppler	[63,65]
Morphea-like reactions	Injection region	• Dermis: echogenicity • Hypodermis: echogenicity	• Loss of definition of the dermal-hypodermal border • Dermal and/or hypodermal hypervascularity	B-mode grayscale + color Doppler	[63,70]

N/A, not applicable. *Consequence of vascular occlusion of the glabellar, nasal, and nasolabial regions. †Can be caused by focal filler accumulations, interaction of absorbable and non-absorbable fillers (overcorrection), and/or an inflammatory reaction (secondary panniculitis or granulomatous reaction).

epimysium. Both the epimysium and fascia appear as hyperechoic bands [46]. Interestingly, vascular flow is not visible in healthy, resting muscles; therefore, color or power Doppler modes will not be useful (Table 44.3) [46]. Imaging skeletal muscle can be challenging, and system settings must be adjusted when muscle tissue properties and echogenicity change based on pathophysiological factors (e.g. weight, increased fibrotic content, or age) [45].

44.4.6 Periosteum

Periosteal deposition is the farthest that CaHA injection will go to enable lifting, elevating effects. Some authors even refer to it as the deep fascia [47], when both the deep fascia and the periosteum become a continuum [39]. The *periosteum* is an outer fibrous membrane providing vascularization to the bone and immediately adjacent to the underlying cortex, whose thickness is inversely related to one's age, progressively thinning as we grow old (Table 44.3) [48]. In normal conditions, the periosteum cannot be recognized sonographically as a separate structure in adults [44]; only the bone surface appears as a highly hyperechoic line with PAS and some reverberation artifacts (Figure 44.4) [49]. Conversely, in children, it does show, but as a thin, hypoechoic band located above the hyperechoic cortex [48]. The Doppler signal is also used in musculoskeletal ultrasound imaging, and despite not showing any vascular flow in the healthy periosteum, the penetrating arteries penetrating the periosteum can be detected entering the bone (Table 44.3) [48].

44.5 ULTRASOUND VISUALIZATION OF CAHA COMPLICATIONS

During follow-up, ultrasound can also be implemented on patient complications and in the treatment of these, i.e., assisting in percutaneous thrombolytic therapy (HA) using ultrasound upon accidental intravascular injection [50]. Possible complications can be categorized by time of onset (early to late) or severity; range from local edema to hyperpigmentation; and can mimic common dermatologic diseases, such as morphea (Table 44.4) [51]. Some of these complications are operator dependent, like superficial depositions resulting in lumps or vascular occlusions posing a threat to patient's safety. The result of intramuscular injections—especially in highly mobile areas such as perioral structures—can also cause the creation of nodules by compression of the filler from a strand into a lump [52]. Major side effects from vascular occlusions can result in vision loss or even stroke, turning ultrasound examination into a useful tool in the management and potentially in the prevention of vascular occlusions [53–55]. The summary of the most common complications after CaHA treatment and the ultrasound signs associated to them can be found in Table 44.4. For a more extensive glimpse at filler complications, please refer to Chapter 45.

REFERENCES

[1] M. Calomeni et al., "Precision of soft-tissue filler injections: An ultrasound-based verification study," *Aesthet Surg J*, vol. 43, no. 3, pp. 353–361, 2023.

[2] K. Malherbe, S. Roberts, "Sonographic principles and techniques," in: *Ultrasound Protocol for Facial Aesthetics*. Springer, 2024, pp. 5–23.

[3] D. Gaitini, "Introduction to color doppler ultrasound of the skin," in: Wortsman, X., ed., *Dermatologic Ultrasound with Clinical and Histologic Correlations*. Springer, 2013, pp. 3–14.

[4] X. Wortsman et al., "Guidelines for performing dermatologic ultrasound examinations by the DERMUS group," *J Ultrasound Med*, vol. 35, no. 3, pp. 577–580, 2016.

[5] O. Catalano, X. Wortsman, "Dermatology ultrasound: Imaging technique, tips and tricks, high-resolution anatomy," *Ultrasound Q*, vol. 36, no. 4, pp. 321–327, 2020.

[6] A. Fernando Alfageme et al., "European Federation of Societies for Ultrasound in Medicine and Biology (EFSUMB) position statement on dermatologic ultrasound stellungnahme der European Federation of Societies for Ultrasound in Medicine and Biology (EFSUMB) zu dermatologischem ultraschall," *Bibliography Ultraschall in Med*, vol. 42, pp. 39–47, 2021.

[7] X. Wortsman, "Technical recommendations, settings, protocols, training, and reports of the dermatologic ultrasound examinations," in: *Textbook of Dermatologic Ultrasound*. Springer, 2022, pp. 3–15.

[8] P. J. Velthuis et al., "The use of ultrasound imaging in aesthetic injectables: A modified Delphi consensus," *J Plast Reconstr Aesthet Surg*, vol. 104, pp. 33–37, 2025.

[9] X Wortsman, "Common applications of dermatologic sonography," *J Ultrasound Med*, vol. 31, no. 1, pp. 97–111, 2012.

[10] L. Schelke et al., "Precision in midfacial volumization using ultrasound-assisted cannula injections," *Plast Reconstr Surg*, vol. 152, no. 1, pp. 67–74, 2023.

[11] F. Urdiales-Gálvez et al., "Ultrasound patterns of different dermal filler materials used in aesthetics," *J Cosmet Dermatol*, vol. 20, no. 5, pp. 1541–1548, 2021.

[12] J. Jia et al., "Superior outcomes with ultrasound-guided hyaluronidase for impending filler-induced facial skin necrosis: A systematic review and pilot meta-analysis," *Aesthet Plast Surg*, pp. 1–7, 2025.

[13] J. A. Kadouch, "Calcium hydroxylapatite: A review on safety and complications," *J Cosmet Dermatol*, vol. 16, no. 2, pp. 152–161, 2017.

[14] L. Schelke et al., "Incidence of vascular obstruction after filler injections," *Aesthet Surg J*, vol. 40, no. 8, pp. NP457–NP460, 2020.

[15] L. Schelke et al., "Ultrasound as an educational tool in facial aesthetic injections," *Plast Reconstr Surg Glob Open*, vol. 10, no. 12, p. e4639, 2020.

[16] L. W. Schelke et al., "Investigating the anatomic location of soft tissue fillers in nonin-flammatory nodule formation: An ultrasound-imaging–based analysis," *Dermatol Surg*, vol. 49, no. 6, p. 588, 2023.

[17] K. Malherbe, S. Roberts, "Clinical indications for facial aesthetic ultrasound," in: *Ultrasound Protocol for Facial Aesthetics*. Springer, 2024, pp. 37–39.

[18] X. Wortsman et al., "Ultrasound imaging of subcutaneous tissue and adjacent structures," in: *Handbook of Non-Invasive Methods and the Skin*, 2nd edn. CRC Press, 2006, pp. 515–530.

[19] X. Wortsman, J. Wortsman, "Clinical usefulness of variable-frequency ultrasound in localized lesions of the skin," *J Am Acad Dermatol*, vol. 62, no. 2, pp. 247–256, 2010.

[20] X. Wortsman et al., "Ultrasonographic patterns of calcium hydroxyapatite according to dilution and mix with hyaluronic acid," *J Ultrasound Med*, vol. 42, no. 9, pp. 2065–2072, 2023.

[21] X. Wortsman, "Technical considerations of the dermatologic ultrasound examination," in: *Atlas of Dermatologic Ultrasound*. Springer, 2018, pp. 23–34.

[22] L. W. Schelke et al., "Use of ultrasound to provide overall information on facial fillers and surrounding tissue," *Dermatol Surg*, vol. 36, no. Suppl 3, pp. 1843–1851, 2010.

[23] X. Wortsman, "Ultrasound in aesthetics," in: *Textbook of Dermatologic Ultrasound*. Springer, 2022, pp. 415–432.

[24] X. Wortsman et al., "Ultrasound detection and identification of cosmetic fillers in the skin," *J Eur Acad Dermatol Venereol*, vol. 26, no. 3, pp. 292–301, 2012.

[25] L. W. Schelke et al., "Nomenclature proposal for the sonographic description and reporting of soft tissue fillers," *J Cosmet Dermatol*, vol. 19, no. 2, pp. 282–288, 2020.

[26] X. Wortsman et al., "Sonographic anatomy of the skin, appendages, and adjacent structures," in: *Dermatologic Ultrasound with Clinical and Histologic Correlations*. Springer, 2013, pp. 15–35.

[27] P. P. Guastalla et al., "Detection of epidermal thickening in GJB2 carriers with epidermal US1," *Radiology*, vol. 251, no. 1, pp. 280–286, 2009.

[28] W. J. Lee, "Skin," in: *Vitamin C in Human Health and Disease*. Springer, 2019, pp. 167–175.

[29] X. Wortsman, "Normal ultrasound anatomy of the skin, nail, and hair," in: *Atlas of Dermatologic Ultrasound*. Springer, 2018, pp. 1–23.

[30] J. C. Luck et al., "Multiple laser doppler flowmetry probes increase the reproducibility of skin blood flow measurements," *Front Physiol*, vol. 13, p. 876633, 2022.

[31] T. Quan, G. J. Fisher, "Role of age-associated alterations of the dermal extracellular matrix microenvironment in human skin aging: A mini-review," *Gerontology*, vol. 61, no. 5, pp. 427–434, 2015.

[32] A. C. Nicolescu et al., "Subepidermal low-echogenic band—its utility in clinical practice: A systematic review," *Diagnostics*, vol. 13, no. 5, p. 970, 2023.

[33] J. de Rigal et al., "Assessment of aging of the human skin by in vivo ultrasonic imaging," *J Investig Dermatol*, vol. 93, no. 5, pp. 621–625, 1989.

[34] J. Czajkowska et al., "High-frequency ultrasound in anti-aging skin therapy monitoring," *Sci Rep*, vol. 13, no. 1, pp. 1–13, 2023.

[35] R. Rayner et al., "Measurement of morphological and physiological skin properties in aged care residents: A test–retest reliability pilot study," *Int Wound J*, vol. 14, no. 2, pp. 420–429, 2017.

[36] M. Gniadecka, "Effects of ageing on dermal echogenicity," *Skin Res Technol*, vol. 7, no. 3, pp. 204–207, 2001.

[37] P. Giavedoni et al., "High-frequency ultrasound to assess activity in connective tissue panniculitis," *J Clin Med*, vol. 10, no. 19, p. 4516, 2021.

[38] V. Mitz, M. Peyronie, "The Superficial Musculo-Aponeurotic System (SMAS) in the parotid and cheek area," *Plast Reconstr Surg*, vol. 58, no. 1, pp. 80–88, 1976.

[39] J. M. Sykes et al., "Upper face: Clinical anatomy and regional approaches with injectable fillers," *Plast Reconstr Surg*, vol. 136, no. 5, pp. 204S–218S, 2015.

[40] A. Ghassemi et al., "Anatomy of the SMAS revisited," *Aesthet Plast Surg*, vol. 27, no. 4, pp. 258–264, 2003.

[41] L. C. Zattar et al., "U-SMAS: Ultrasound findings of the superficial musculoaponeurotic system," *Radiol Bras*, p. e20240035, 2024.

[42] S. Desyatnikova, "Ultrasound-guided temple filler injection," *Facial Plast Surg Aesthet Med*, vol. 24, no. 6, pp. 501–503, 2022.

[43] L. Minelli et al., "The deep fascia of the head and neck revisited: Relationship with the facial nerve and implications for rhytidectomy," *Plast Reconstr Surg*, vol. 153, no. 6, pp. 1273–1288, 2024.

[44] K. H. Cho et al., "Sonography of bone and bone-related diseases of the extremities," *J Clin Ultrasound*, vol. 32, no. 9, pp. 511–521, 2004.

[45] A. Ashir et al., "Skeletal muscle assessment using quantitative ultrasound: A narrative review," *Sensors*, vol. 23, no. 10, p. 4763, 2023.

[46] D. Orlandi et al., "Muscles," in: Martino, F. et al., eds., *Musculoskeletal Ultrasound in Orthopedic and Rheumatic Disease in Adults*. Springer, 2022, pp. 49–60.

[47] A. H. Charafeddine et al., "Facelift: History and anatomy," *Clin Plast Surg*, vol. 46, no. 4, pp. 505–513, 2019.
[48] A. Moraux et al., "Ultrasound features of the normal and pathologic periosteum," *J Ultrasound Med*, vol. 38, no. 3, pp. 775–784, 2019.
[49] S. J. Erickson, "High-resolution imaging of the musculoskeletal system," *Radiology*, vol. 205, no. 3, pp. 593–618, 1997.
[50] X. Wortsman, "Sonography of dermatologic emergencies," *J Ultrasound Med*, vol. 36, no. 9, pp. 1905–1914, 2007.
[51] X. Wortsman, J. Wortsman, "Sonographic outcomes of cosmetic procedures," *Am J Roentgenol*, vol. 197, no. 5, pp. W910–W918, 2011.
[52] G. Lemperle, D. M. Duffy, "Treatment options for dermal filler complications," *Aesthet Surg J*, vol. 26, no. 3, pp. 356–364, 2006.
[53] W. Lee et al., "Safe glabellar wrinkle correction with soft tissue filler using doppler ultrasound," *Aesthet Surg J*, vol. 41, no. 9, pp. 1081–1089, 2021.
[54] L. W. Schelke et al., "Early ultrasound for diagnosis and treatment of vascular adverse events with hyaluronic acid fillers," *J Am Acad Dermatol*, vol. 88, no. 1, pp. 79–85, 2023.
[55] V. C. Doyon et al., "Update on blindness from filler: Review of prognostic factors, management approaches, and a century of published cases," *Aesthet Surg J*, vol. 44, no. 10, pp. 1091–1104, 2024.
[56] R. K. Mlosek et al., "High-frequency ultrasound in the 21st century," *J Ultrason*, vol. 20, no. 83, p. e233, 2020.
[57] D. E. Goertz et al., "High-frequency 3-D color-flow imaging of the microcirculation," *Ultrasound Med Biol*, vol. 29, no. 1, pp. 39–51, 2003.
[58] T. Tansatit et al., "Ultrasound evaluation of arterial anastomosis of the forehead," *J Cosmet Dermatol*, vol. 17, no. 6, pp. 1031–1036, 2018.
[59] T. Phumyoo et al., "Anatomical and ultrasonography-based investigation to localize the arteries on the central forehead region during the glabellar augmentation procedure," *Clin Anat*, vol. 33, no. 3, pp. 370–382, 2020.
[60] D. Jaguś et al., "Usefulness of doppler sonography in aesthetic medicine," *Pediatria i Medycyna Rodzinna*, vol. 20, no. 83, pp. e268–e272, 2020.
[61] P. J. Velthuis et al., "A guide to doppler ultrasound analysis of the face in cosmetic medicine. Part 1: Standard positions," *Aesthet Surg J*, vol. 41, no. 11, pp. NP1621–NP1632, 2021.
[62] C. Pirri et al., "Ultrasound imaging of head/neck muscles and their fasciae: An observational study," *Front Rehabilit Sci*, vol. 2, p. 743553, 2021.
[63] X. Wortsman, "Sonography of dermatologic emergencies," *J Ultrasound Med*, vol. 36, no. 9, pp. 1905–1914, 2017.
[64] M. Antonio Munia et al., "Doppler ultrasound in the management of vascular complications associated with hyaluronic acid dermal fillers," *J Clin Aesthet Dermatol*, vol. 15, no. 2, p. 40, 2022.
[65] X. Wortsman, "Ultrasound of common inflammatory dermatologic diseases," in: *Atlas of Dermatologic Ultrasound*. Springer, 2018, pp. 279–342.
[66] A. Durkin et al., "Single-center, prospective comparison of calcium hydroxylapatite and bycross-20L in midface rejuvenation: Efficacy and patient-perceived value," *J Cosmet Dermatol*, vol. 20, no. 2, pp. 442–450, 2021.
[67] R. K. Mlosek et al., "High-frequency ultrasound-based differentiation between nodular dermal filler deposits and foreign body granulomas," *Skin Res Technol*, vol. 24, no. 3, pp. 417–422, 2018.
[68] S. R. Cohen et al., "Radiesse rescue: A preliminary study for a simple and effective technique for the removal of calcium hydroxyapatite–based fillers," *Aesthet Surg J*, vol. 43, no. 3, pp. 365–369, 2023.
[69] C. Gonzalez et al., "Ultrasonographic features of nonvascular complications of hyaluronic acid fillers: A retrospective study at a reference center for dermatologic ultrasonography," *Clin Dermatol*, vol. 42, no. 5, pp. 538–546, 2024.
[70] X. Wortsman, "Top advances in dermatologic ultrasound," *J Ultrasound Med*, vol. 42, no. 3, pp. 521–545, 2023.

Complication Management and Prevention

45

JONATHAN KADOUCH, PHILIPPE SNOZZI, PEEROOZ SAEED, AND JANI VAN LOGHEM

Injection with calcium hydroxylapatite (CaHA) to male and female patients is generally safe and well tolerated. To date, there are relatively few serious adverse events (SAEs) or other clinically significant product-related adverse events reported.

Adverse events (AEs) can be classified in various ways. An overview can be found in Table 45.1, where we classify CaHA-related AEs on the basis of clinical presentation (skin discoloration, edema, infection nodules, and vascular AEs).

45.1 SHORT-TERM SAFETY

The most frequent reported adverse events are local, and they are most often referred to as "injection site reactions", such as bruising, edema, erythema, pain, pruritus, and infection (Figures 45.1–45.7) [2–4]. These AEs are transient and mild in intensity, and usually no medical intervention is needed. In most cases, they are not assessed as related to CaHA but are deemed a result of the injection trauma and/or injection technique. AEs have also been reported with other types of fillers, such

Table 45.1 Common Classification of AEs after Filler Injection (from ref 1 with permission).

Early-Type AEs(Onset Less Than 2 Weeks)	Late-Type AEs(Onset More Than 2 Weeks)
Technical mishap:	***Infection (biofilm):***
• Non-inflammatory nodule	• Erythema
• Asymmetry	• Edema
• Contour irregularity	• Pain
Infection:	• Inflammatory nodule
• Erythema	• Ulceration
• Edema	***(Granulomatous) Type IV hypersensitivity reaction:***
• Tenderness or pain	• Erythema
• Inflammatory nodule	• Edema
• Abscess	• Pain
Type I hypersensitivity reaction:	• Inflammatory nodule
• Erythema	• Ulceration
• Edema/angioedema	***(Granulomatous) Foreign body reaction:***
Type IV hypersensitivity reaction:	• (Non-)inflammatory nodule
• Erythema	• Erythema
• Edema	• Edema
• Tenderness or pain	• Pain
• Inflammatory nodule	• Ulceration
• Ulceration	***(Pseudo-)abscess:***
Vascular occlusion:	• Fluctuating inflammatory swelling
• Tissue necrosis	***Migration (dislocation) of filler material:***
• Blindness	• Non-inflammatory nodule
Skin discoloration:	***Persisting skin discoloration:***
• Tyndall effect	• Hyperpigmentation
• Hyperpigmentation	• Erythema/telangiectasis
• Erythema	

Source: From 1. Kadouch JA. Calcium hydroxylapatite: A review on safety and complications. *J Cosmet Dermatol* 2017 Jun;16(2):152–161, with permission.

Reproduced with permission from Kadouch JA. Calcium hydroxylapatite: A review on safety and complications. *J Cosmet Dermatol* 2017 Jun;16(2):152–161 [1].

DOI: 10.1201/9781003617129-45

as hyaluronic acid fillers. In the early trial comparing CaHA suspended in carboxymethyl cellulose gel and collagen-treated patients, there was no significant difference in adverse event rates or duration [3,4].

45.2 LONG-TERM SAFETY

CaHA is currently the second most often chosen filler after hyaluronic acid fillers [5]. A review on the safety and complications of CaHA concluded that CaHA

Diagnosis	Hematoma	Neovascularization	Hyperpigmentation	Tyndall effect/Skin brightening/visible product	Ischemia
Time of occurrence	• Within minutes to hours	• Within days to weeks	• Within days to weeks	• Within days	See *Vascular Compromise algorithm*
Clinical presentation	• Deep hematoma may appear as a subacute swelling, with no visible bruises • Temporary or permanent hemosiderin deposits are possible	• Telangiectasia days to weeks after intradermal filler treatment • Often in the upper nasolabial fold region	• Post-inflammatory hyperpigmentation • Especially with Fitzpatrick skin types IV-VI	• Yellow discoloration	
Differential diagnosis	• Erythema (several possibilities) • Ischemia (blue-gray phase) • Post-inflammatory hyperpigmentation	• Rosacea • Dermatitis	• Hemosiderin deposits	• (Malar) edema	
Therapy	• Heparin- or Vit. K-containing ointment • IPL • Hemosiderin deposits: alpha hydroxy acid, or laser	• Mostly self-limiting in 3-12 months without therapy • Laser • IPL	• Sun protection SPF50 • Bleaching agent • Chemical peels • IPL (skin type I-IV) • Nd:YAG laser (Skin type V-VI)	• Expression / CO_2 laser	
Prophylaxis	• Apply immediate compression when visible bleeding • Use blunt cannulas • Beware of patients using oral anticoagulants	• By placing fillers only subcutaneously (cannula) • Increased risk of rosacea patients possible	• By placing fillers only subcutaneously (cannula) • Beware skin type Fitzpatrick V / VI	• Selecting the right filler • Avoid too superficial placement of filler	

Figure 45.1 Differential diagnosis of skin discoloration.

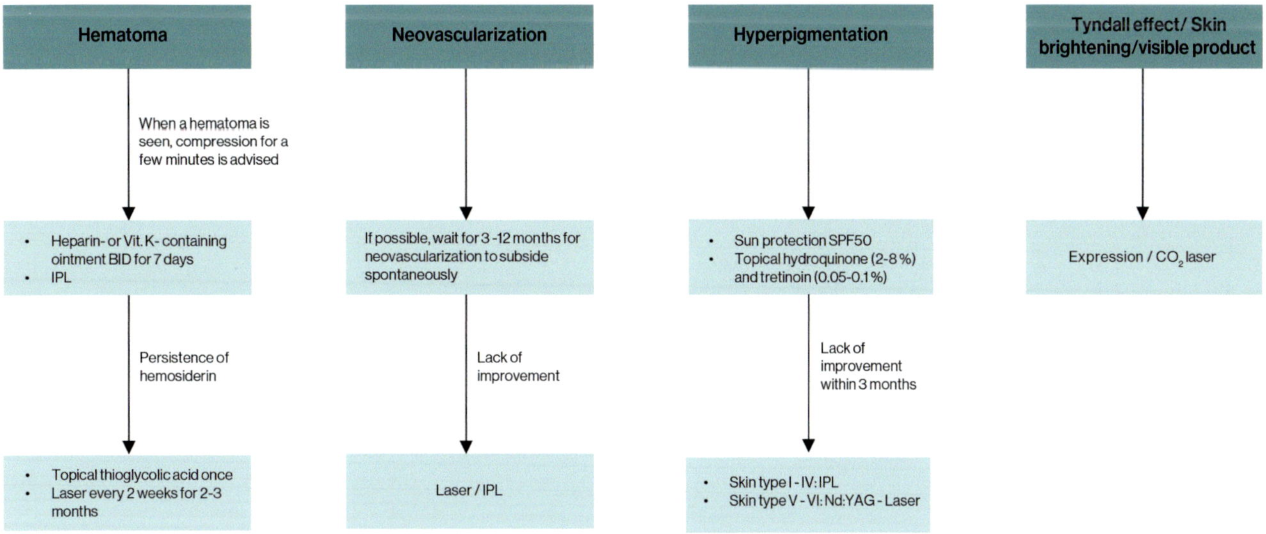

Figure 45.2 Skin discoloration detection and treatment algorithm.

Diagnosis	Post-interventional edema	Malar edema	Immediate type allergy (type I)	Delayed type allergy (type IV)	Acute Infection, LIRS
Time of occurrence	• Within hours	• Within days	• Within minutes to hours	• Within days	See ***Nodules and Infections algorithm***
Clinical presentation	• Edema without inflammatory signs (with the exception of slight erythema) • Maximum 24 -48 hours after treatment	• Malar edema after tear trough treatment, or treatment of the mid-face	• Erythema, eritema, pruritus • Local or generalized swelling of the face • Urticaria • Beware of two-phased course	• Induration, erythema, edema, nodules • Appearance: between 1 day (already sensitized) to several weeks (sensitizing phase is 5 -7 days)	
Differential diagnosis	• Overcorrection • Type I – allergy • Physical urticaria • Hereditary or acquired angioedema	• Overcorrection	• Physical urticaria • Hereditary or acquired angioedema • Post-interventional edema	• Infection • Transition into a chronic granulomatous reaction through permanent immune stimulation may be possible (see section on nodules)	
Therapy	• Cooling • Keep head in elevated position at night • Bromelain	• Keep head in elevated position at night	• Cooling • Antihistamines • Prednisone	• Prednisone	
Prophylaxis	• Split the treatment over multiple sessions • Patients with rosacea have an increased risk of erythema/edema after the treatment	• No superficial injections in the area of the malar septum • Beware of personal or family history of malar edema	• Take caution with patients with a history an "allergic reaction" to hyaluronic acid • In unclear cases: perform a skin test	• Take caution with patients with a history an "allergic reaction" to hyaluronic acid • In unclear cases: perform a skin test	

Figure 45.3 Differential diagnosis of edema.

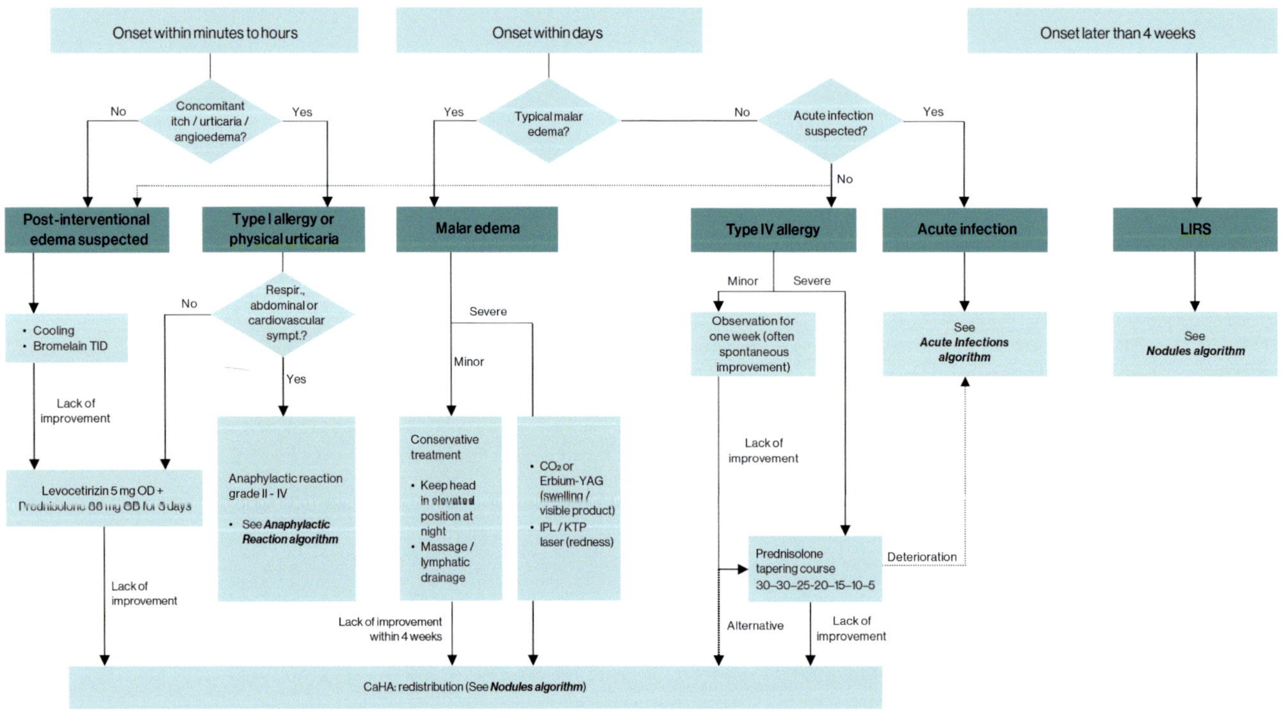

Figure 45.4 Edema treatment detection and treatment algorithm.

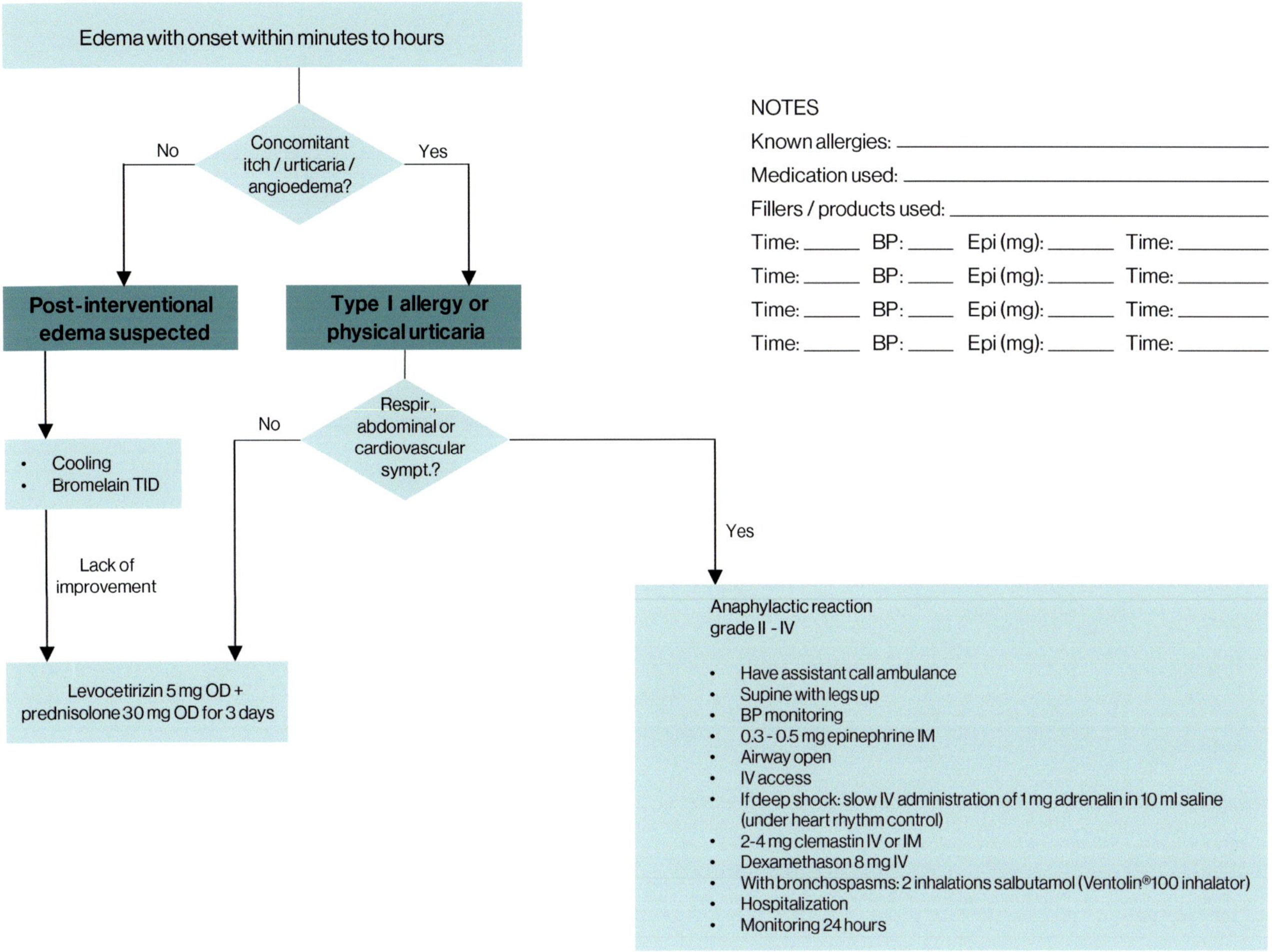

Figure 45.5 Anaphylactic reaction detection and treatment algorithm.

appears to have a good safety profile [1]. The review included a cohort of 5,081 treatments performed on 2,779 patients, and nodules were the only late-type AEs reported, with an incidence of 3% (166 of 5,081). However, it must be stated that a large percentage of the assessed 166 nodule cases occurred in old reports after injection at highly dynamic facial areas, such as lips, peri-orally, and peri-orbitally. Currently, such dynamic regions are contraindicated since the muscular activity can lead to product accumulation and nodule formation [6]. If such indications had not been included, the nodule incidence would have been much lower. Nonetheless, it appears that CaHA causes the lowest amount of foreign body granulomas among all fillers [7,8]. In comparison, the incidence of nodules and papules in patients treated with poly-L-lactic acid is believed to be around 10–16% [9].

While vascular compromise and occlusion can occur with any dermal filler, the risk increases with particulate filler substances [10]. Furthermore, the consequences may be more severe for those fillers without a reversal procedure. The care provider must be aware of the type of adverse events that can occur and how to treat them. A comprehensive understanding of facial anatomy and dermal filler characteristics is essential. Given the rarity of vascular compromise, physicians might not have any experience in the recognition or management of these complications. In this chapter, the management algorithm for CaHA-induced vascular occlusion is discussed in detail [11].

45.3 NODULES

Nodules are slightly elevated lesions on or in the skin but can also develop in deeper tissues or internal organs. They are larger than papules—over 5 mm in diameter. It is a clinical description as opposed to granuloma, which is a histological diagnosis [12,13]. The diagnosis nodule does not indicate anything on the cause. It can be caused by incorrect positioning of filler material or overcorrection, accumulation or migration of the product, type IV hypersensitivity reaction, infection, or a foreign body reaction [14,15]. Granulomatous foreign body reactions have been demonstrated after CaHA injection, but only a handful of case reports have been documented to date [12,16–18]. The incidence of granuloma formation after CaHA is the lowest compared to all other soft tissue fillers on the market [8].

	Erysipelas, cellulitis	Abscess	Herpes lesions	Biofilm
Diagnosis	Acute (within days)			Subacute (within weeks to months)
Time of occurrence	• *S. pyogenes*, *S. aureus* • When developing later than two weeks after the injection atypical bacteria may be involved	• *S. aureus* • When developing later than two weeks after the injection atypical bacteria may be involved	• Herpes Simplex Type I or II	• *Pseudomonas* species, *S. epidermidis*, *P. acnes*, *Acinetobacter*, other
Clinical presentation	• Sharp (erysipelas) or non-sharply defined (cellulitis) inflammatory swelling • Sometimes fever or malaise • Sometimes lymphadenopathy	• Like cellulitis, but with a palpable, fluctuating mass	• Herpes typical vesicles • Sometimes lymphade-nopathy	See ***Nodules algorithm***
Differential diagnosis	• Type IV immune reaction • Edematous granuloma (early onset unusual)	• Cystic granuloma (early onset unusual)	• Vascular compromise (necrosis)	
Therapy	• Antibiotics • In severe cases, referral to a hospital	• Swab for culture • Antibiotics • In severe cases, referral to a hospital	• Anti-viral therapy	
Prophylaxis	• Take care to create an aseptic environment during treatments • Use only high quality products	• Take care to create an aseptic environment during treatments • Use only high quality products	• Regular history of herpes: valciclovir 500 mg BID for 3 days as a prophylaxis	

Figure 45.6 Differential diagnosis of infection.

45.4 MANAGEMENT OF NODULES

In the management of CaHA nodules, it is important to define the type and the onset of the nodule, as this will determine the therapy (Figure 45.8). Early onset nodules are most likely the result of the injection technique, whereas late onset nodules may be the result of accumulation/migration of the filler product or a foreign body reaction [15]. Early onset nodules can be managed with massaging or intralesional injection with saline or sterile water. Late onset nodules can be treated with intralesional injection of a corticosteroid (Figure 45.9) [19–21]. The risk of an inflammatory reaction is extremely low, as CaHA has good biocompatibility with human tissue [22,23]. CaHA is identical to the mineral component of the bony structures in humans, leading to minimal immune responses [23–25].

Nodule formation after CaHA injection has most often been reported at the lips (45%), the peri-oral area (4%), and the nasolabial fold (3%) [1]. Per the manufacturer's recommendation, CaHA should not be injected in the lips, oral mucosa, and glabella. To minimize the risk of nodule formation, the authors recommend avoiding the perioral area, as this is a mobile area in the face. A non-inflammatory nodule may be corrected by direct massage (manually or with a vibrating device) in an attempt to redistribute the nodule over a larger surface area, resulting in about 20% reduction if treated after three weeks after injection. Injection of saline or sterile water intralesionally prior to massage may increase the effectiveness to 25% and 35%, respectively [26] (see Video 45.1). In more severe cases, a blend of dexamethasone, triamcinolone, 5-fluorouracil, and lidocaine may be injected directly into the nodule, followed by massage [27].

Video 45.1 Nodule redistribution.

45.4.1 Step-by-Step Protocol for Treating Nodules

1. Palpate the nodule and fix it between the fingers of the non-dominant hand.
2. Inject saline or sterile water blended with lidocaine into the nodule (here, for a nodule of approximately 0.1 mL, a total of 1 ml saline and 0.1 ml lidocaine 2% was used).
3. Apply a firm massage, pressing against the bone. If the nodule is located over the oral cavity, one finger inside the mouth and one outside is recommended in order to squeeze and flatten the nodule between two fingers.
4. If needed, a vibrating device can be used for additional redistribution of the nodule.

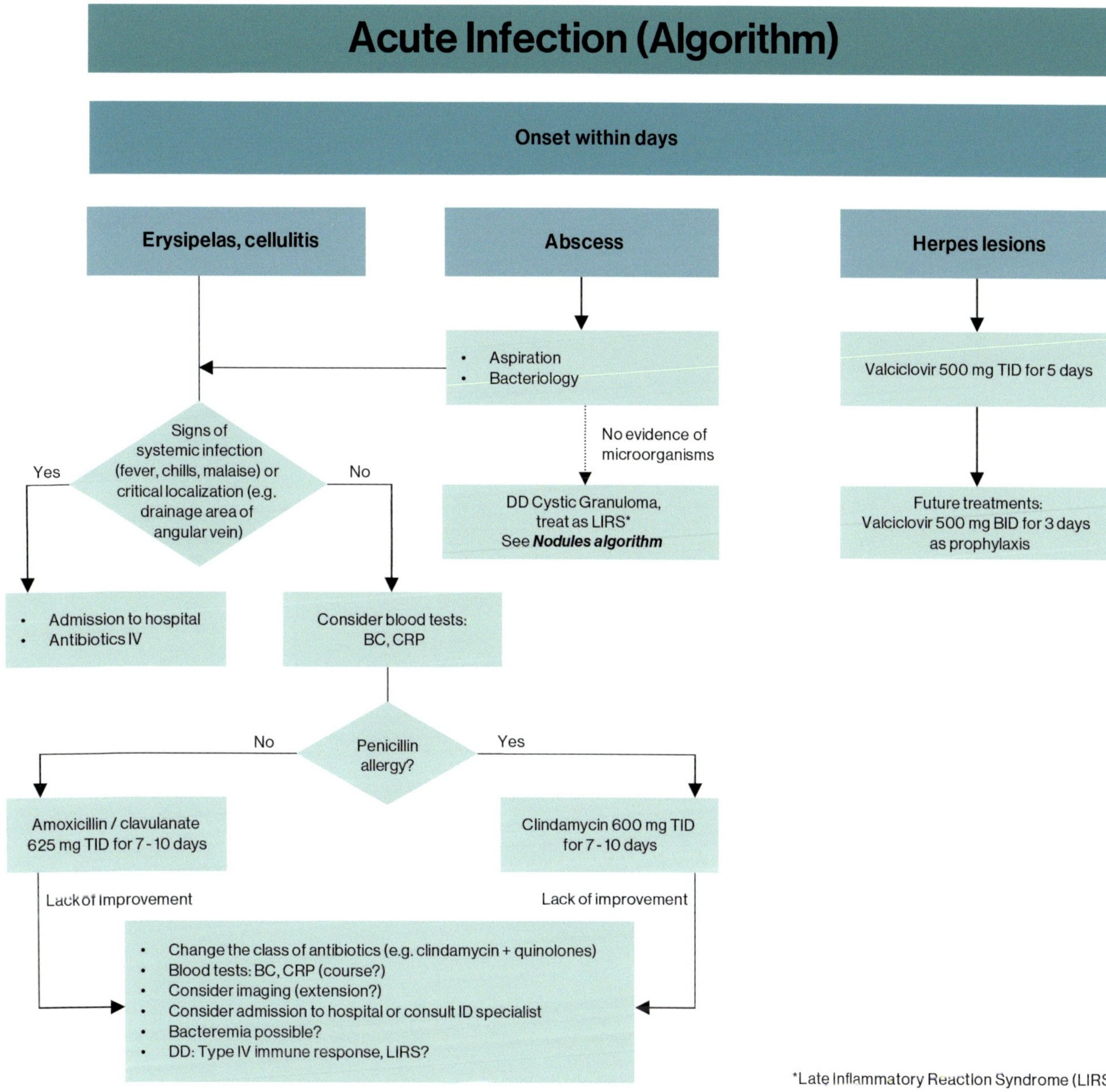

Figure 45.7 Acute infection detection and treatment algorithm.

45.5 VASCULAR COMPROMISE

Blindness may result from injections anywhere in the face, but there are several anatomical danger zones which are more prone to occlusion of the central retinal artery. A thorough understanding of the vascular anatomy is vital. The glabella has been reported as the most common filler injection site triggering blindness [28], followed by the nose and the forehead [29]. Small vessels branching from the supratrochlear and supraorbital arteries provide the blood supply to the glabellar region, and the collateral circulation is limited. Injections to the nasal area have been reported as the main cause of tissue necrosis and the second cause of visual loss after the glabella zone, as this area has little vascular collaterals. Injection into the nasolabial fold or nasal dorsum may therefore accidentally deliver product intra-arterially, and if plunger pressure is greater than arterial pressure, product can move proximally into the central retinal artery [30–35]. Finally, vascular occlusion is more likely to occur in areas with extensive anastomoses between vascular territories, because of the risk of occluding adjoining smaller diameter arteries, for example, the central retinal artery [36].

45.6 RECOGNIZING THE SYMPTOMS OF VASCULAR OCCLUSION

The incidence of necrosis due to vascular compromise following dermal filler treatment (any type of filler) has been estimated at 1 in 2,000 to 1 in 10,000

	Non-inflammatory	Inflammatory	
Diagnosis/ type	**Accumulated filler material/ implant nodule**	**Biofilm possible** → (Genetic factors, Product factors, Immunological factors) →	**Chronic granulomatous reaction**
		Late Inflammatory Reaction Syndrome (LIRS)	
Time of occurrence	• Usually immediate • Sometimes delayed occurrence due to migration of the filler material	• After weeks to months, sometimes years	
Pathophysiology	• Accumulated filler: overcorrection, migration • Implant nodule: mild foreign body reaction to the filler is physiological; excessive reaction may lead to a fibrotic, encapsulated implant nodule	• Biofilm seems pivotal by inducing a permanent immune response, thus leading to a chronic granulomatous reaction • Other immunological phenomena may play a role (e.g. excessive foreign body reaction, Type IV reaction, etc.) • Occasionally another infection (e.g. flu, gastroenteritis) may precede and trigger LIRS • Product factors and patient factors play a role	
Clinical presentation	• Painless, non-sore resistance	• Inflammatory, tender nodules	• Inflammatory nodules, plaques or seldom cysts • All areas where the filler is present may react • Histology: sclerosing, edematous or cystic granuloma • Progression of fibrosis over time
Differential diagnosis	• Deep situated hematoma, encapsulated hematoma • Abscess	• Fluctuating nodule: abscess • Sarcoidosis	
Therapy	• Accumulated filler material: redistribution by massage or saline/sterile water injection • Encapsulated implant nodule: intra-lesional corticosteroids often not successful, excision may be required	• Consider broad spectrum antibiotics	• Intra-lesional corticosteroids • Intra-lesional 5-FU • Oral methotrexate (MTX)
Prophylaxis	• Avoid overcorrection	• Creating an aseptic environment during treatments • Avoiding products that seem to be more prone than others to cause a LIRS	

Figure 45.8 Differential diagnosis of nodules.

(0.05–0.01%) [37], particularly among less experienced injectors and when sharp needles are routinely used. Disproportional pain, pallor, and blanching are the usual initial symptoms of vascular compromise or occlusion. However, in some cases patients may not complain of symptoms or show signs of ischemia during the filler injection or even on the day of the procedure [33,38]. A livedo reaction (mottled discoloration) may follow in 1–10 min, which may progress to hemorrhagic changes, blisters, and necrosis in the days after. Finally, secondary infection may occur.

Retinal artery occlusion can also occur after injection in almost any area of the face and leads to a sudden onset of impairment/loss of vision and often complaints of severe pain (ocular, facial, and/or headache). Furthermore, symptoms such as aphasia or even contralateral hemiparesis might present when a cerebral infarction accompanies a retinal artery occlusion [39]. An overview can be found in Figure 45.14.

45.7 PREVENTION OF VASCULAR OCCLUSIONS

CaHA should be injected slowly, with a low injection force, and with the smallest amount of product necessary (Figure 45.15). For deep injections, the periosteum remains the preferred level, but with caution, as there is no guarantee that injections will be extravascular. Large boluses should be avoided, especially in the periorbital area, where the amount should not exceed 0.025 mL. Also, in other facial areas, caution should be taken, and it is advised to limit boluses to a maximum of 0.1 mL.

When using a needle in a danger zone, material should be deposited at the pre-periosteal level with the needle in contact with the bone and at a slightly oblique angle. Small needle caliber increases plunger pressure and the likelihood of clogging, which may cause the injector to increase the pressure on the plunger and provoke vascular events. Large gauge needles increase the risk of bruising but might decrease the risk of intravascular injections. If unexpected resistance is detected, blanching observed, or the patient indicates pain, the injection must be stopped immediately.

Other options to decrease the risk of vascular compromise include injecting in a retrograde fashion so as not to deliver a large deposit in one location. The use of adrenaline/adrenaline-containing local anesthesia promotes arterial constriction, reducing the size of vessels and therefore the risk of filler entry.

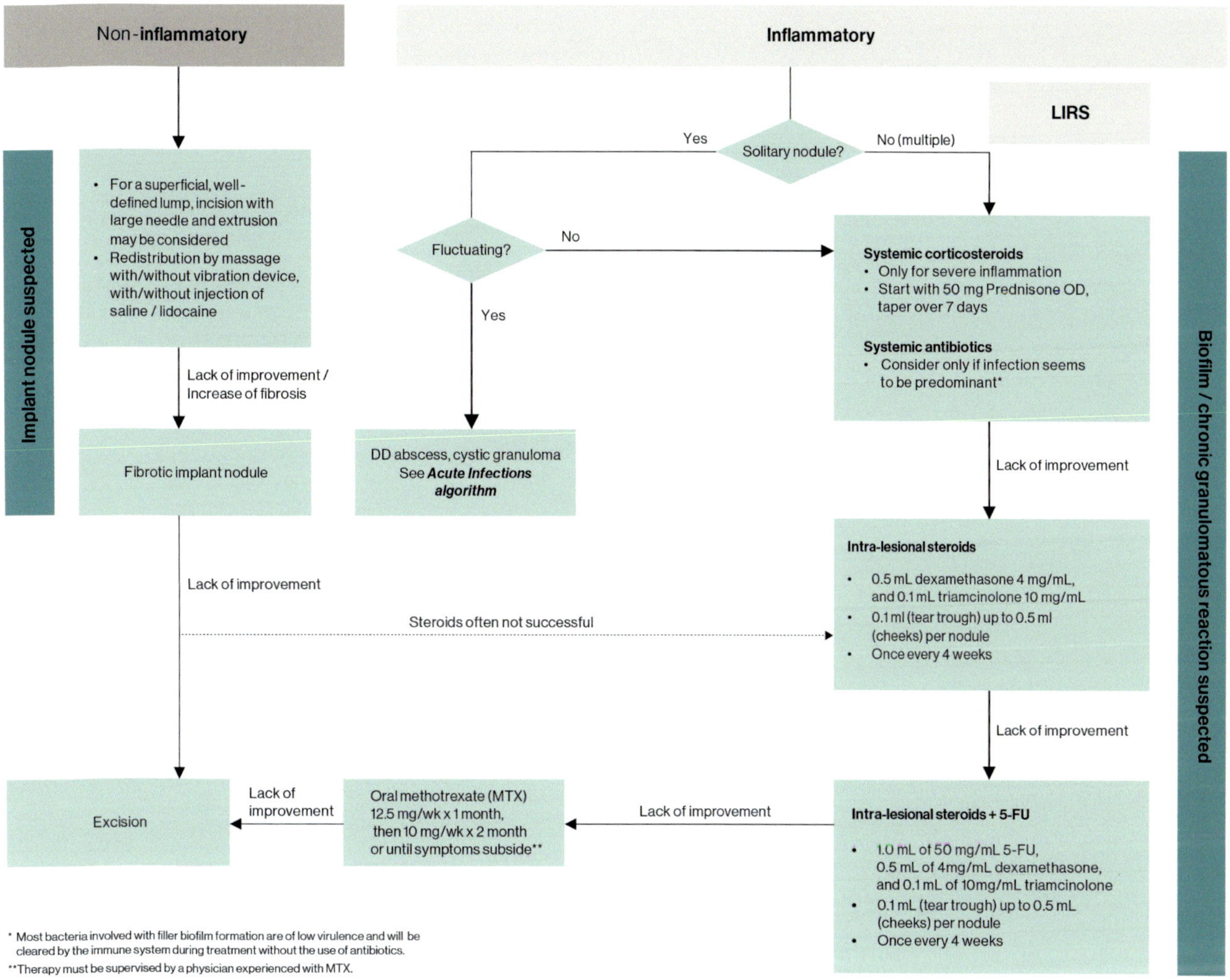

Figure 45.9 Nodules detection and treatment algorithm.

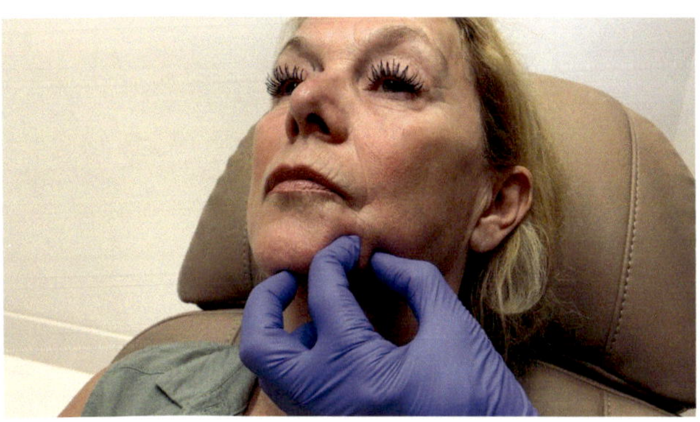

Figure 45.10 Palpation and fixation of the nodule between the fingers.

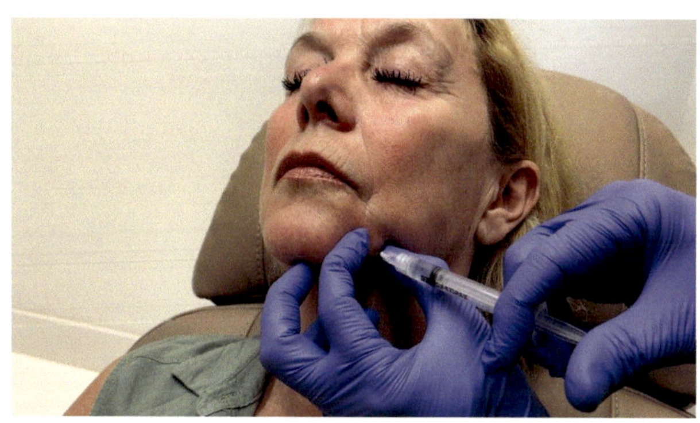

Figure 45.11 Injection of vehicle with lidocaine to anesthetize the nodule.

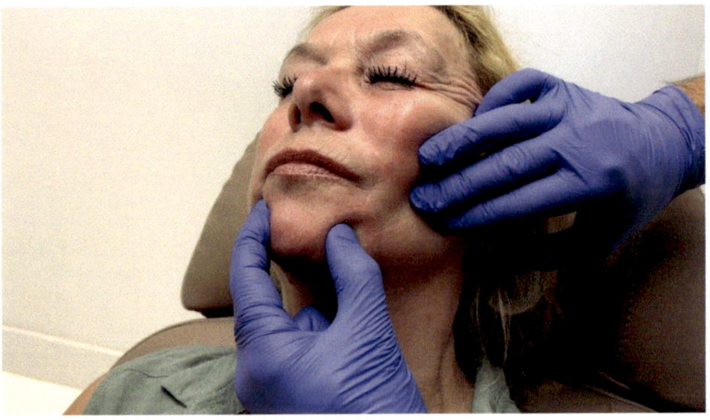

Figure 45.12 Massage firmly to flatten the nodule.

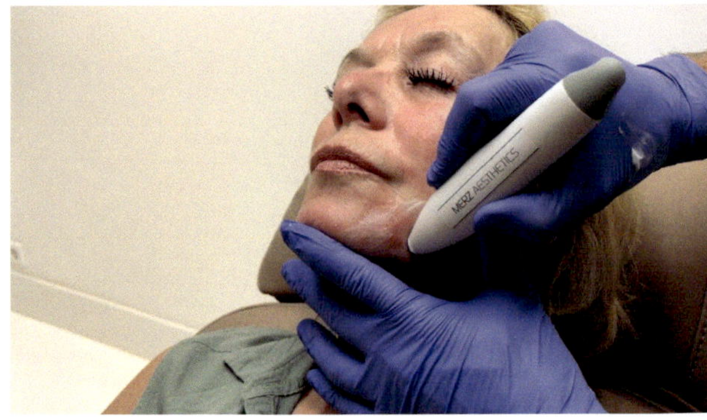

Figure 45.13 Vibration device used to redistribute the nodule.

Diagnosis	Peripheral ischemia with impending necrosis	Retinal ischemia
Clinical presentation and time of occurrence	1. Blanching phase • Immediate onset, duration < 1min; sometimes painful 2. Livedo reticularis phase (marbling) • After a few minutes (seldom within a few hours), due to lack of oxygen resulting in venous dilation, virtually pathognomonic 3. Blue-gray phase • Tens of minutes to hours, due to sustained lack of oxygen. May appear more rapidly in the vermillion 4. Blister phase • After 1-2 days, as a first sign of skin necrosis 5. Demarcation and ulceration phase • After days to weeks, healing by secondary intention	• During Injection or immediately after injection: loss of vision, sometimes concurrent eye pain • Over the course, sometimes ophthalmoparesis
Differential diagnosis	• Vasoconstriction due to epinephrine containing local anesthetics (blanching phase) • Hematoma (blue-grey phase) • Herpes simplex / herpes zoster lesions (blister phase)	• Transient vision loss following exposure to examiner's light
Therapy	• High dose hyaluronidase within a few minutes to hours • Warm compresses • Aspirin • Further therapeutic options: low-molecular weight heparin (LMWH), pentoxyfillin, hyperbaric oxygen therapy (HBOT)	• In the office: pressure lowering eyedrops, HYAL at the supraorbital notch and affected skin areas; Consider retrobulbar injection if well trained • Hospitalization and referral to stroke unit / ophtalmologist • MRI of the brain to rule out any cerebral ischemia
Prophylaxis	• Use blunt cannulas (25G) in high-risk areas • Small boluses (max. 0.05mL / bolus) in high-risk areas • Slow injection • Aspiration (needle) • Consider manual compression of the angular artery during injection • Risk factors: previous surgery, scars (including acne scars!), small gauge needles / cannulas	

Figure 45.14 Differential diagnosis of vascular occlusion.

However, products containing adrenaline may mask blanching produced by occlusion [40]. Tumescent injection, also known as saline hydrodissection, has been used successfully when performing CaHA injections of the forehead [41,42]. The tumescent solution for tissue hydrodissection creates a pocket of space for filler placement.

In the periorbital area, injectors should compress the nasion where the supraorbital/supratrochlear/dorsal nasal arteries are with the fingers of the nondominant hand in an effort to prevent retinal embolization [43]. In addition, the authors advise not to exceed 0.025 mL per injection volume (the so-called "Jani van Loghem bolus") in the area close to the supratrochlear notch [11,44,45].

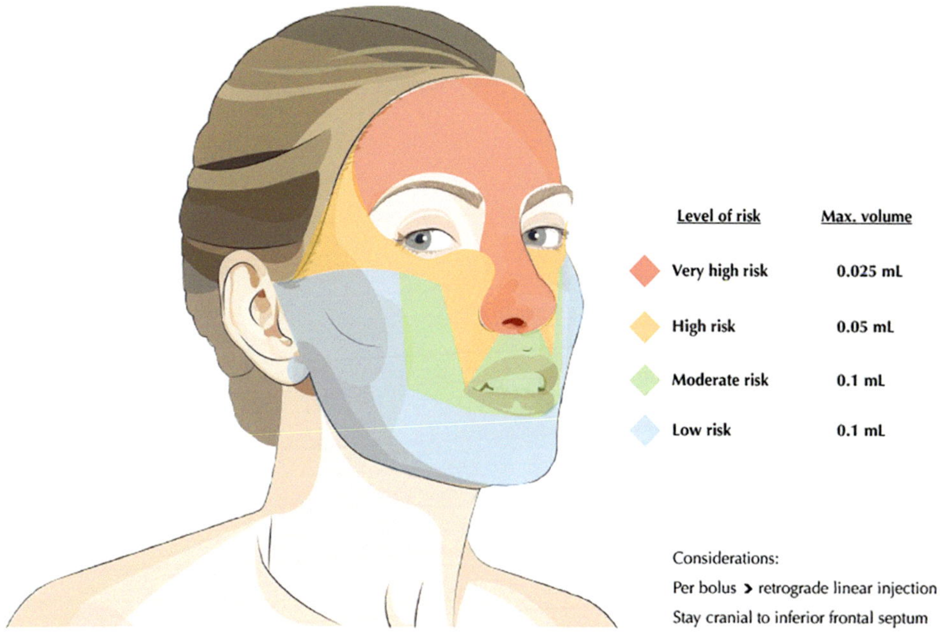

Figure 45.15 Injection strategy for reducing the risk of blindness.

45.8 MANAGEMENT OF VASCULAR COMPROMISE

Management should be focused on a rapid reinstatement of the blood flow; see Figure 45.14 for an overview. Recommendations for impending necrosis after injection with CaHA are mostly similar to the consensus recommendations for the treatment of hyaluronic acid filler-induced impending necrosis [46–49].

Injection should be stopped immediately when the patient complains of a disproportional sudden pain and/or skin discoloration or as soon as the injector suspects the blood supply has been compromised. An attempt should be made to aspirate the product and to improve the blood flow. Warm compresses should be applied and the area massaged to promote vasodilation.

Hyaluronidase reconstituted in 2% lidocaine (without adrenaline) should be injected in the area of vascular compromise due to its edema-reducing and vasodilating properties [11,50,51]. The hyaluronidase may be injected directly into the affected site, with doses of 600 units per 0.1 mL of intravascular CaHA [11]. If no improvement (e.g. less blanching, improvement of capillary refill) is seen within one to two hours, additional quantities of a hyaluronidase should be injected every two hours (repeat three to four cycles).

Sodium thiosulphate (STS) is an inorganic sodium salt used to treat heavy metal poisoning in humans [52]. Due to its chelating properties, STS is thought to remove calcium from CaHA and assist in the dissolving of the microspheres [53–55]. This hypothesis has been tested experimentally, resulting in CaHA dissolution in some reports [26,56–59], although Yankova *et al.* showed limited efficacy in dissolving intraarterial CaHA, and further research for vascular complications is deemed necessary [58]. Moreover, these studies were lacking robust samples sizes or control arms. In fact, researchers are inclined to attribute the treatment of CaHA with STS and the significant volume decrease to a dispersion effect more than to degradative properties and would not recommend it for the treatment of vascular occlusions [54]. Additionally, Danysz and others also pointed out that significant necrosis and hemorrhages after STS treatment should not go unnoticed [54], whereas Kreymereman *et al.* did not register such AEs at all [54,56]. Given the degree of conflicting results, some researchers have proposed the use of STS as treatment for overcorrection or nodule formation only in small boluses, spaced in several treatment sessions and followed by a massage [55,60,61], whereas others have not seen any improvement when adding STS [62].

Aspirin at 500 mg should be used to limit platelet aggregation, clot propagation, and further compromise [36]. Drugs such as sildenafil and tadalafil can be used to induce smooth muscle relaxation, dilate blood vessels, and increase blood flow [10]. Finally, subcutaneous injection of a low molecular weight heparin such as nadroparin (fraxiparine) can be used to prevent thrombus formation proximal to the embolus and should be done within four hours of the intravascular event [30].

45.9 MANAGEMENT OF OCULAR OCCLUSION/VISION LOSS

Once the retinal artery has been occluded, only a short window of opportunity of 60 to 90 minutes to reestablish blood flow to the retina exists before blindness is irreversible [63]. The patient must be transferred immediately to the nearest ophthalmologist with as much information as possible regarding the product, injection site(s), and volume of injection.

Rapid reduction of intraocular pressure is the first goal of treatment (Figure 45.16–45.17). This will allow the emboli to dislodge downstream and improve retinal perfusion. To promote a lowering of the intraocular pressure as well as to advance the embolus through the retinal vessels, an ocular massage should be started as soon as possible. The technique involves small rapid changes of intraocular pressure over a period of one to three hours until all retinal emboli have been cleared from the vessel. Ocular massage is performed with the patient in a supine position, looking down with their eyes closed. Gentle pressure is applied to the sclera of the anesthetized eye with two fingers, indenting the globe by a few millimeters and then suddenly releasing at a frequency of two to three times a second [64]. The prolonged, rapid small changes in intraocular pressure have been found to be more conducive to dislodging emboli than a brief high-pressure aggressive massage of the eye. The procedure should be continued until the patient reaches the treating ophthalmologist in the hospital.

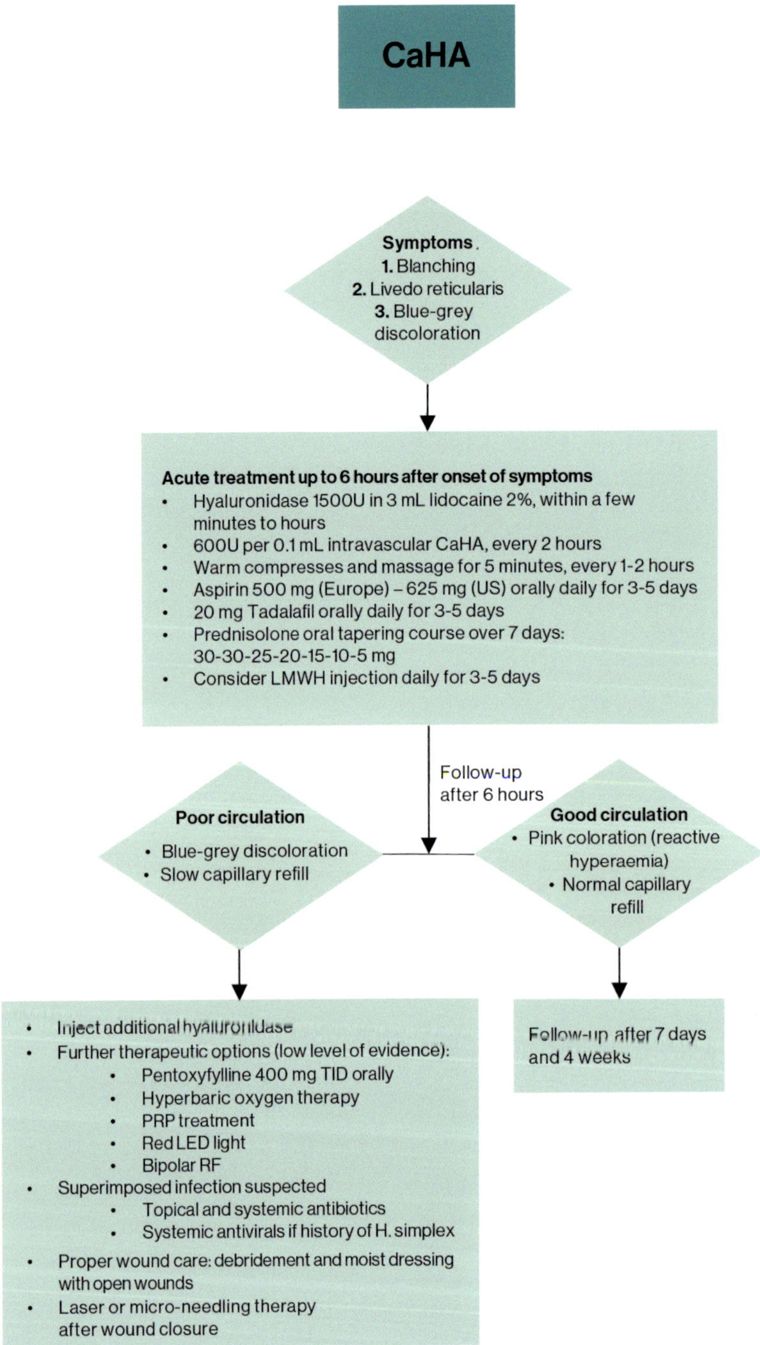

Figure 45.16 Peripheral ischemia with impending necrosis algorithm.

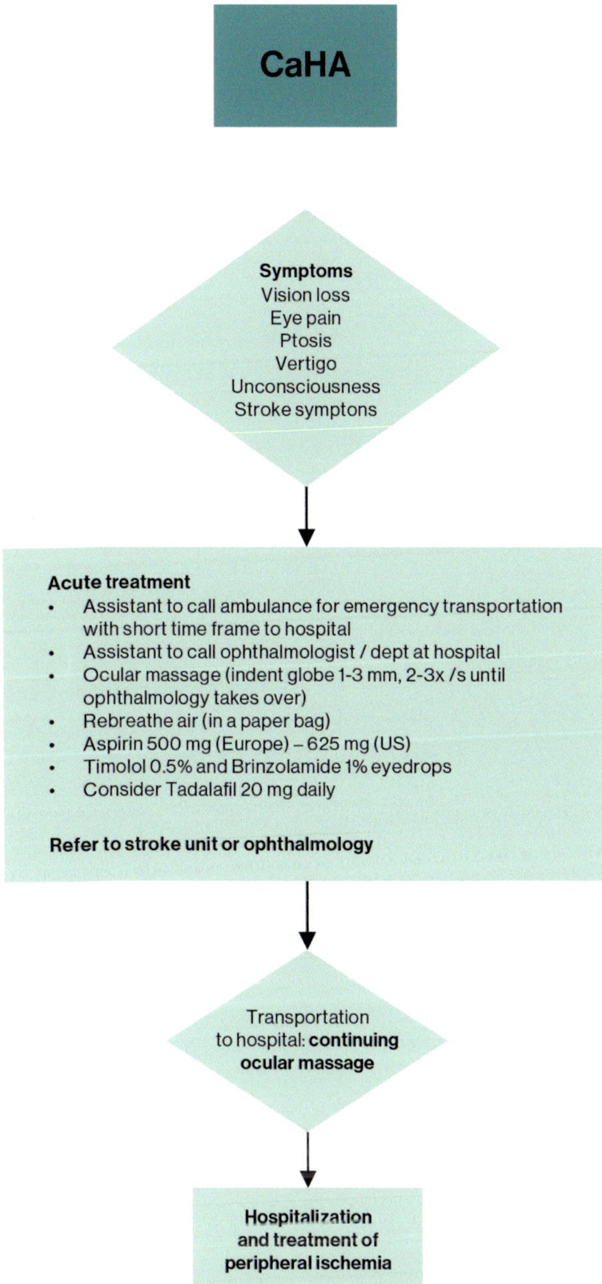

Figure 45.17 Acute blindness caused by retinal ischemia algorithm.

Administration of a β-adrenergic antagonist in the form of eye drops (e.g. Timolol 0.5%), brinzolamide, or azetazolamide will also help to reduce intraocular pressure; azetazolamide may be of greater benefit if administered intravenously. Aspirin (500 mg) should be prescribed to reduce the risk of blood clotting, and intravenous dexamethasone should be used to decrease inflammation. An additional acute measure is to encourage the patient to "re-breathe" in a paper bag to increase carbon dioxide levels in the blood, which will cause the retinal arteries to vasodilate and could help dislodge the blockage [65]. A consensus paper on treatment of vascular complications after CaHA has been published discussing both early as well as late intervention strategies after CaHA vascular compromise [11].

REFERENCES

[1] J. A. Kadouch, "Calcium hydroxylapatite: A review on safety and complications," *J Cosmet Dermatol*, vol. 16, no. 2, pp. 152–161, 2017.

[2] S. L. Silvers et al., "Prospective, open-label, 18-month trial of calcium hydroxylapatite (Radiesse) for facial soft-tissue augmentation in patients with human immunodeficiency virus-associated lipoatrophy: One-year durability," *Plast Reconstr Surg*, vol. 118, no. Suppl 3, pp. 34S–45S, 2006.

[3] S. Smith et al., "A randomized, bilateral, prospective comparison of calcium hydroxylapatite microspheres versus human-based collagen for the correction of nasolabial folds," *Dermatol Surg*, vol. 33, no. Suppl 2, pp. S112–S121, 2007.

[4] J. Van Loghem et al., "Calcium hydroxylapatite: Over a decade of clinical experience," *J Clin Aesthet Dermatol*, vol. 8, no. 1, pp. 38–49, 2015.

[5] The Aesthetis Society, "Cosmetic surgery National Data Bank: Statistics 2013," [internet], 2023: www.theaestheticsociety.org/media/procedural-statistics (accessed Apr. 2025).

[6] G. Casabona, M. S. Sato, "Calcium hydroxylapatite to treat the face," in: Issa, M., Tamura, B., eds., *Botulinum Toxins, Fillers and Related Substances*, vol. 4. Cham: Springer, 2018, pp. 327–347.

[7] G. Lemperle et al., "Foreign body granulomas after all injectable dermal fillers. Part 1: Possible causes," *Plast Reconstr Surg*, vol. 123, no. 6, pp. 1842–1863, 2009.

[8] G. Lemperle, N. Gauthier-Hazan, "Foreign body granulomas after all injectable dermal fillers. Part 2: Treatment options," *Plast Reconstr Surg*, vol. 123, no. 6, pp. 1864–1873, 2009.

[9] C. G. J. C. A. De Vries, R. E. Geertsma, "Clinical data on injectable tissue fillers: A review," *Expert Rev Med Devices*, vol. 10, no. 6, pp. 835–853, 2023.

[10] K. Beer et al., "A treatment protocol for vascular occlusion from particulate soft tissue augmentation," *J Clin Aesthet Dermatol*, vol. 5, no. 5, p. 44, 2012.

[11] J. van Loghem et al., "Managing intravascular complications following treatment with calcium hydroxylapatite: An expert consensus," *J Cosmet Dermatol*, vol. 19, no. 11, pp. 2845–2858, 2020.

[12] T. Daley et al., "Oral lesions associated with injected hydroxyapatite cosmetic filler," *Oral Surg Oral Med Oral Pathol Oral Radiol*, vol. 114, no. 1, pp. 107–111, 2012.

[13] J. A. Kadouch et al., "Granulomatous foreign-body reactions to permanent fillers: Detection of CD123+ plasmacytoid dendritic cells," *Am J Dermatopathol*, vol. 37, no. 2, pp. 107–114, 2015.

[14] P. J. Nicolau, "Long-lasting and permanent fillers: Biomaterial influence over host tissue response," *Plast Reconstr Surg*, vol. 119, no. 7, pp. 2271–2286, 2007.

[15] J. A. Kadouch et al., "Delayed-onset complications of facial soft tissue augmentation with permanent fillers in 85 patients," *Dermatol Surg*, vol. 39, no. 10, pp. 1474–1485, 2013.

[16] L. Requena et al., "Adverse reactions to injectable soft tissue fillers," *J Am Acad Dermatol*, vol. 64, no. 1, pp. 1–34, 2011.

[17] I. Moulonguet et al., "Foreign body reaction to Radiesse: 2 cases," *Am J Dermatopathol*, vol. 35, no. 3, pp. e35–e40, 2013.

[18] S. Shahrabi-Farahani et al., "Granulomatous foreign body reaction to dermal cosmetic fillers with intraoral migration," *Oral Surg Oral Med Oral Pathol Oral Radiol*, vol. 117, no. 1, pp. 105–110, 2014.

[19] D. A. Jansen, M. H. Graivier, "Evaluation of a calcium hydroxylapatite-based implant (Radiesse) for facial soft-tissue augmentation," *Plast Reconstr Surg*, vol. 118, no. Suppl 3, pp. 22S–30S, discussion 31S–33S, 2006.

[20] D. Roy et al., "Clinical trial of a novel filler material for soft tissue augmentation of the face containing synthetic calcium hydroxylapatite microspheres," *Dermatol Surg*, vol. 32, no. 9, pp. 1134–1139, 2006.

[21] N. S. Sadick et al., "A multicenter, 47-month study of safety and efficacy of calcium hydroxylapatite for soft tissue augmentation of nasolabial folds and other areas of the face," *Dermatol Surg*, vol. 33, no. Suppl 2, pp. S122–S126; discussion S126–S127, 2007.

[22] P. Flaharty, "Radiance," *Facial Plast Surg*, vol. 20, no. 2, pp. 165–169, 2004.

[23] T. Pavicic, "Calcium hydroxylapatite filler: An overview of safety and tolerability," *J Drugs Dermatol*, vol. 12, no. 9, pp. 996–1002, 2013.

[24] J. Stein et al., "Histopathologic study of alternative substances for vocal fold medialization," *Ann Otol Rhinol Laryngol*, vol. 109, no. 2, pp. 221–226, 2000.

[25] E. S. Marmur et al., "Clinical, histologic and electron microscopic findings after injection of a calcium hydroxylapatite filler," *J Cosmet Laser Ther*, vol. 6, no. 4, pp. 223–226, 2004.

[26] R. Voigts et al., "Dispersion of calcium hydroxylapatite accumulations in the skin: Animal studies and clinical practices," *Dermatol Sur*, vol. 36, no. Suppl 1, pp. 798–803, 2010.

[27] S. Bay Aguilera et al., "Successful treatment of calcium hydroxylapatite nodules with intralesional 5-Fluorouracil, dexamethasone, and triamcinolone," *J Drugs Dermatol*, vol. 15, no. 9, pp. 1142–1143, 2016.

[28] J. F. Scheuer et al., "Anatomy of the facial danger zones: Maximizing safety during soft-tissue filler injections," *Plast Reconstr Surg*, vol. 139, no. 1, pp. 50e–58e, 2017.

[29] G. J. Goodman et al., "A consensus on minimizing the risk of hyaluronic acid embolic visual loss and suggestions for immediate bedside management," *Aesthet Surg J*, vol. 40, no. 9, pp. 1009–1021, 2020.

[30] A. S. Glaich et al., "Injection necrosis of the glabella: Protocol for prevention and treatment after use of dermal fillers," *Dermatol Surg*, vol. 32, no. 2, pp. 276–281, 2006.

[31] L. D. Grunebaum et al., "The risk of alar necrosis associated with dermal filler injection," *Dermatol Surg*, vol. 35, no. Suppl 2, pp. 1635–1640, 2009.

[32] C. N. Ozturk et al., "Complications following injection of soft-tissue fillers," *Aesthet Surg J*, vol. 33, no. 6, pp. 862–877, 2013.

[33] L. Tracy et al., "Calcium hydroxylapatite associated soft tissue necrosis: A case report and treatment guideline," *J Plast Reconstr Aesthet Surg*, vol. 67, no. 4, pp. 564–568, 2014.

[34] X. Li et al., "A novel hypothesis of visual loss secondary to cosmetic facial filler injection," *Ann Plast Surg*, vol. 75, no. 3, pp. 258–260, 2015.

[35] H. M. Rayess et al., "A cross-sectional analysis of adverse events and litigation for injectable fillers," *JAMA Facial Plast Surg*, vol. 20, no. 3, pp. 207–214, 2018.

[36] C. DeLorenzi, "Transarterial degradation of hyaluronic acid filler by hyaluronidase," *Dermatol Surg*, vol. 40, no. 8, pp. 832–841, 2014.

[37] L. Schelke et al, "Incidence of vascular obstruction after filler injections," *Aesthet Surg J*, vol. 40, no. 8, pp. NP457–NP460, 2020.

[38] B. S. F. Bravo et al., "Delayed-type necrosis after soft-tissue augmentation with hyaluronic acid," *J Clin Aesthet Dermatol*, vol. 8, no. 12, p. 42, 2015.

[39] D. Lazzeri et al., "Blindness following cosmetic injections of the face," *Plast Reconstr Surg*, vol. 129, no. 4, pp. 995–1012, 2012.

[40] R. S. Narins et al., "Clinical conference: Management of rare events following dermal fillers—focal necrosis and angry red bumps," *Dermatol Surg*, vol. 32, no. 3, pp. 426–434, 2006.

[41] Y. Y. Y. Chao, "Saline hydrodissection: A novel technique for the injection of calcium hydroxylapatite fillers in the forehead," *Dermatol Surg*, vol. 44, no. 1, pp. 133–136, 2018.

[42] J. Kim, "Novel forehead augmentation strategy: Forehead depression categorization and calcium hydroxyapatite filler delivery after tumescent injection," *Plast Reconstr Surg*, vol. 6, no. 9, p. e1858, 2018.

[43] T. Tansatit et al., "Verification of embolic channel causing blindness following filler injection," *Aesthetic Plast Surg*, vol. 39, no. 1, pp. 154–161, 2015.

[44] T. T. Khan et al., "An anatomical analysis of the supratrochlear artery: Considerations in facial filler injections and preventing vision loss," *Aesthet Surg J*, vol. 37, no. 2, pp. 203–208, 2017.

[45] J. A. J. Van Loghem, "Use of calcium hydroxylapatite in the upper third of the face: Retrospective analysis of techniques, dilutions and adverse events," *J Cosmet Dermatol*, vol. 17, no. 6, pp. 1025–1030, 2018.

[46] C. Delorenzi, "Complications of injectable fillers, part I," *Aesthet Surg J*, vol. 33, no. 4, pp. 561–575, 2013.

[47] J. L. Cohen et al., "Treatment of hyaluronic acid filler-induced impending necrosis with hyaluronidase: Consensus recommendations," *Aesthet Surg J*, vol. 35, no. 7, pp. 844–849, 2015.

[48] M. King et al., "This month's guideline: The use of hyaluronidase in aesthetic practice (v2.4)," *J Clin Aesthet Dermatol*, vol. 11, no. 6, pp. E61–E68, 2018.

[49] C. DeLorenzi, "New high dose pulsed hyaluronidase protocol for hyaluronic acid filler vascular adverse events," *Aesthet Surg J*, vol. 37, no. 7, pp. 814–825, 2017.

[50] A. Engstrom-Laurent et al., "Raised serum hyaluronate levels in scleroderma: An effect of growth factor induced activation of connective tissue cells?," *Ann Rheum Dis*, vol. 44, no. 9, pp. 614–620, 1985.

[51] S. H. Dayan et al., "Management of impending necrosis associated with soft tissue filler injection," *J Drugs Dermatol*, vol. 10, pp. 1007–1012, 2011.

[52] P. L. McGeer et al., "Medical uses of sodium thiosulfate," *J Neurol Neuromedicine*, vol. 1, no. 3, pp. 28–30, 2016.

[53] W. C. O'Neill, K. I. Hardcastle, "The chemistry of thiosulfate and vascular calcification," *Nephrol Dial Transplant*, vol. 27, no. 2, pp. 521–526, 2012.

[54] W. Danysz et al., "Can sodium thiosulfate act as a reversal agent for calcium hydroxylapatite filler? Results of a preclinical study," *Clin Cosmet Investig Dermatol*, vol. 13, pp. 1059–1073, 2020.

[55] A. D. McCarthy et al., "A structured approach for treating calcium hydroxylapatite focal accumulations," *Aesthet Surg J*, vol. 44, no. 8, pp. 869–879, 2024.

[56] P. Kreymereman, W. Miller, "Sodium thiosulfate injection dissolves calcium hydroxylapatite particles: An animal study," *J Am Acad Dermatol*, vol. 79, no. 3, p. AB265, 2018.

[57] D. M. Robinson, "In vitro analysis of the degradation of calcium hydroxylapatite dermal filler: A proof-of-concept study," *Dermatol Surg*, vol. 44, no. Suppl 1, pp. S5–S9, 2018.

[58] M. Yankova et al., "Intraarterial degradation of calcium hydroxylapatite using sodium thiosulfate—an in vitro and cadaveric study," *Aesthet Surg J*, vol. 41, no. 5, pp. NP226–NP236, 2021.

[59] E. A. Merkel et al., "In vitro and ex vivo investigation of intralesional sodium thiosulfate as a reversal agent for calcium hydroxylapatite soft tissue filler," *J Invest Dermatol*, vol. 142, no. 11, pp. 3125–3127, 2022.

[60] P. P. Rullan et al., "The use of intralesional sodium thiosulfate to dissolve facial nodules from calcium hydroxylapatite," *Dermatol Surg*, vol. 46, no. 10, pp. 1366–1368, 2020.

[61] I. Aksenenko et al., "A method for treating complications developed following countour correction with calcium hydroxylaptite-based filler," *J Clin Aesthet Dermatol*, vol. 15, no. 3, pp. 38–43, 2022.

[62] M. D. Nipshagen et al., "Non-inflammatory nodule formation after hyperdiluted calcium hydroxyapatite treatment in the neck area," *Dermatol Ther*, vol. 33, no. 6, p. e14272, 2020.

[63] K. T. D. Loh et al., "Prevention and management of vision loss relating to facial filler injections," *Singapore Med J*, vol. 57, no. 8, pp. 438–443, 2016.

[64] D. L. Baker, "Gentle, prolonged ocular massage can restore vision after retinal artery occlusion," *Ocular Surgery News* [online], Healio, 2004: www.healio.com/news/ophthalmology/20120331/gentle-prolonged-ocular-massage-can-restore-vision-after-retinal-artery-occlusion (accessed Apr. 2025).

[65] L. Walker, M. King, "This month's guideline: Visual loss secondary to cosmetic filler injection," *J Clin Aesthet Dermatol*, vol. 11, no. 5, pp. E53–E55, 2018.

Index

Note: Page numbers in *italics* indicate a figure and page numbers in **bold** indicate a table on the corresponding page.